Seeking the Light

Seeking the Light

The Lives of Phillips and Ruth Lee Thygeson, Pioneers in the Prevention of Blindness

BERET E. STRONG

Foreword by
G. RICHARD O'CONNOR, M.D.

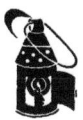

McFarland & Company, Inc., Publishers
Jefferson, North Carolina, and London

All of the photographs are from the Estate of Phillips Thygeson, M.D., and Ruth Lee Thygeson.

LIBRARY OF CONGRESS CATALOGUING-IN-PUBLICATION DATA

Strong, Beret E., 1961–
  Seeking the light : the lives of Phillips and Ruth Lee Thygeson, pioneers in the prevention of blindness / Beret E. Strong ; foreword by G. Richard O'Connor.
    p.   cm.
  Includes bibliographical references and index.

  ISBN 978-0-7864-3673-6
  softcover : 50# alkaline paper ∞

  1. Thygeson, Phillips, 1903–2002. 2. Thygeson, Ruth Lee, 1904–1994. 3. Ophthalmologists — United States — Biography. 4. Blindness. 5. Trachoma. I. Title.
  [DNLM: 1. Thygeson, Phillips, 1903–2002. 2. Thygeson, Ruth Lee, 1904–1994. 3. Ophthalmology — Biography. 4. Blindness. 5. History, 20th Century. 6. History, 21st Century. 7. Ophthalmology — history. 8. Trachoma. WZ 100 T549S 2008]
  RE31.S77   2008
  617.7092'2 — dc22 [B]   2008033564

British Library cataloguing data are available

©2008 Beret E. Strong. All rights reserved

No part of this book may be reproduced or transmitted in any form or by any means, electronic or mechanical, including photocopying or recording, or by any information storage and retrieval system, without permission in writing from the publisher.

On the cover: *clockwise* Phillips Thygeson doing trachoma research in his laboratory at the Pasteur Institute in Tunis, 1931; Vision abstract ©2007 Shutterstock; Ruth Lee Thygeson as a young married woman

Manufactured in the United States of America

*McFarland & Company, Inc., Publishers
  Box 611, Jefferson, North Carolina 28640
  www.mcfarlandpub.com*

In memory of Elizabeth S. Rosenfield

Acknowledgments

This book would not exist in its present form and might not exist at all were it not for the great labors of G. Richard O'Connor, M.D. Months were devoted by Dr. O'Connor to building an archive of documents, letters, essays, and photographs from the tumultuous ocean of papers that Phillips and Ruth Lee Thygeson left behind when they died. He chose, organized and, above all, salvaged previous materials. Throughout the research and writing of this book, he served as content expert, interviewee, advisor, and editor. He is the sine qua non and the shepherd of this book, and I am deeply grateful to him.

Sally Smith Hughes, Ph.D., created an invaluable oral history of Phillips Thygeson and thus provided the chronology and a great deal of material that has been generously made available to this book. Both were friends and colleagues of Phillips and Ruth Lee.

I would like to thank the board of directors of the Alta California Eye Research Foundation, and especially its president, Thomas Lietman, M.D., for making this book possible and helping shape its content and purpose. The Thygesons' children, Fritjof and Kristin, devoted uncounted hours to telling personal stories and offering editorial input. Special thanks go to my friend and fellow writer-editor, Bruce Petty, for an abundance of insightful editing and advice; and to Mary Leihy for supporting this project and befriending Thygesons across the generations. Ann Lottridge went an extra mile as a photo editor, Morgen Warner transcribed interviews and read a draft of the manuscript, and the interlibrary loan system across the nation provided hard to find materials. The American Academy of Ophthalmology (AAO) and the Regional Oral History Office at the University of California at Berkeley generously granted permission to use key oral history materials from the 1980s and 1990s. Jenny E. Benjamin, director of the Museum of Vision at the AAO, had tapes turned into transcripts and was helpful in many other ways.

I would like to thank the interviewees for being generous with their time and memories: Mathea Allansmith, M.D.; Emmett Cunningham, M.D.; Earlene Chapman, Chandler Dawson, M.D.; Jan and Sam Harwood; Gary Holland, M.D.; Sally Smith Hughes, Ph.D.; Jeffrey Day Lanier, M.D.; Margot and Gerry Lawrence; Ralda Lee, Ph.D.; Mary Leihy; G. Richard O'Connor, M.D.; Paul Riordan-Eva, M.D.; Fritjof Thygeson; Kristin Thygeson; Mara Thygeson; Marcus Thygeson, M.D.; and the late Daniel Vaughan, M.D.

As will become clear to the reader, Phillips and Ruth Lee Thygeson told their own story through the medical publications, letters, essays, and photographs they left behind. Although they would not agree with everything to follow in these pages, I believe they would be glad to have their story told, for they loved history and storytelling. They also were excited to have lived through nearly an entire century of dramatic change in medicine and in human history.

I bear responsibility for all errors in and shortcomings of this book. Thank you to the many people who have done their best to help me get it right, and my apologies for errors that remain.

Finally, I wish to thank my husband, John Tweedy, who gave me every kind of support possible, including his excellent editorial skills. And a sweet, special thank you to Paige and Marcus, who are ever so patient with their research and writing loving mother.

Table of Contents

Acknowledgments	vii
Foreword (by G. Richard O'Connor, M.D.)	1
Introduction	3

1. A Minnesota Childhood — 7
2. A San Francisco Childhood — 18
3. A Death in the Family — 28
4. Genteel Poverty and a Pandemic — 33
5. Meeting at Stanford — 36
6. Courtship, a Wedding, and Victorian Values — 43
7. Married and in Medical School — 47
8. Frontier Medicine in Colorado — 53
9. Building a Real Log Cabin — 63
10. To Egypt in Search of Trachoma — 72
11. Learning from a Nobel Laureate in Tunisia — 78
12. Research Idyll in Iowa City — 90
13. Fort Apache and the Great Experiment — 101
14. The New York Chapter: Two Kinds of Politics — 110
15. World War II in the Army Air Corps — 132
16. California and an Experiment in Private Practice — 149
17. The Francis I. Proctor Foundation for Research in Ophthalmology — 153

18. Father and Son: From San Quentin to Steroids	158
19. Mother and Daughter: World Federalist and Equestrienne	166
20. The Glory Days of Academic Medicine	170
21. World Health Organization and World Class Editing	179
22. International Fellows and Fellowship	193
23. Lake Tahoe and the Alta California Eye Research Foundation	199
24. Ripened Souls Tend Their Orchard	203
25. The End of the Journey	210
Chapter Notes	225
Bibliography	243
Index	249

Foreword

In the pages that follow, the reader will encounter a most unusual story. It concerns Dr. Phillips Thygeson and his devoted wife, Ruth Lee, both of whom I knew for a period of over forty years. The story is one of extraordinary accomplishment including, among other things, the discovery of both the cause and the cure of trachoma, a potentially blinding disease affecting millions of people throughout the world. The tale is one of steadfast determination in all things, reflecting Phillips Thygeson's strong personal sense of right and wrong. He had to lock horns with eminent scientists of his day, including Nobel Prize winners such as Charles Nicolle. This story is definitely not a joy ride. It is filled with conflicts and confrontations. Thygeson's strong feelings about national politics, about the proper rearing of children, and about the preservation of the nation's natural resources were reflected in several unpleasant episodes. Even some members of his own family regarded him as an unyielding curmudgeon.

With regard to his contributions to ophthalmic education, everyone is agreed that they were superb. For a time, no one in the United States had a greater knowledge of external diseases of the eye. Thygeson was an excellent observer, and he transmitted his clinical skills to medical students, residents, and research fellows alike. He emphasized the crucial importance of early accurate diagnosis, and he stressed that eye doctors must know the expected natural course of a given disease before prescribing potentially damaging medications such as broad-spectrum antibiotics or corticosteroids. He did not believe in shotgun therapy for the treatment of an undiagnosed red eye, and history has proven him to be right! All of us owe him heartfelt thanks.

G. Richard O'Connor, M.D. • Director Emeritus
Francis I. Proctor Foundation for Research in Ophthalmology
University of California, San Francisco

I beseech you to take interest in these sacred domains so expressively called laboratories. Ask that there be more and that they be adorned, for these are the temples of the future, wealth and well-being. It is here that humanity will grow, strengthen and improve.

— Louis Pasteur

It is vitally important to know the natural history of disease. An ophthalmologist should not treat an eye infection just to relieve pain. He must think of the future.

— Phillips Thygeson

Introduction

In 1927, a young married couple drove a Ford Model T over alpine passes and across the high deserts of the American West. Their journey from San Francisco to Denver took nine days on narrow gravel roads. Early in the trip, they camped among the spruces and firs in the Sierra Nevada mountains. Inside a heavy canvas tent, they lay between thick layers of blankets held together by large pins. Phillips Thygeson, the young husband, who had not yet graduated from Stanford Medical School, began to hemorrhage profusely near the inside corner of his eye. For his wife, Ruth Lee Thygeson, the uncontrolled bleeding was terrifying.[1] There was no hospital or emergency care for hours in any direction. Phil was calm, as he believed he could stop the hemorrhage. "It was eventually easy to control by pressure.... It didn't scare me because I knew that I could control it by pressure," he said. They spent seven more days crossing the arid, yet beautiful expanses of Nevada, Utah, and western Colorado.

Phil had dacryocystitis, a painful inflammation of the tear sac often caused by blockage of the duct that drains tears from the tear sac to the nose. These were the days when surgical remedies were often drastic and too frequently used. Phil had undergone surgery, had caught an infection, and underwent a second operation that led to his hemorrhage.[2] Upon their arrival in Denver, Phil arranged to see Dr. William C. Finnoff, a highly respected ophthalmologist and professor at the University of Colorado. Finnoff removed the rest of the tear sac and Phil's wound finally began to heal.

Phil and Ruth Lee had come to Denver for Phil's medical internship. His plan was to become a microbiologist, and he soon accepted an appointment from the chief of microbiology at the University of Colorado to become an instructor of bacteriology. Dr. Finnoff talked him into a different path, however — ophthalmology. Phil joked about this: "They say everybody who goes into medicine, if they have anything wrong with them, they go into that specialty." And so he did.

Not long after the adventure on the high Sierra pass, Phil and Ruth Lee entered into a life-long collaboration. Phil did laboratory research and Ruth Lee helped him write and edit many important medical papers. The goal of a large number of these papers was to understand and reduce the incidence of the leading cause of preventable blindness worldwide, trachoma. As a disease of poverty and lack of access to clean water, trachoma is said even now to put 10 percent of the world's population at risk of blindness. It is highly contagious, is easily spread by flies, and is responsible for much blindness in Asia and Africa. In the heyday of European immigration to the United States, trachoma was the eye disease most looked for by medical inspectors at Ellis Island.

An infection caused by the *Chlamydia trachomatis* bacterium, trachoma affects primarily the eyelid and cornea, is intensely painful, and can cause permanent corneal scarring. Unlike the quiet stealth of the leading causes of noninfectious blindness worldwide, glaucoma and cataracts, a person can be reinfected many times in the course of his or her life. Trachoma is a great cause of human misery, as scarring can be so intense on the inside of the eyelids that it causes them to contract, making the eyelashes scratch against the cornea. The advanced, scarring stage of the disease is called trichiasis. It is intensely painful and has been described as feeling like sand scraping against one's eye. In untreated people, the disease will blind slowly and inexorably, a cruel, gradual dimming of the light.

Trachoma is endemic in 55 countries and nearly a hundred million people are thought to have the active disease at any given moment. Phil and Ruth Lee chose to devote their lives to understanding and eradicating it. Although they were from the wealthy, developed part of the world, their efforts were dedicated to the world's less fortunate, especially the rural poor on continents far away. In addition to trachoma, Phil and Ruth Lee worked on a number of other external eye diseases. Although external eye disease has plagued human beings since the dawn of our species, it came into its own as a field of research in the twentieth century, when Phil Thygeson made himself into a leading expert in the field, demarcated its boundaries, and began to train other ophthalmologists in its unique issues. In this way, he was a pioneer. Now, of course, the field is much too vast for one person to master.

In 1947, with funding from Dr. and Mrs. Francis I. Proctor, who chose Phil as their protégé in research on trachoma, Phil helped found the prestigious Francis I. Proctor Foundation for Research in Ophthalmology at the University of California at San Francisco. At the Proctor Foundation, through a fellows program, Phil trained many young ophthalmologists from around the world in the best research and clinical skills he could offer — his own. After their residencies, the young eye doctors came to the Proctor Foundation for a year or two of research-oriented training. They researched and wrote papers, saw patients, refined their clinical skills, and learned how to teach others as they were being taught.

Phil had a passion for the microscope that he would never outgrow. His fascination with microbiology and bacteriology became the backbone of his research on trachoma and other infectious external diseases of the eye. The legacy of Phil Thygeson is both his seminal research on the cause and treatment of trachoma, and his training of young doctors who would return to their home countries and train other doctors as they had been trained. Ruth Lee's legacy is that she did an incalculable amount of work to help Phil be successful as a researcher and writer, and she taught many other ophthalmologists to express themselves clearly and elegantly in writing.

Phil and Ruth Lee Thygeson shared a unique life adventure. It included living in North Africa, building a log cabin with their own hands, and engaging in an unending quest to conquer preventable blindness around the world. Their lives spanned nearly the entire twentieth century. Ruth Lee Spilman was a young child in San Francisco at the time of the great 1906 earthquake, and she lived through the Loma Prieta earthquake in 1989. She grew up to be a free-thinking and very talented woman who could have pursued any number of careers, and who chose to become her husband's invaluable assistant in writing and publishing research findings on external diseases of the eye. Born at the dawn of the twentieth century, Phil grew up loving his father, scouting, and ham radio. He came to embrace California, a career in medical research, and a life of building things with his bare hands. At age ninety-six, while bedridden, Phil wrote dozens of essays about his life experiences.

Theirs was an era of pioneering in medicine and in life, of modernization, political upheaval, two world wars, and revolutionary changes in pharmacology and the art and practice of medicine. On a personal level, theirs is a story of a shared work ethic, a profound belief in the gifts of science, and a unique love affair characterized by sustained collaboration between two intrepid, tireless, and deeply committed people.

Phil always talked about his "good old days" and was glad to have been born when he was. His research work, which spanned half of the twentieth century, has helped save the eyesight of millions of people around the world. As colleagues and later generations of ophthalmologists point out, the Thygesons' work will continue to influence the field of external eye disease for generations to come.

1. A Minnesota Childhood

Phillips Baker Thygeson was born March 28, 1903, in St. Paul, Minnesota, to a Norwegian-American father and a rabble-rousing suffragette mother. He was named after a woman friend of his mother's, but at a young age Phillips decided he hated his first name. At times he hated his mother, though those feelings took longer to develop. He asked to be called "Phil" and that's what his family, colleagues, and friends called him. He was proud of his Norwegian heritage and confided to others that he wished he were a full-blooded Norwegian-American, like his father, Nels Marcus. He admired the Norwegian people — their hardiness and resourcefulness and even what he thought of as their Viking spirit. He loved the color red and identified with those who were warriors, raiders, farmers, and settlers.

Phil's paternal grandfather, Elling, was from the fishing town of Bergen on the west coast of Norway. The family was originally from Denmark, but spent about a century in Norway before a few members emigrated to the New World. To this day, the town of Bergen smells of fish and features brightly painted houses. Elling emigrated to the United States with his brother in the 1840s or early 1850s.[1] His brother went to North Dakota and all traces of him and his descendants are now lost. Elling chose to be a farmer in Wisconsin, living with his family near the town of Martell in Pierce County, Wisconsin. He bought an 80-acre farm there in 1854.[2] Elling was not an educated man, and was "of farm stock, peasant stock."[3] His wife, Mary Nelson, came from a family that valued higher education. Through her influence, her son embarked on a path that led to an advanced university degree and two professions, geology and law.

There were so many Norwegians in the community that Elling's son Nels Marcus grew up hearing and speaking only Norwegian.[4] At the "normal school" Nels Marcus attended starting at the age of ten, he excelled in English and went on to be a "real English scholar" who wrote beautiful legal briefs.[5] In the Norwegian tradition, Nels Marcus skied on long skis to school in the winter, and rode a horse to school in the autumn and spring. Before and after school, he worked extremely hard on the farm, helping his parents.

Later, Nels Marcus had to go to River Falls, Wisconsin, to finish his schooling. When he was ready for college, there was no money to pay his expenses at the University of Wisconsin, so he worked his way through doing all kinds of odd jobs. He appreciated work of most kinds and later in life regaled his son, Phil, with stories of what he did during his college years in Madison. After he completed a degree in geology, he joined the U.S. Geodetic Survey. However, as Phil said, "he didn't like the nomadic life" because it wasn't compatible with raising a family.[6] Since he didn't want to be a wandering geologist, he completed a law degree at the University of Minnesota, and became district attorney for Ramsey County. Nels Marcus then went into private practice in St. Paul and specialized in the taxation issues of railroads, including the railways of St. Paul, Minneapolis, and Chicago. He became a "corporation lawyer."[7] Nels Marcus's father could speak no English; his children would speak no Norwegian.[8] Phil loved his father and felt deeply loved by him. "I remember wanting to grow up to be just like him.... I listened to every word my father said and when he asked me to do something I did it. He was a bit of a philosopher.... Father's philosophy of life became my philosophy of life."[9]

Phil's mother was likewise no stranger to hard work and self-sufficiency. She was born Sylvie Grace Thompson in June of 1868, in the small town of Forreston, Illinois. She described it as "a beautiful little town," with white painted buildings with green shutters, beautiful elm trees, and flowers everywhere.[10] Her mother, Mary Thompson, bore eleven children, three of whom died at birth or in early childhood. Sylvie's minister grandfather had been involved with the Underground Railroad that helped slaves escape to northern states. As a child, Sylvie's father stayed briefly at one of the safe houses on the Underground Railroad "as they were coming along the Mason-Dixon Line."[11] For two or three days during one of those visits, her father was in the company of a little girl — a slave — from Louisiana who was escaping to the North with her parents and siblings. The little girl's name was Sylvie. When Sylvie Grace Thompson was born, she was named in memory of that girl. Sylvie believed that when she came along, the fourth child, her parents had "no special name"[12] picked out for her, and that was why her father used a childhood memory to choose her name.

Sylvie's mother had married at the tender age of fifteen and so had had a relatively short childhood. She was an adventuresome person who heard Abraham Lincoln deliver the Gettysburg Address and who traveled by covered wagon across the plains to Illinois from the East Coast.[13] Sylvie's mother's great passion was reading and she often read several books at a time. Sylvie said,

> The only sad thing I remember about my mother was that she was an inveterate reader. If she got a book to read maybe we had to wait around for our meals in a very sad kind of way while our mother was absorbed in this book. One time we did a terrible thing, we bought a set of Dickens. It was six volumes, I remember so well, green-bound with three columns on the page. We paid fifteen cents a month to buy this set of Dickens, and when we got that set, oh how we suffered![14]

They suffered because their mother paid so little attention to her children when she was engaged in reading books. But there was also great benefit to their mother's addiction to reading; she taught her children to love books and become avid readers. They read for pleasure, borrowing books from the local school library and the Lutheran Church library. Sylvie remembered reading George Eliot, Charles Dickens, and German and British literary classics.

In spite of being surrounded by Lutherans, the family had no religion. In fact, "In the whole town we were the only family that were atheists."[15] The family was atheist by choice—they had decided to reject God. Sylvie's paternal grandfather was a Presbyterian minister and her mother's parents were religious as well. The minister and his five-year-old son were killed in a prairie fire while out ministering to a dying member of their congregation.[16] According to a story that has been passed down through the generations, the family never forgave God for taking the lives of this father and son while they were engaged in an errand of mercy.[17] "I never in the world could have had any religion after that, hearing that story," Sylvie said.[18] Being atheists was a problem for the Thompson children in a town where everyone else attended church and believed in God. The children compensated by consistently winning top honors at school.[19] In spite of her views on organized religion, Sylvie believed in the Bible as a great work of literature and once said that if you read a chapter of the Bible every day and seven chapters every Sunday, you could read the whole Bible in a year.[20]

Sylvie described her father as a "small town lawyer," akin to a justice of the peace.[21] He had grown up poor in rural Iowa, and never prospered. "We often had a precarious living," she recalled. "We never went hungry because we always had a big garden in summer time.... We raised chickens and everything."[22] Their mother was very careful with money and sewed her daughters' calico dresses. She even made their winter wear—for Sylvie, two woolen suits and a winter coat.[23] And though their means were limited, they subscribed to the Chicago daily newspaper and bought a secondhand piano.[24] Sylvie enjoyed her childhood a great deal and loved having a lot of siblings with whom to play and interact.

Sylvie began high school at age twelve. After graduating at the age of sixteen, she taught school at the local country school, but only briefly, because her father died when she was a newly hired teacher. Her father had fought in the Civil War under General Ulysses S. Grant, where "he was wounded in the head ... and had to have a silver plate" inserted. When he died, a special tomb was built for him because of his war service.[25] Sylvie's uncle, Seymour Dwight Thompson, an appellate court judge in St. Louis, Missouri, took his favorite niece straight from her father's funeral to St. Louis and put her to work doing typing, stenography, and even a bit of research and writing for his legal cases.[26] After her lean childhood, Sylvie had the pleasure of living in a large, fancy house with servants and a complete, beautifully illustrated set of Shakespeare. Her uncle's success was an inspiration to Sylvie, though she cared more about learning than she did about money. When a rich suitor tried to marry her and take her off to the wilds of Nebraska, her uncle quickly put a stop to it by saying she was unsuited for life on the frontier.

Judge Thompson was an editor of the *American Law Review*, and Sylvie learned citation checking and other legal skills working for him. She took shorthand and then typed up the "the opinions of the court" that her uncle dictated to her.[27] His intention was to give her an intellectual life and help her become a self-sufficient woman who could earn her own living. He was entirely successful in his effort. She recalled that period as "a wonderful time of mental and spiritual awakening."[28] She went with her cousin George to lectures on theosophy and other spiritual topics. They even attended séances together, including one where the spirit of a three-year-old boy who had died was called forth and made to float above the table.[29] In time, Sylvie came to miss her family and moved to St. Paul, Minnesota, to be with her siblings and mother.

Sylvie was, in her own words, a "cripple." She had sprained her ankle at the age of twelve and later broke a bone in that same ankle. As good medical care was not available, she had a slight limp and wore stiff boots that laced up well above her ankles for the rest of her life.[30] The injury doesn't appear to have affected Sylvie's sense of possibility for her own life in any way. She got a job in St. Paul for the "fabulous sum" of $100 a week doing stenography and typing.[31]

Sylvie Thompson and Nels Marcus Thygeson were thus launched in the world. What remained was for them to meet and marry. They met by chance in an elevator in St. Paul in 1891. Sylvie, age 23, was attending a lecture on Shakespeare with a friend. Into their elevator stepped Nels Marcus, already a partner in the law firm of Munn, Boyesen, and Thygeson. Sylvie's friend whispered to Sylvie, "That's Mr. Thygeson." Nels Marcus later told Sylvie that when he caught his first glimpse of her that night, he thought to himself that this was the woman he was going to marry. Sylvie was skeptical about this story, but they did marry within five weeks of that first meeting.[32] She admired him throughout her life. "Of all the people in the whole world, there never was a nicer, kinder or more capable man than my husband," she said.[33]

With eleven children, Sylvie's mother probably lacked access to birth control. Sylvie, on the other hand, insisted on family planning from the start. Their first child, Ruth, was born in 1895, and son Elling was born in 1898. Phil was born in 1903. Sylvie always said that she planned her children, except for the baby, Mary, born in 1906.[34] By the time Mary was born, Sylvie was deeply involved in political activity. Sylvie's mother had always been interested in women's rights, but was too busy with her children to pursue her interest. Sylvie, in contrast, was an officer in the Women's Welfare League and worked tirelessly on behalf of women's suffrage and access to birth control. She didn't mind that people knew she was engaged in illegal activities. At the time, even disseminating information about birth control was illegal. "I stood out. I was a little more aggressive than some of the people that I was associated with.... [W]hen Margaret Sanger ... publicly worked for it on a large scale, it was the most natural thing in the world for me to join it and to go along with it as I did.... My husband was always progressive."[35]

Sylvie helped establish a birth control clinic with the aid of two male doctors, though her own work was mainly in educating women about contraception and family planning. "We didn't advertise. We were entirely secret and had no name."[36] They distributed a birth control device Margaret Sanger particularly believed in and that Sylvie described as "very ingenious."[37] Sylvie held socials and teas as a way to lecture on birth control and suffrage. She was the first vice president of the Woman's Welfare League and helped host a hundred women at each of a series of Saturday luncheons for which they charged twenty-five cents per person.[38] Their purpose was to advocate and lobby for women's suffrage. They invited important people to lecture, including, in 1891, David Starr Jordan, a strong advocate of universal suffrage who went on to become the first president of Stanford University.[39] Sylvie had a large Cadillac that could hold seven people and she took to driving important out-of-town guests around in her car.

Nels Marcus made Sylvie proud when he spoke out publicly on behalf of women's suffrage. His role as general counsel for the Twin City Rapid Transit Company[40] kept her from being arrested for her illegal activities promoting birth control.[41] "I had my name written up editorially in the big newspaper of St. Paul ... denouncing me," she said. "It was a criminal offense in those days to practice birth control. Our clinic was against the law.... I had to rely on my husband's prestige in the community. He had real prestige. They would have thought a long time before arresting me on birth control with my husband in the position he was."[42]

Sylvie was egalitarian in her view of the sexes — women and men were equally capable and equally fallible. She remained politically active and left-leaning all of her life. She later visited Soviet Russia and had an extensive correspondence with Stokely Carmichael,[43] who coined the term "black power" and served as prime minister of the Black Panthers.[44] When she was 104 years old, she reflected on women's suffrage, saying, "It was inevitable that women were to vote. They were human beings endowed with certain, as we say the old words, 'inalienable rights.'"[45] She didn't believe in "sexes" but rather in "human beings."[46] She also lamented that even late in her life the United States was still racially segregated in many ways and far from electing a woman president. She instructed her young great-grandchildren to be engaged citizens of their democracy and to register to vote as soon as they were of age.[47] Sylvie believed in what people actually accomplished, not in the prestige of their bloodlines. "Unless they make good, unless they do the work and accomplish things, what their ancestors did doesn't count at all."[48]

Phil Thygeson's parents — Nels Marcus and Sylvie — had a tremendous impact on him, one positive and one negative. He cleaved unto his father and rejected his mother. He believed that his father loved him dearly and his mother did not love him at all. Sylvie had reproached her mother for ignoring her in favor of books, but became like her, neglecting Phil and her other children to pursue her intellectual and social passions. Phil's younger sister Mary said she believed her mother could not possibly love her given the cruel things she said.[49] For example, a very important early love affair of Mary's ended with her Parisian beau dying of pneumonia. Mary was heartbroken. Sylvie said to her, "If you had taken better care of him, he would not have died." Sylvie also told Mary numerous times that she thought she was ugly.[50]

For Phil, "Mother was a figure I only saw at meals. She and father had separate rooms and romance seemed to have vanished. Nowadays of course there would be divorce."[51] He was convinced that he and his sister Mary were unplanned children, that their mother disliked all forms of physical labor, and that she was "too busy with her women's suffrage, birth control, leftist politics, Unitarian church affairs, civic clubs, etc., to pay much attention to unplanned children."[52]

On the other hand, Phil loved his father, who called him the Norwegian term for "good boy." He also loved his nurse, nicknamed "Lala." Miss Anna Larsen, a Norwegian with an R.N. degree, was present to assist the family physician when Phil was born at his parents' home in St. Paul. Unmarried and with no children of her own, she stayed on as an employee of the Thygeson family from Phil's birth in 1903 until 1917. She doted on Phil and

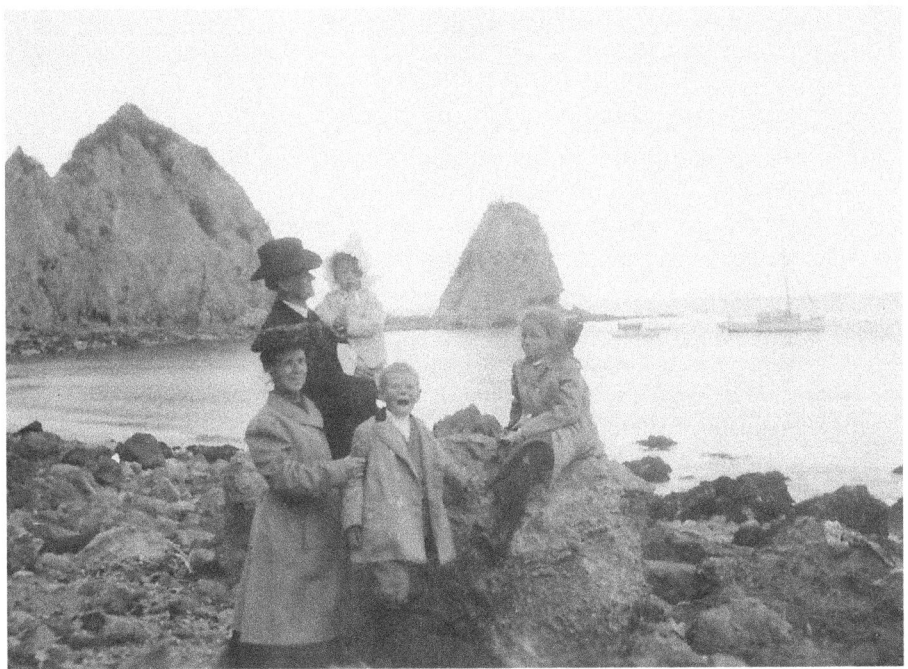

Sylvie and Nels Marcus Thygeson with three of their children on a trip to Catalina Island, 1905. Phillips Thygeson is held by his father, Nels Marcus.

even went into quarantine with him when he was stricken with scarlet fever at the age of three.[53] He credited Lala with pulling him through that life-threatening illness. By his own account, he had a somewhat obsessive attachment to her. "The first person I saw in my life at age three was Lala, my wonderful nurse. She was my surrogate mother and I loved Lala with all my heart. I could not bear to let her out of my sight.... I needed her for my existence.... And ever since Lala, I have been attached to women. I cannot do without them."

Poor Lala was not allowed any respite from her young charge. When she took short vacations to visit her family, Phil insisted on going with her. She relented and took him along every time.[54] Lala was part of the family and did much of the work traditionally assigned to "the lady of the household." She managed the hired help — the cook, the gardener, the "wash ladies"— and the family accounts.[55] She also helped manage Phil's life. "It may seem strange but at age 13, I was dependent on Lala for advice and help in all my little problems of adolescence."[56]

Young Phil's hobbies were inspired by his father's interests. His father worked for the streetcar and railway company, so Phil loved trams and trains.

Phil was a late talker who didn't speak at all until he was three years old. On his third birthday, his father gave him a "little steam train, complete with an engine, cars, caboose, and lots of track. The little steam engine was powered by an alcohol burner [and] had a steam whistle."[57] Phil was so excited, his first reported words were a complete sentence: "Roll up the rugs!" His father added bridges, tunnels, depots, and special crossings to the set. He also introduced Phil to other kinds of engines — a hot air engine, a steam engine, and, later, an electric engine. At a young age, Phil decided he wanted to grow up to be an engineer — ideally, an electrical engineer.[58]

Nels Marcus turned the vacant lot next door to their house into a winter skating rink for neighborhood use. The Thygeson kids had skates and hockey sticks. Phil also pursued his father's interests in "electricity, telegraphy, telephone, and amateur radio."[59] The house at 894 Laurel Avenue in St. Paul was roomy enough to have a sleeping porch, a finished attic, and, remarkably, "a big basement that was converted into a rifle range for .22 rifle target practice."[60] Phil disliked there being only one bathroom for three adults and four children. The fact that baths were customary — indeed, allowed — only once a week, on Saturday nights, helped decrease the demand on the bathroom.[61]

Phil enjoyed his schooling except for his first year of high school, when his father decided to send him to a "posh private school, the St. Paul Academy, a school for rich kids."[62] Norwegian kids were considered immigrant kids and were not high in the social pecking order.[63] Nor were they good at street fighting. When they got into scrapes with other kids, they often lost the battle. Phil had rocks thrown at him a number of times.

Phil overheard a number of political arguments between his parents. Nels Marcus was an admirer of Abraham Lincoln, but was in many ways conservative. Sylvie was by nature a radical. The two of them loved to engage in spirited discussions of the daily news. Nels Marcus believed that corporations benefited the country because they encouraged development, innovation, risk taking and collective enterprise. Sylvie believed that corporations were amoral exploiters of workers. Phil described his mother as a "left wing socialist," but wrote that he, his siblings, and Lala were amused by their parents' vocal differences of opinion.[64] Phil was convinced that his father was right and his mother was wrong and something of a hypocrite: "Mother was down on corporations, but she dearly loved the money that the corporations produced."[65]

Nels Marcus and Phil had a spirited connection. Phil recalled wanting to keep his little boy's bobbed haircut — a bowl cut. Nels Marcus thought it high time his son got a big boy's haircut. "I put up a real fight," Phil said. "Father solved the matter by bringing in the town constable whom he knew very well. When I saw the constable I quieted down immediately. I had a great respect for the law. The haircut cost 35 cents."[66] Nels Marcus implicitly trusted his son. While Nels Marcus was one of the first people in St. Paul to drive a car, he was not comfortable behind the wheel. One day, he stalled the car while he and Phil were crossing some railroad tracks. He got out, handed the keys to Phil, and said, "You drive." Phil loved driving from the very beginning, and he was a great driver.

Phil's most cherished memories of childhood concern the family "farm" at Woodside on Lake Minnetonka. His parents bought a large parcel of land sometime around 1906,[67] perhaps as much as 20 acres, which gave them an extensive stretch of lakefront.[68] Sylvie, Lala, and the children spent entire summers at the farm on the lake, and Nels Marcus commuted back and forth to his job in St. Paul on a "fast, electric car" and then on the steamer that delivered people and goods around the lake.

At Lake Minnetonka, Phil learned how to help tend a small family farm of fruits and vegetables. He learned all sorts of skills by watching and helping his father.

> Father was a builder and a worker, and he found real pleasure in making improvements on the farm. He enlarged the house by building a modern bathroom, a sleeping porch and converting the attic into a dormitory. And he built a modern water system with a windmill, an elevated water tank and a modern kitchen. And then he had to improve the barn, build a little house for the hired man, a little house for the acetylene gas generator and an ice house.[69]

Though the rest of the family didn't awaken until 6 a.m., Nels Marcus was always up at 4 A.M., starting the chores for the day.[70] There was an apple orchard; plots of corn, barley, and wheat; and grapes, blackberries, raspberries, pumpkins, and squash.[71] They drank their one cow's unpasteurized milk, churned butter, whipped cream, and made hand-cranked ice cream on Sundays.[72] They had pigs named John and Mary, a friendly horse named Jim, laying hens, and a flock of pigeons. There were also many forms of recreation — a grass tennis court, a croquet court, and two rowboats.

"One feature of the lake that we specially enjoyed was the annual visit of an Indian family. Lake Minnetonka had been an Indian lake with the Sioux on one side and the Chippewa on the other side.... Because of the Indians I developed an interest in Indian lore," Phil wrote.[73] The visiting family was from the Shakopee Reservation on the Minnesota River. "They didn't ask permission, but their ancestors had always camped there." The Thygesons gave them buckets of raspberries and the Indians gave tiny tomahawks and birchbark canoes in exchange.[74]

Phil's idyllic childhood began to darken around 1913 when the Minnetonka property was sold back to the family that had sold it to the Thygesons.

Sylvie could not resist the siren song of a huge cash offer and so she sold the farm. Unfortunately, the money was "badly invested and entirely lost."[75] Nels Marcus had only two weeks of vacation a year, so he got left behind in subsequent summers when Sylvie took the kids on trips to Banff in the Canadian Rockies and to Old Orchard, Maine.[76]

Phil had a big adventure with his mother during the winter of 1915, when he had severe bronchitis and doctors recommended a warmer, drier climate. Sylvie took advantage of the recommendation to propose a mother-son trip to Southern California. That, at least, is one version of the story. Another is that Sylvie wanted to go on a trip to California and she needed a chauffeur and companion, so she conjured up the story that he had bronchitis.[77] In any case, off they went. They took a horse-drawn sleigh taxi to the train station and boarded a Pullman for Kansas City. There, they changed to the Atchison, Topeka and Santa Fe line, where they had a sleeper compartment. For Phil, the trip became interesting when they arrived in Albuquerque. The local Native Americans sold beautiful Navajo rugs, jewelry, and pottery at the train station. The next stop was Isleta Pueblo, the first traditional southwestern pueblo Phil had ever seen. He was interested in the indigenous language and in a community that appeared to him to be little affected by the Anglos of Arizona. After that, they visited the south rim of the Grand Canyon, where Phil had a fabulous time taking photographs with his Brownie camera.[78] He liked the Hopi culture and dances, the wild turkeys of the desert, and the scent of orange blossoms when he and his mother arrived at their final destination of Los Angeles.

They rented an apartment close to the ocean in Long Beach, the bronchitis cleared up as predicted, nobody mentioned school, and Phil was left to explore a whole new area. Sylvie busied herself with social engagements and political activities — she already had friends there — and Phil felt himself inexorably drawn to the lure of the budding film town of Hollywood. He had been a self-described movie buff in St. Paul, and in Hollywood he found that the studios would actually let him watch them film. He saw D. W. Griffith filming *Intolerance* and *The Fall of Babylon*, enjoyed the Keystone Cops, and even got to watch Mary Pickford and Douglas Fairbanks in action.[79] He begged for film cuttings in the editing rooms, reassembled clips as best he could, and took his sutured-together reels back to Minnesota to show to his friends and siblings. He and his mother took a memorable trip up El Camino Real on the California coast, visiting the Spanish missions from San Diego all the way to Mission Dolores in the heart of San Francisco.[80] Phil always remembered the winter of 1915 with fondness, for he got to see the major cities of California while they were still small and uncrowded.

During these years, life on Laurel Avenue in St. Paul during the school year was sweet — until Phil's father got sick. He was diagnosed with cancer of the pancreas, one of the more deadly kinds of cancer. He went to the Mayo Clinic for surgery and was operated on by one of the Mayo brothers, who judged the tumor to be inoperable.[81] Nonetheless, he was able to go back to work for a few months, settle a major tax case for the Canadian Northern Railroad, and earn a handsome $25,000 fee.[82]

What followed was a turning point for the entire family. "Father never let me down," Phil wrote about his early childhood. "He was never too busy or too sleepy to talk to me. And I must have been quite a bit of a nuisance."[83] However, when Phil went into his father's sickroom late in his father's illness and spoke to him, for the first time in Phil's life, his father could not respond and turned his face to the wall. It was a devastating experience for Phil, a trauma from which he would never fully recover. Sylvie, the dying Nels Marcus, and their four children moved to Palo Alto, California, in preparation for what would soon be a fatherless and husbandless life.

Phil was only fourteen when his father died, and was still a young boy in many ways. As a young child, he had slept in an alcove next to his father's bedroom and was allowed to crawl into his father's bed and be comforted when distressed. Phil lost Lala when he lost his father, as the family was no longer able to afford to employ her. "Unfortunately," Phil wrote, "Father had thought that he would live forever as a big earner, and neither he nor my mother had saved any money."[84] When Nels Marcus died, Phil's happy childhood died as well.[85]

2. A San Francisco Childhood

When Phil Thygeson was learning to walk, his future wife Ruth Lee Spilman was born in San Francisco. Born September 20, 1904, she was the second daughter and youngest child of James Spilman and Elizabeth Brewer Spilman. She was named in part after Robert E. Lee, the most famous general of the Confederate army during the Civil War. Most likely, it was her father who gave her this name, as he was the Southerner of the family. Her name was always intended to be "Ruth Lee," not "Ruth." All her life, she refused to answer if someone called her "Ruth." Less is known of these two than of the parents of Phil Thygeson, but they had a huge impact on their children. Elizabeth came to the United States via Canada. Her ancestral lines are said to trace to a princess of Bohemia, a principality in what became Czechoslovakia. According to the story, in Bohemia long ago, "the barrel maker of the palace ran away with the young princess to the New World, going into the primitive Canadian wilderness together." Family lore further has it that the granddaughter of the princess may have been Elizabeth's grandmother.[1] Ruth Lee's maternal great-grandfather was said to be Captain King, who fought for Admiral Nelson at Trafalgar. Some descendants believe the British crown gave King a handsome parcel of land in Canada, which is how Elizabeth Brewer came to be born there three generations later.[2]

The family was cultivated and well-read. Many of the family were Quaker and there is a surviving photograph of three pairs of severely dressed Quakers — all identical twin sisters. The family ethic was: "Dress plainly and do good works.... Care for the world at large."[3] The family was not always so austere, however. Elizabeth's mother, Esther, was a sharp dresser who liked to wear stylish clothing and the latest fashion in hats. She learned to use a treadle sewing machine and make her own clothes.[4]

James Spilman was born into the tradition of the old-fashioned southern gentleman, and lived it in spite of his family's fallen fortunes. He loved the English language and wrote beautiful letters and legal briefs. He "came from the Southern grand style, the southern plantation family."[5] However, his family in Virginia lost a great deal — especially in family wealth — during the devastation of the Civil War. The date of James Spilman's birth is unknown, but his wife was born in 1869 and it is likely that his parents owned slaves before the war.

Family history, passed through the generations, claims an ancestor of James Spilman was with Captain John Smith at the first English settlement of Jamestown, Virginia, in 1607.[6] Smith's *The Generall Historie of Virginia, New England & The Summer Isles* tells of a massacre near Jamestown during the winter of 1609 while he was away in England. A trading party headed by Captain Sickelmore was slain by Chief Powhatan's warriors. Of that party, only one boy and one man survived, according to John Smith. "Sickelmore upon the confidence of Powhatan, with about thirtie others as carelesse as himselfe, were all slaine, onely Jeffrey Shortridge escaped, and Pokahontas the Kings daughter saved a boy called Henry Spilman, that lived many yeeres after, by her meanes, amongst the Patawomekes."[7]

Another account of the young Henry Spilman, penned by William Box, tells of "finding an English boy, one Henry Spilman, a young Gentleman well descended, by those people preserved from the furie of Powhatan, by his acquaintance had such good usage of those kinde Salvages, that they fraughted his ship with Corne, wherewith he returned to James towne."[8] There is another Spilman in the Jamestown narrative, Thomas Spilman, who owned 50 acres of Virginia land in the Corporation of Elizabeth City, as noted in *The Complete Book of Emigrants, 1607–1776*.[9] He arrived in Jamestown from England in 1616 on the *George*, a ship that carried a 15-year-old girl named Hanna, who was to become his wife. He was a landowner with servants, a possible ancestor of James Spilman.[10]

Whatever the truth of his lineage, James was schooled in old-fashioned manners. To his eyes, men were very different from women and their roles were to be meted out accordingly. "Men took care of their women in a grand manner and always provided for them and treated them as beautiful, important — but to some extent — as objects."[11]

The union of Elizabeth Brewer and James Spilman happened against the odds. First, James had to successfully woo Elizabeth. In 1890, he was living in Sacramento and wrote her a letter on beautiful cream-colored parchment paper addressed to "Dear Friend Libbie."

> When we parted last, you will remember that I had been very much depressed for some time, and you asked me the reason. I will tell you. The conviction came upon me with greater force than ever before, that our companionship, which means so much to me, cannot last forever.

> Oh Libbie! When I say that I love you, it is not a new confession. I know that you have not been blind, but have read my heart as you have my mind. How long my love has been written on my face, word and action, I do not know, but I do know that I have loved you ever since the first evening spent in your company, two years ago.... I am strong in your friendship, in your confidence in me, in your influence upon my life; an influence that will guide me long after you have given your heart and life into the keeping of one more worthy of the priceless gift than I, when our friendship and our long, beautiful hours together will exist only as a holy memory of something that has passed away. No, I won't say that, for we will always be friends, will we not? Sometimes I am mad enough to hope that you love me. A wild, beautiful dream surges through my soul, a dream of our lives spent together in the sublime harmony that would make a perfect life. But this is too beautiful to be true, for even if I filled the place in your heart that you do in mine, we would be parted by material considerations, at least for a long, long time.

James closed his declaration of love by asking her to write to him soon, to "say that you forgive my presumption, and that you will always be my friend."[12]

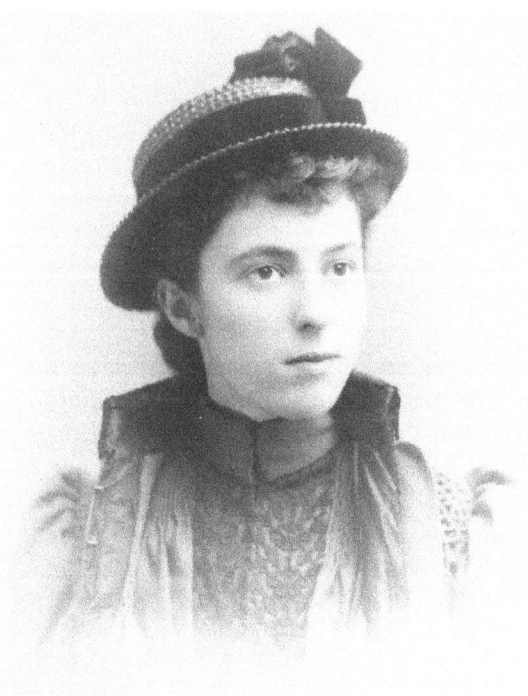

Elizabeth Brewer (Spilman) in the 1890s.

Four days later, he had his answer. He responded with another letter, thanking her for responding with "an overflow of your grand noble self" and declaring himself glad to have unburdened himself of his ill-kept secret. "You know my love, you have seen me suffer; you have probed the depths, there is nothing more." Her answer, as he anticipated, was "No." "I am not disappointed," he wrote. "I had no reason to expect or hope for your love, and when I did hope, it was but vaguely, without a foundation of faith.... Libbie, I say this solemnly, and it comes from the heart: your friendship is to me more than would be

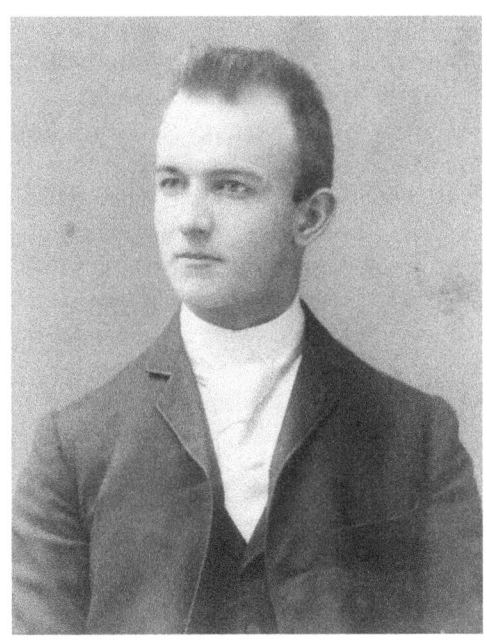

James Spilman in the 1890s.

the love, the life devotion of any other woman in the universe...." He added, "So let us resume our old friendship, which I can promise will never be marred by reference to my helpless, hopeless love, which dies tonight on lip and pen but not in the heart."[13]

Like those of most ardent lovers, lip and pen must have followed heart, because the following summer, he wrote to her yet again. All had changed somehow in the intervening months. "My Darling" was the salutation of a letter of courtship: "Oh my dearest loved one, words refuse to speak for my heart today. They would seem barren indeed if I did not know — for you have told me — that they are as music to you. Life would be so dull and flat without your love."[14] The two were clearly getting to know each other better — she told him by letter that he didn't yet know her as well as he thought he did. In another, written from her family's home in Kingston, Ontario, Canada, she confided that she considered herself a little bit "spoiled." A deep conversation unfurled over the ensuing months and years. He was at that time in Sacramento doing legal work, and acknowledged wishing that he had a fine house and a good business so that they might be together. He seemed only somewhat tongue in cheek when he wrote, "Ah my queen, I do not fear your rule of love. It shall be my duty to make your realm, as far as possible, worthy of its sovereign. How deeply I realize the magnitude of this task."[15] He alluded to the struggle, the joy of success, and his fear of failure.

There are several more years of letters written back and forth between the engaged couple. Through much of the 1890s, the two were in California, but as yet unmarried due to lack of funds. He wrote to "Miss Brewer" until late in the decade, when he began addressing her as "Mrs. Spilman." He wrote whenever they were apart, it seems, and the letters became full of the business of daily living but no less full of love and devotion. Theirs was a happy match; Elizabeth and James loved each other dearly and had a great deal in common. They were always civil to each other — disputes were worked out through gentle, polite discussion. James was a lawyer and Elizabeth a gentleman's wife. He forbade her to earn money with her piano, though she commanded a high price for lessons before they married, on the grounds that a gentleman is the sole responsible party for his wife and family's maintenance.

Elizabeth and James moved to San Francisco in the last years of the nineteenth century. James established a law office downtown and the young couple were excited by all of the cultural and commercial activity in the dynamic, young port city. Their first child, a beautiful blond baby named Elizabeth, was born in 1899 when her parents were well into their thirties. It was such a hard birth, the doctor advised the couple not to risk having any more children.[16] In addition, the baby nearly died. It is not clear whether breastfeeding was attempted, but baby "Lib" was very allergic to the cow's milk they tried to feed her. They tried everything they could think of as the baby grew weaker. Finally, they were able to save her with goat's milk.[17] For the next few years, her parents made sure not to risk another pregnancy. In 1904, either intentionally or accidentally, they had another baby, a cherubic, blond, curly-headed, outgoing child — Ruth Lee.

Ruth Lee's older sister Lib grew up being a bit of a tomboy, happy to dress in male clothing and be athletic. Lib and Ruth Lee were said to have very different temperaments. The former was analytical, quiet, thoughtful, and prone to moments of irritability; the latter was sunny, sociable, and irrepressibly optimistic. Lib was told by their mother over and over again to work on her disposition and make it more like Ruth Lee's. Whether their mother's campaign ever effected real change and made the firstborn daughter more like the lastborn daughter is debatable.

When Ruth Lee was eighteen months old, the San Francisco earthquake and fire of 1906 devastated their city. Although we have no direct account from James or Elizabeth of the terror of the moment, other residents of San Francisco who survived the earthquake that rocked the city shortly after five A.M. on April 18 recorded their experiences. Emma M. Burke, wife of a San Francisco attorney, lived near Golden Gate Park. Her experience is undoubtedly like that of many other families:

> The shock came, and hurled my bed against an opposite wall. I sprang up, and, holding firmly to the foot-board managed to keep on my feet to the door. The shock was constantly growing heavier; rumbles, crackling noises, and falling objects already commenced the din.... It grew constantly worse, the noise deafening: the crash of dishes, falling pictures, the rattle of the flat tin roof, bookcases being overturned, the piano hurled across the parlor, the groaning and straining of the building itself, broken glass and falling plaster, made such a roar that no one noise could be distinguished. We never knew then the chimney came tearing through.... [T]he floor moved like short, choppy waves of the sea.... I never expected to come out alive.[18]

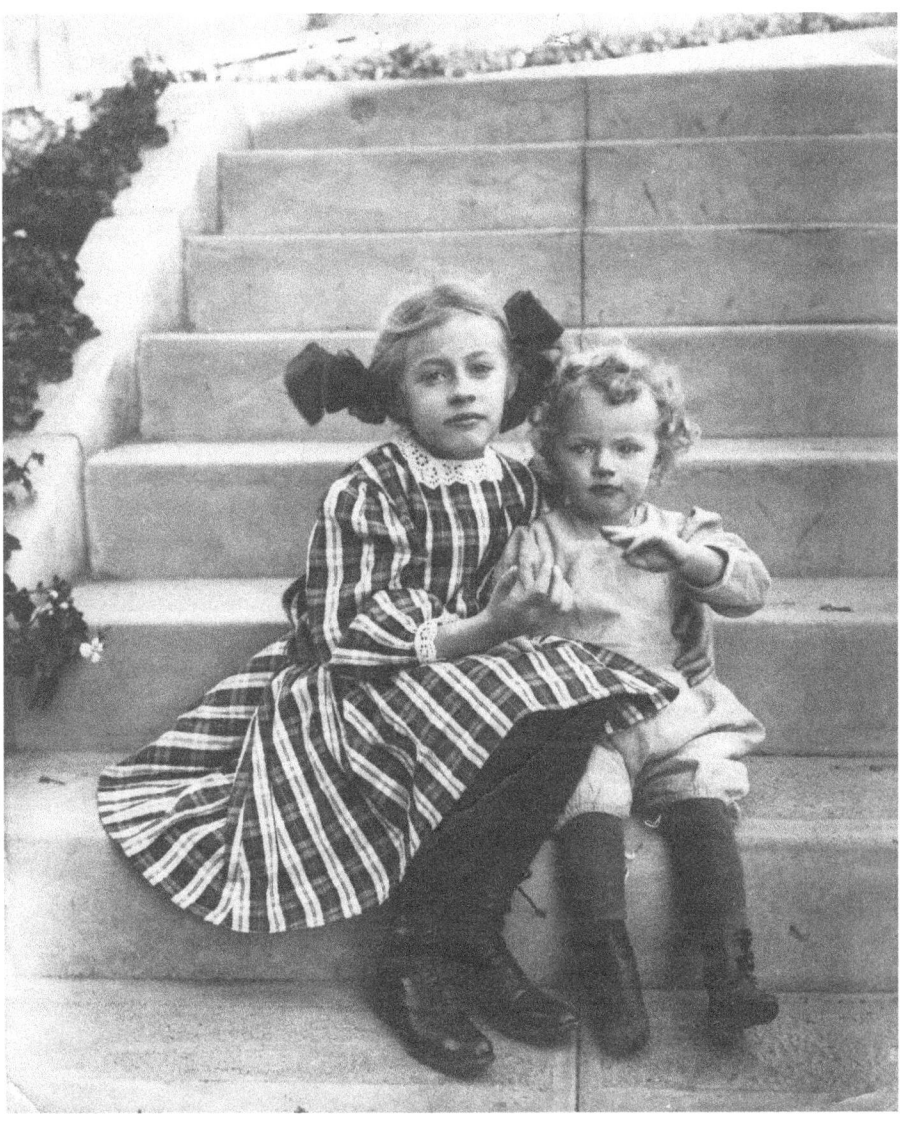

Elizabeth (Lib), left, and Ruth Lee Spilman, soon after they survived the 1906 San Francisco earthquake.

For those who survived the 48 terrifying seconds, more fear and hardship lay ahead. The calculus of life changed dramatically in that minute. As Burke described it, "All estimates of value were annihilated. Human life seemed the only thing worth consideration." The struggle to survive was not over. "The spirals of smoke now began to ascend from various places in the business section, and we realized how completely we were at the mercy of fire, with the broken water-mains, the reservoirs perhaps destroyed."[19] Gas mains were broken and leaking, which quickly led to ravaging fires across the city. That first night, as thousands of homeless, hungry people took refuge in the relative safety of Golden Gate Park, "immense fires ... now made such a ruddy glow that it was easy to see everything, although the flames were two miles away." People in the park reported ash falling on them as if it were snow. It took nearly two hours of standing in line to get a precious drink of water.[20]

The fire turned out to be more distressing than the earthquake for the Spilman family. Their house at 1309 O'Farrell Street, though damaged, was still standing. When fires moved closer to their neighborhood, James saw his family to the comparative safety of Golden Gate Park. Ruth Lee was little more than a babe in arms. The family walked all the way to the park, with Ruth Lee being carried most of the way and Lib losing her shoes and having to walk barefoot, the soles of her feet blistering from the hot streets. In Golden Gate Park, they slept on the open ground for days with thousands of others who feared damaged buildings collapsing and the uncontrolled spread of fire. Other San Franciscans walked through the smoldering embers of downtown to the ferry at the foot of Market Street in the hope of catching a boat to anywhere out of the city. Famed missionary Donaldina Cameron remembers "that weary, unwashed, and uncombed procession on the long tramp through stifling, crowded streets near where the fire raged, and through the desolate district already burned, where fires of yesterday still smoldered."[21]

Lib would always remember how the sky glowed orange in the middle of the night and how she worried about her father, who had set off on foot in the direction of his downtown law office in the desperate hope that it could be saved. A fellow survivor recalled, "As we gazed with feelings of indefinable dread over the blocks below, there passed at full gallop a company of United States Cavalry. The city was under martial law."[22] The cavalry could not save the city, but it let people know that some vestige of civil society must be preserved. Looters were shot on sight, and signs were hung on their corpses to warn others to avoid making the same mistakes.

The only means to prevent fire from burning down the entire city — given the gas leaks and the awful lack of water — was to dynamite house after house, as fire spreads much less quickly through rubble. Even the mansions on Nob Hill burned to the ground. James Spilman's office was located in the beautiful, ten-story Mills Building at 200 Montgomery Street in the financial district. Built in 1892, the building suffered only minor damage to its exterior in 1906. The interior, however, was devastated — "virtually gutted" — by the fire.[23] James Spilman's legal files went up in smoke. Emma Burke described "the great, pulsing commercial heart of the town in ashes."[24] Another eyewitness wrote, "Buildings were tumbled over on their sides, others looked as though they had been cut off short with a cleaver, the whole front having fallen through the sidewalk into the basement."[25]

Even for those lucky families whose houses were left standing, no one was allowed to cook indoors for fear of the risk of open flame. A boy of eight remembered people cooking in the middle of the street because of the prohibition on lighting candles or matches inside of buildings. "Mother felt that she just had to have some warm milk for my baby sister, Virginia, who was just six months old," he wrote. "Cautiously Mother struck a match to light a Sterno. Soon enough an officer knocked at our door and said, 'Madam, put out the light and if you do that again I have to shoot you.'"[26] The family was forced to evacuate as the fire approached their house on Dolores Street, in what is now the Mission District. Other houses, dynamited to rubble, were sacrificed to save theirs.

The Spilman family left San Francisco in a matter of days. They separated—Elizabeth and the young girls took refuge in East Auburn in the foothills of the Sierra Nevada, while James went first to Sacramento and then prowled around Oakland, looking for office space and lodging for his family. On April 27, 1906, he wrote rather plaintively to his wife about the situation: "If I find a suitable house I shall have to take it. I can't think of any other solution of the great difficulty. We must have a place that will do if I stay in Oakland for some time, and from which we should not *have* to move immediately on my return to S.F. I do hope you are better today, sweetheart. We must be strong because of our love and what we *haven't* lost."[27]

James wrote from Sacramento, but was soon receiving his mail at the North American Dredging Co. in Oakland. It got harder from there. On April 29, he wrote: "I spent the entire day, after my arrival, looking for an office. Everything in that line is terribly congested, of course. People on side streets, and even far out into the residence districts, are renting their front rooms for offices.... Everybody is advancing rents and there is not much at any price."[28] In another letter posted soon thereafter, he wrote: "The towns are almost literally packed. The streets of staid, old bedroom Oakland, suggest the early days of a boom town."[29]

James alluded to the emotional distress his wife was suffering: "My dearheart: I hope you feel much better than you were when I left you. You showed so much strength and character, I do not wonder at a temporary reaction.... [T]he essentials are saved, and energy and courage will replace everything else.... 'Nil desperandum' must be our working motto, and there can be no failure. Kiss our babies for their 'Boppa.'"[30] Their former home in San Francisco did not burn, but the roof was so damaged that rainwater leaked in and threatened the furniture they left behind.[31] On May 3, James reported that he had found a house to rent in Berkeley.[32] Many letters went back and forth between Oakland and Berkeley, and it appears that the young couple were often apart, separated by what in those days was the insurmountable distance of eight miles. Nonetheless, life began to settle back into a kind of routine.

Ruth Lee's parents were apart quite often over the next few years, as James traveled extensively on business. The letters came from New York, Chicago, Los Angeles, and Oregon, and they were replied to from as many places, most of them in Northern California. After sojourns in the East Bay of the San Francisco Bay area and in Sacramento, the Spilmans moved down the peninsula from San Francisco to San Mateo. They were able to afford a cook and a maid, at least for some years. Business was a struggle for James at times. In 1909, he wrote from New York: "I am busy most of the time, and have no real privacy any of the time.... The deal is in very doubtful condition just now. We are up against a hard formation — big capitalists, who are accustomed to deal with small fry like us on their own terms. And there are some inherent difficulties that strengthen their position and weaken ours."[33]

Elizabeth home-schooled Ruth Lee because she didn't believe the local school was good enough in the early grades for their very bright daughter.[34] At age eight, Ruth Lee finally attended a regular school. The school insisted she be put in the youngest class, since this was her first school experience, but she was bumped up quickly through several grades before the school staff decided she was in the right classroom. She was always younger than her classmates, however, because of her home schooling and academic precocity. Ruth Lee was still wearing pinafores, which none of the other girls wore, until not long before she went to college.[35] She was also out of step with her peers socially during her school years, probably because of the age gap.[36]

Ruth Lee had a happy childhood, and the family eventually moved to Palo Alto, which they considered a "village." It was an era when the local green grocer, butcher, and dairyman stopped by your house to take your order and delivery carts brought fresh food daily. Lib played tennis and followed baseball games with her father. Everyone read copiously and enjoyed one another's company. Elizabeth and James loved English literature and the English language, a love the girls would grow to share and pass on to the next two generations. A huge dictionary, kept right next to the family dining table, would land in the middle of that table nearly every meal as they discussed the usage, meaning, history, or etymology of a word.

At some point, James Spilman began struggling financially in earnest. Perhaps it was always a struggle, as his early courtship letters suggest. He was a good lawyer, but he wasn't as good a businessman. He quietly grew despondent and was humiliated by the public and private nature of what he considered to be his failure. His wife was an excellent household manager and

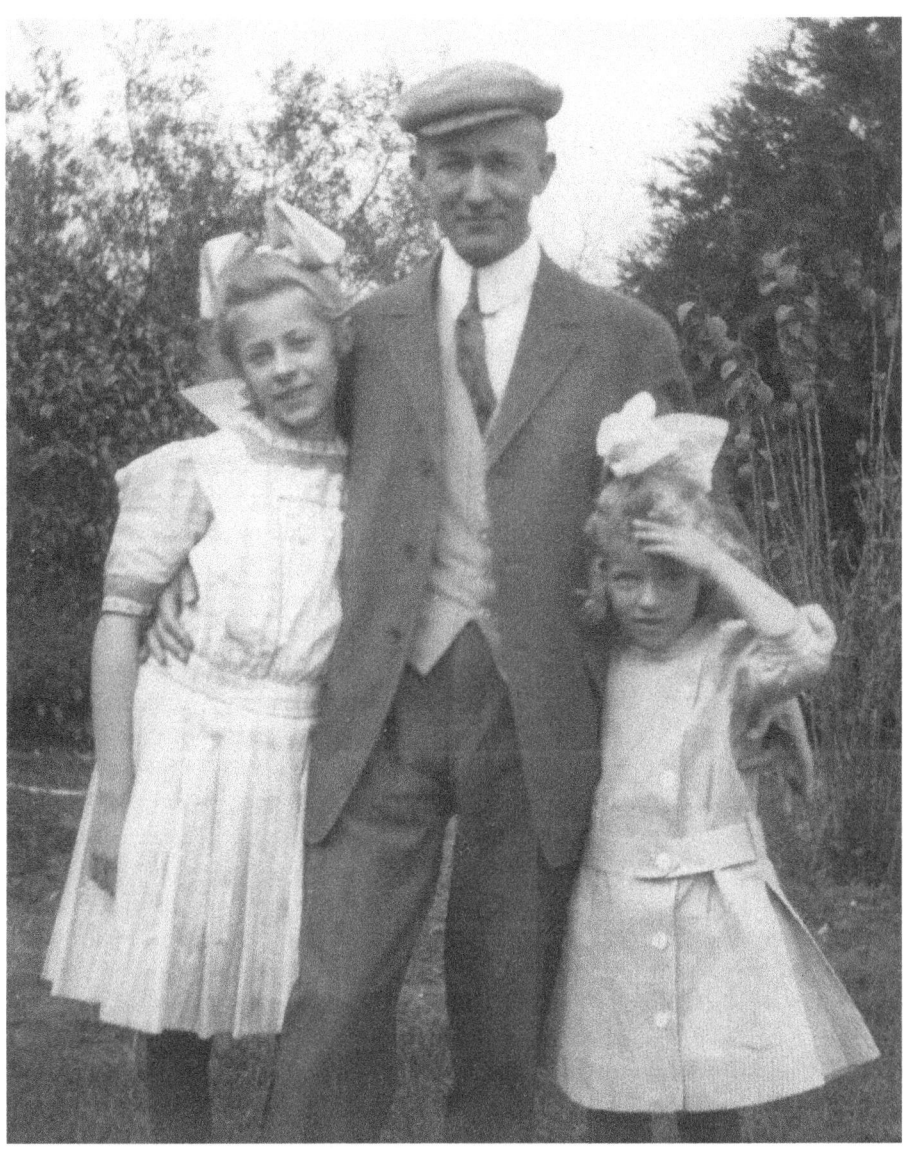

Lib, James, and Ruth Lee Spilman, circa 1910.

watched every penny. The family took steps to avoid looking as poor as they were. Still, for these years, the daughters were happy, excelling at their school work, learning to play tennis, and feeling lucky to have been born to loving parents and raised in an environment full of ideas, books, good manners, and kindness.

3. A Death in the Family

Phil's idyllic childhood ended when he lost his father at the tender cusp of his adolescence. In spite of this tragedy, he was resourceful in exploring new passions, engaging with people, and learning what he could. He had already started his involvement with scouting and ham radio in St. Paul, and he carried these interests with him when they moved to Palo Alto. He matriculated at Palo Alto High School, which he affectionately called Pali High. His family moved to Palo Alto in April 1917, so he didn't have a complete year at the prestigious St. Paul Academy or at Palo Alto High. The public high school made him take the whole year over. He ended up spending five years in high school, which was perfectly fine with him. Phil's best friend was Chinese American. The students, many of whom were the children of Stanford faculty, were motivated and engaged, and very few were rich or spoiled.[1] Although Phil was the kind of kid who did not get into trouble, he nonetheless spent a night in jail during his high school years. He was one of several passengers in a car driven by a high school friend when they were stopped for a traffic violation. One thing led to another, and they all spent the night in jail.[2]

All things considered, the Thygeson family were lucky. Stanford's first president, who went on to become chancellor, was David Starr Jordan, whom Nels Marcus had known through their shared connection to the University of Wisconsin. Jordan came in the 1890s to Minneapolis to speak at one of Sylvie Thygeson's grand suffrage-advocacy events. During Nels Marcus's struggle with cancer in the spring of 1917, President Jordan invited the Thygeson family to live on the Stanford campus. They rented half a duplex there from Professor Burlingame, who taught botany. The Hoover family lived in the other half.[3] Nels Marcus died that summer, at a moment when the family were away from home and out touring in a motor car. The children had not expected him to die so suddenly. Sylvie may have known her husband was dying and could not face having the children watch him breathe his last.

Whatever the case, Phil felt deeply betrayed by his mother's choice — he felt they had all abandoned their father in his hour of need. He never forgave his mother for not preparing them better and for failing to offer Nels Marcus the comfort and companionship he needed in his dying. As they adjusted to the shock of losing Nels Marcus, the Thygeson family decided not to return to St. Paul. After all, the older Thygeson children were nearly ready for college. Sylvie sold their beautiful three-story house in St. Paul and used the money to buy a house in Palo Alto for four thousand dollars.[4]

Phil became seriously involved in wage labor for the first time. As he described the aftermath of his father's death, "there was a complete change in economic status. We were four children with an income of about $100 a month. So everybody had to get out and work. Previously the children in the family didn't work. [Now] we all worked weekends and after school...."[5] Phil was responsible for earning money to help pay for his clothes and books; he also had to support his ham radio habit and his scouting. During high school, he got paid to deliver groceries to local families. Later, he was very popular as a handsome young chauffeur for Stanford faculty wives.

In St. Paul in the days before telephones were common, Phil built his own radio set and spent countless hours relaying messages for other people. "He built his own radio shack in the backyard.... He'd sleep out there to monitor his radio. And then, all the rest of his life, he had the radio going all night."[6] Ham radio operators had to pass a licensing test. Phil began his involvement with ham radio in 1915, a year after the formation of the American Radio Relay League, a national association of ham radio operators. As with many of his other pursuits, Phil was a pioneer. He obtained his first license in St. Paul in 1916, but he had to give up his radio rig soon thereafter because of World War I, when all amateur radio was forbidden for fear it would be infiltrated by spies. He bought his own vacuum tubes and equipment when the war ended in 1918, and began operations under the call letter 6BU.[7]

Phil was willing to stay up all hours of the night to perform public service, using frequencies designated for ham operators.[8] This often nocturnal work may have been Phil's first taste of internationalism, as ham radio was an effective way to reach ham operators from all over the world. To obtain even an amateur license, ham operators had to be able to communicate using Morse code. The code can be described as a pattern of dots and dashes, or short and long signals, that form the letters of the alphabet. The letter A, for example, is short-long, and B is long-short-short. Phil kept a telegraph key on his desk and heard the unusual "song" that is Morse code in his head all of the days of his life.

The date of Phil's involvement with the Boy Scouts is unclear, but it was near the beginning of the organization's history. The Boy Scouts of America was founded in 1910 and issued its first handbook in 1911. It was a perfect fit for Phil, given the skills and values he learned at his father's hands, especially during the family's summers on the shore of Lake Minnetonka. The values of the Scouts were respect, obedience, and service. Ernest Thompson Seton was the first chief scout of the Boy Scouts of America. In 1910, he wrote that scouting was created in part to remedy the ills of modernity:

> It is the rare exception, now, when we see a boy that is handy with tools and capable of taking care of himself under all circumstances. It is the very, very rare exception when we see a boy whose life is absolutely governed by the safe old moral standards.... To combat the system that has turned such a large proportion of our robust, manly, self-reliant boyhood into a lot of flat-chested cigarette-smokers, with shaky nerves and a doubtful vitality, I began the Woodcraft movement here in America.[9]

In this era before television and the ubiquitous use of motor cars, it's hard to know exactly what threatened American boyhood, but Seton clearly felt that too many boys were losing the frontier spirit and becoming overly effete and lazy. The United States had become industrialized, and millions of children under the age of sixteen were laboring on farms and in factories. Knowledge of how European Americans wrested the vast American West from indigenous Native Americans and settled the plains and mountain states was also fading. Phil embraced the history as well as the skills taught in the Scouts and he became an Eagle Scout — the top rank for boys his age — in the fastest possible time. His scout master and main adult male role model was a Unitarian minister.

Robert S. S. Baden-Powell, the founder of the international scouting movement, was an English war hero who fought on behalf of the British Empire.[10] He believed in adventure, collaboration, taking responsibility, self-sufficiency, and learning by doing.[11] Phil not only committed wholeheartedly to these values, he also carried them throughout his life. In his youth, he found surrogate fathers in the form of Scout leaders.[12] Phil liked the notion of chivalry, of a scout being a sort of modern-day knight and of carrying on in the tradition of Abraham Lincoln, ideas that were set forth in the first Boy Scout handbook.[13]

Like Seton, Baden-Powell believed that boys in wealthy countries in the early twentieth century were too soft. He was shocked by the lack of fitness of young British army volunteers during the Boer War. One report suggested that only two of every nine prospective soldiers were fit enough to fight.[14] This was attributed to poor living conditions, inadequate diet, urban crowding, and excessive child labor. In his public speeches, Baden-Powell liked to tie physical degeneracy to moral degeneracy, and to argue that scouting was a remedy for societal ills.[15] He did not want to turn his efforts into a proto-military operation focusing on drilling boys and trying to get them to act like junior soldiers. Rather, he wanted to teach them how to observe, reflect, solve problems, and work together.

Phil was an easy sell; Baden-Powell's values became his values. Phil's older brother Elling was less scout-like in his inclinations. Elling spent too much money, ran up gambling debts, smoked tobacco, and even went AWOL for several days from the U.S. Army Air Corps during World War I. His straight arrow younger brother was scandalized, in part because he knew that their late father would have been distressed by Elling's behavior. In one famous episode, Sylvie and her children were out in a motor car near Yosemite. Elling was at the wheel. He managed to get the car stuck in loose sand on the side of the road. When Sylvie upbraided Elling, he flew into a rage, got out of the car, and began the 200-mile walk home. Phil had to take over.[16] Phil's view was that Elling had been spoiled by the family money and was anything but "thrifty," as scouts were supposed to be. He felt himself lucky to have been born later and to have had to earn his own pocket money as a teenager. But neither Phil nor his brother followed the Scouts' dictum to believe in God. Phil also failed to live up to the Boy Scout values of being consistently cheerful and friendly — no one in the Thygeson family was after Nels Marcus died.

Phil developed a passionate commitment to scouting. He took up its credo of contributing to society, collaborating across socioeconomic class lines, and learning skills for self-reliance. Early on, scoutcraft was defined as "a combination of observation, deduction, and handiness, or the ability to do things," whether the subject was life saving, tracking, campcraft, patriotism, or seamanship.[17] Phil loved the Boy Scout uniform: a khaki flat-brimmed Stetson, similar to that worn by the Canadian Mounted Police, a rustic button-down coat, a neckerchief, shorts that gave way in his late adolescence to jodhpur-like breeches, and knee-high boys' socks in knee-high leather boots. In the early days, the uniform cost about four dollars.[18] Phil was still wearing a version of this uniform in the 1930s as he climbed a number of Rocky Mountain peaks that ranged up to 14,000 feet.

Scouts were supposed to know how to tie knots, build a shelter from the sparsest of materials, start a fire with a bow and spindle, apply life-saving first aid, and even build things such as the "Wind-turned meat-roaster," which consisted of a pole anchored in the ground and bending over the campfire. From it, a cut of meat was hung.[19] Phil liked the scouting badges and enjoyed earning them to rise up through the ranks. He also was deeply attracted to the military spirit that infected the entire country during World War I. Scout troops helped support the work of the American Red Cross, sold vast numbers of Liberty Loan bonds, and were asked to plant gardens in the spirit of "Every scout to feed a soldier."[20] Scouts also collected peach pits to help make gas mask filters for the soldiers in the trenches of France.²¹ They staffed soup kitchens and inventoried black walnut trees, whose precious wood was used for airplane propellers and gun stocks.²²

It was an easy transition for Phil to become a high school cadet in Palo Alto. His involvement was short but exciting. "I advanced to the status of corporal and I took it all very seriously. I really thought I was aiding the war effort!" They carried mock wooden guns and drilled and marched every afternoon, "dressed in regular army uniforms with puttees and boots." Germans were often reviled and Phil was ashamed of being one-quarter Pennsylvania Dutch on his mother's side.²³ Though he was eager to serve his country and supported it through all the wars and military engagements of his life — he came pretty close to subscribing to the credo of "my country, right or wrong" — his deeper love was for what E. T. Seton had in mind when he organized woodcraft activities for America's boys.²⁴ Phil subscribed to the dictum in the first Boy Scout Handbook that said, "It is horrible to be a coward. It is weak to yield to fear and heroic to face danger without flinching."²⁵ He also believed in the value and necessity of wage labor. He got summer jobs at local power companies, the San Joaquin Light and Power Company and Pacific Gas and Electric. The days of feeling like a wealthy man's son were long gone.

4. Genteel Poverty and a Pandemic

During Phil's high school years, Ruth Lee's happy home life grew more complicated, worrisome, and difficult. Her parents' financial struggles worsened, but James refused to let Elizabeth offer piano lessons to private students. Before they married in the 1890s, Elizabeth commanded the princely sum of $10 an hour for her lessons. She was willing to do it again — in fact, she wanted to teach — but her old-fashioned southern gentleman of a husband said no. To him, it was humiliating and dishonorable to have one's wife in the workforce. Soon, however, both of his daughters were out in the working world helping to pay for their educations and support the family. One wonders what they thought of their father's stubbornly held position. A classic "generation gap" probably arose, with the daughters taking their mother's side. Ruth Lee and Lib went on to become fervent supporters of women's suffrage, affordable family planning, social justice, the dismantling of institutional racism, and equal pay for equal work. They quickly became progressive women of the twentieth century.

In late 1918, when Ruth Lee was just fourteen, her beloved sister Lib was infected in the global influenza pandemic that killed millions of people worldwide. Ruth Lee, who was always perceived as having the stronger constitution, escaped her sister's fate and most likely helped nurse her sister.[1] The influenza pandemic was swift and deadly. It is estimated that between 20 and 40 million people died worldwide, making it the most devastating pandemic in human history.[2] Over 25 percent of Americans came down with the virus, sometimes known as the "Spanish flu," though it didn't originate in Spain. An astounding 20 percent of the population of the world got sick or died.

What was unusual about this particular pandemic was that it killed young, healthy adults in abundance, not just the elderly, the infirm, and the very young.[3] Sometimes death came so fast, the infected person barely had time to feel sick. There is a story of four women playing bridge long into the evening. By morning, three were dead of influenza.[4] The origin of this killer pandemic was a mystery to many people. Some thought it was a new biological weapon developed by the Germans as they lost the war. Some thought it was a by-product of mustard gases and other horrors of trench warfare.[5] In fact, the virus was so virulent and its spread so hard to contain that there existed three different waves of influenza in different parts of the world over the course of two years. The first wave spread through the United States in March 1918, followed by a second wave that circled the world from September to November of that year.[6]

The medical situation in the United States was dire for a number of reasons. Many doctors and nurses were in Europe serving in World War I, leaving inexperienced medical students to take their places in hospitals back home. Medical school classes shut down so that their students could try to serve as the doctors they in fact were not. Public health officials resorted to desperate measures. It was understood that the virus was transmitted by airborne droplets, so people were urged to wear masks, avoid gathering in groups, especially in indoor spaces, and keep themselves as well fed, rested, and healthy as possible. Funerals were kept short and private, many towns would not let train passengers disembark unless they carried proof of health certificates, and thousands of schools shut down around the world.[7] The American Public Health Association determined that "saloons, dance halls, and cinemas should be closed" and church services should be kept short, uncrowded, and well ventilated.[8] Quarantine was required for the severely ill, home quarantine for the rest. The latter was Lib Spilman's fate. She had just turned nineteen when she fell ill and she spent most of the coming year in bed.

Through the pandemic, many people got their first taste of modern science and the medical revolution that characterized the twentieth century. It was widely understood by then that germs were deadly and, in this case, easily transmissible. British surgeon Joseph Lister, an admirer of Louis Pasteur, had experimented with different methods of antisepsis and published an article in 1867 in *The Lancet* on the use of a carbolic acid solution to disinfect surgical wounds, surgical instruments, and surgeons' hands.[9] During the 1918–1919 influenza epidemic, his ideas were put into practice in the form of masks, hand-washing, disinfection of dishes and bedding, and ventilation of sickrooms. Gauze face masks were mandatory for all San Franciscans for a time, and everyone in Ruth Lee's family wore them at home.[10] Some people gargled or rinsed their nasal passages with boric acid and sodium bicarbonate.[11]

The *Journal of the American Medical Association* reported that patients who died tended to develop toxemia and vasomotor depression not long before death.[12] Lib had access to white blood cell counts, measures of albumin, and the Wasserman test for antibodies in the blood, but therapy was not nearly so advanced.[13] Aside from bed rest, patients were given aspirin, epinephrine, hot packs, cold packs, intravenous "digitalis," and salt of quinine. Lib developed the common and often deadly secondary bacterial infection that stalked the influenza victims — pneumonia. She ran a high fever and may have been one of many victims who found herself coughing up blood. She was nursed tenderly at home by her mother and sister. Finally, she returned to Stanford a year behind her class, still weak but glad to be alive.

5. Meeting at Stanford

As young college students, Ruth Lee and Phil turned out for a freshman football rally for what was called the Big Game, the annual match of Stanford and the University of California at Berkeley. High up in the amphitheater, Phil saw a "blue-eyed blond girl ... in the balcony yelling her heart out for dear old Stanford.... I looked up and saw her, and I thought that she was the most beautiful woman in the world. And she was!"[1] In lower division courses, students were seated alphabetically. Ruth Lee's last name was Spilman, so she was always about two rows ahead of Phil. He could see the back of her neck, but that did not help him meet her. He had to find another way.

Phil matriculated at Stanford University in 1920 or 1921, for he reports different starting years in different written documents. Ruth Lee matriculated at the age of sixteen, which means she entered in 1921, weeks before her seventeenth birthday.[2] It was an empowering moment for young women, as the Nineteenth Amendment guaranteeing women the right to vote was finally ratified in 1920.

Former California governor Leland Stanford and his wife Jane Lathrop Stanford established the university in 1891, in memory of their only child, Leland Jr., who had died at age fifteen.[3] Leland had worked as a child, gathering bushels of chestnuts to sell when he was only seven years old. He became a lawyer who, like James Spilman, lost his law files and library to a devastating fire. He moved west and joined his five brothers in their mercantile enterprise in the gold fields of the Sierra Nevada. The brothers ran a store where Leland "slept on the counter under buffalo robes with his boots for a pillow...."[4] As soon as he was able, he bought out his brothers' interest in the store and went back to New York for Jane, whom he had left behind during this experiment in the West.

Leland Stanford was a lot like Phil and Ruth Lee — fearless, undaunted, and willing to take on huge new challenges. He campaigned on behalf of

5. Meeting at Stanford

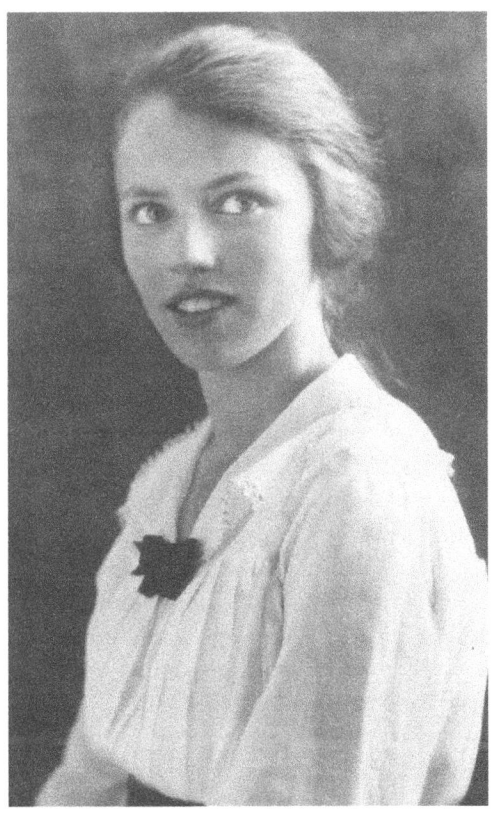

Ruth Lee Spilman as a Stanford University student, early 1920s.

Abraham Lincoln in 1860, and in 1861 was elected governor of California. In 1885, he was elected to the U.S. Senate. He also had a key role in completing the nation's first transcontinental railroad against all odds.[5] Not a few people considered him to be an anti-labor, anti-socialist "robber baron." It all depended on one's political perspective. Soon after the dream of a transcontinental railroad was a reality, the Stanfords' only child, Leland, Jr., celebrated his first birthday. As a teenager, Leland, Jr. was a natural scholar and was interested in French, archaeology, and the fine arts. His parents took him frequently to Europe. In 1884, he came down with typhoid fever while they were traveling in Italy. He died two months shy of his sixteenth birthday, plunging his parents into deep grief.[6]

The Stanfords decided that they wanted to create a memorial in his honor—a major university, technical school, or museum. After some research into their options, they chose a university, intended especially to benefit young men. Leland Stanford envisioned the university as a school where practical skills in addition to classical areas of study would be taught and that would not be affiliated with any religious entities. He wanted costs to be kept low enough that students of limited means could enroll. In addition, he insisted publicly, "females shall have equal advantages."[7] The university opened in 1891 in what Easterners considered rather primitive circumstances.

Even before he came to Stanford, President and then Chancellor David Starr Jordan spoke often and publicly about the value of a college education. He believed that everyone could find his or her way to a college education. He had been a ditch digger, corn husker, waiter, and carpenter's assistant on his way through Cornell, and he issued a clarion call to young people to find their own way forward.⁸ As President Jordan said in his opening day address, "Our University has no history to fall back upon.... It is hallowed by no tradition; it is hampered by none."⁹ The pioneer spirit that infused Stanford would infuse Ruth Lee and Phil.

In spite of the Stanfords' best-laid plans, Leland, Sr. died before even the most basic campus was completed. His estate was soon caught up in a prolonged probate battle with the federal government. Salaries at Stanford were cut and no new faculty were hired. "Chalk came to be doled out by the stick. Pages left blank in examination books served for interdepartment letters. Classrooms went unswept."¹⁰ The local coal seller, whose son was a Stanford student, let the university buy coal on credit.¹¹ In 1896, the U.S. Supreme Court ruled in favor of the estate, but the probate process dragged on. Jane Stanford sold the family's railroad assets to keep the university going.¹² She died two years after Memorial Church was dedicated and a year before it and other buildings were devastated by the 1906 earthquake.

Stanford developed a relationship of mutual support, trust, and assistance with the community around it. It has stood by its faculty and students through all manner of crisis, and the community has rallied around its university. In 1906, though several almost brand-new buildings at Stanford were damaged or destroyed, the university encouraged students and staff to stop everything to help the people of San Francisco. They offered manual labor and all of the supplies that could be spared, from yeast for bread to tins of hastily sterilized milk to tools for digging in the rubble.¹³ The president's office issued a proclamation: all classes were suspended until the fall quarter.¹⁴ "Within the week, the campus was empty except for faculty and for a hundred or so working students whose summer was to be given over to sorting rubble, chipping mortar from bricks, serving as guards around the roped-off buildings...."¹⁵

Faculty lived in the small towns of Palo Alto and Menlo Park. Menlo was described as having a ratio of saloons to churches that ran nearly ten to one in favor of saloons, tap water that was full of silt and had a nasty odor, and cooling cupboards that served as inefficient substitutes for ice boxes.¹⁶ Many students were not wealthy — fully half worked their way through school.¹⁷ Students worked for fifteen cents an hour and could buy a rather humble meal for twenty cents. Some students lived in the attics of faculty houses, washing dishes and doing chores to earn their keep.¹⁸

The academic performance of the Thygeson kids at Stanford was somewhat uneven. The oldest sister, Ruth, was a stellar student who graduated Phi Beta Kappa and went on to become a physician. Elling flunked out of medicine, but became a successful petroleum engineer. Mary excelled in the social sciences, became a social worker in Harlem, and later a highly respected anthropologist. As a teenager, Phil decided he wanted to be an electrical engineer, and he focused on engineering during his first year as a Stanford undergraduate.[19] When he matriculated, the price was just right for the Thygeson family. Tuition was forty dollars a quarter, plus fees.[20] This was the first formal tuition at Stanford, which had previously cost nothing, and it shocked the student body.[21] Stanford put out a call for scholarship fund donations and allowed students to use "tuition notes," which were essentially student loans due within seven years.[22] As historian of Stanford Edith R. Mirrielees wrote, "From being a poor man's school, Stanford in the twenties was a middle-income one. Far fewer undergraduates earned while they learned, though the tuition was resented nonetheless."[23] Still, as then–Stanford president Ray Lyman Wilbur said, "If anybody will give me an explanation to offer to a faculty man who rides a bicycle why we should teach for nothing a boy who has his own automobile, I should like to hear it."[24]

Moreover, costs were higher than expected; an average salary of an associate professor was three thousand dollars a year in 1914.[25] The president of the university in the early 1920s didn't want spoiled rich students on campus and penned a letter to parents with the following admonition:

> We particularly regret that students are often given too large an allowance of money and some are given or loaned automobiles by their parents or others. A student's principal business is his studies.... A surplus of money is one of the biggest handicaps possible for the youth who expects to be a good student.... Please look over the booklet ... sent with this letter, and if you do not feel that it expresses the right attitude towards alcohol, hazing, self-control, payments of debts, etc., it would be better to keep your son or daughter at home or send them elsewhere.[26]

Jane Stanford was more succinct. Her edict was simple: "No automobile beyond the entrance gates."[27] Her will did not prevail and soon there were many Stanford students with beautiful cars. At the same time, there were many rejected applicants because of the number of qualified high school graduates who wanted to attend. Stanford held firm, at least for a time, raising its admissions requirements and generally demanding more of its students.[28]

There were approximately 2,000 male students and 500 female students when Phil and Ruth Lee were enrolled. This ratio suited the Spilman sisters fine, as both of them enjoyed being with young men.[29] Jane Stanford wanted the number of enrolled women to be well below that of men. She felt that because women matured earlier and were more likely to excel academically, they might crowd out the men.[30] Stanford was, after all, a school founded to honor a boy and to serve the educational and vocational needs of boys on their way to becoming men.

Jordan was an outspoken advocate for peace. His vehement objection to

World War I put him at odds with many faculty and staff at Stanford, but he persevered. Fortunately, he was no longer chancellor of Stanford when he spoke out, because his position was the opposite of the one the university chose.[31] Herbert Hoover, a key donor and supporter of Stanford, helped the Stanford Board of Directors issue its own statement of support soon after the United States openly declared war. Stanford allowed students to take leaves of absence to serve in the American Ambulance Corps in Europe, Belgian relief, and the Reserve Officers Training Corps. It offered a military training course, and in some cases gave students academic credit while they were on active duty in the military. The university also permitted professors to take paid leaves of absence in order to serve the government during the war.[32]

When soldiers returned from World War I, they were welcomed in the classroom regardless of their previous academic situation. Lib met her future husband at Stanford's law school, where she was one of a mere handful of female students. Her beau, Milton Snyder Rosenfield, would come to class on crutches one day. The next, he might walk in, painfully, on his prosthetic leg. This back and forth between no leg and prosthetic leg irritated Lib, who wanted him to make up his mind which it was going to be. It ended up being the crutches. Milton was shot in the foot in no-man's-land in France, and lay abandoned between the lines for two days before he was rescued by his own men. His foot was amputated, and, due to creeping gangrene, he underwent numerous other surgeries before the tiny remainder of his leg was judged healthy.

Lib's marrying Milton was brave in more ways than one. He was Jewish and she was not. They were told that no one would attend their wedding in protest of the match, and so they married quietly. Not even their parents attended. As a young married couple, Lib and Milton were offered jobs as librarians at a small college. They probably would have enjoyed working together, but instead Milton devoted his career as a lawyer to working for the Veterans' Administration (VA) and helping disabled veterans obtain government benefits and assistance. His job was not altogether a good match for his values, though, as his duties included "adjudication" where, as a VA attorney, he sometimes had to deny benefits to veterans he personally believed deserving of them. When Franklin Delano Roosevelt cut military pensions — and Milton was forced to watch his clients suffer — Milton never forgave him. He also had to commute to San Francisco on the train, spending long days in the city.

Lib and Milton never had children. They gave different explanations for their decision. Milton's explanation was that since he could not walk without crutches, he could not save a child from a burning house. Lib said that she could not care for a child and care for Milton, her widowed mother, and her aging grandmother, all of whom were under her roof in the 1930s. Because of Lib's selfless choices, Ruth Lee was the sister who had the gift of freedom to explore the world and have a career.

Though they were born over two thousand miles apart and had very different childhoods, Ruth Lee and Phil had similar feelings about Stanford University. They admired its academics, rooted for Stanford in its great football and academic rivalry with Berkeley, and maintained their affection for the school all through their lives. They especially admired the pull-yourself-up-by-your-bootstraps ethos of its founders, Leland and Jane Stanford. Ruth Lee said, "We usually called Harvard the Stanford of the East."[33] She and Phil enjoyed looking down their noses at UC Berkeley, Stanford's academic and football archrival. They also always loved the notion that Stanford was intended to be what they called a "poor boys" school.[34] They lived long enough to see Stanford become something quite different from what it was when they were students, but some of their loyalty and affection remained.

Phil's initial interest in becoming an electrical engineer was scuttled by his inability to do the math required. He claimed that as a sophomore, he was lured into zoology and thus into biology by Professor Harold Heath, whose courses he loved. Ruth Lee couldn't resist teasing him: "There was a little something about mathematics?" Because Phil had skipped the sixth grade to go on the fabulous trip through the southwest to Los Angeles (the winter he had terrible bronchitis), he missed months of school. He liked to say that that was why he was always weak in math. Ruth Lee responded, "That's been his excuse all his life. I tried to tell him that sixth grade could have been covered in a month."[35] Whatever the cause, Phil always considered math his hardest subject. He liked to make fun of himself. He did not mind confessing that he didn't have all A's in high school and that at Stanford in the 1920s, "the admission requirements for medicine were practically nonexistent.... It never occurred to me that I would have any trouble getting into medical school; I just signed up...."[36]

Ruth Lee studied chemistry and was quite good at it. She was an excellent student. In fact, most female Stanford students excelled over their male counterparts. Not long before Ruth Lee and Phil matriculated, the academic failure rate for women was about 1 percent, while it was closer to 14 percent for men.[37] Not a great deal is known about Ruth Lee's coursework or activities at Stanford except that she was a top student, was involved with her sorority, and had a lot of friends. She had trouble deciding on a major. "I took a lot of chemistry," she said. "I really couldn't make up my mind."[38]

Ruth Lee had to work her way through college. She worked as a receptionist-typist-stenographer for Dr. Clelia Mosher, a female physician on the Stanford staff, to pay tuition and help support her family. She was quite fond of Dr. Mosher and admired her progressive way of thinking about women's health and women's rights. In a rebuttal to the prevailing ideas of the time, Dr. Mosher taught Ruth Lee that there was nothing physically debilitating about menstruation, that it didn't make women sick or unable to function in any way. She also served as a model for how competent and hard-working women could be as professionals, and argued for an egalitarianism of gender to which Ruth Lee and her sister Lib would subscribe all of their lives.

One of the reasons Phil had such a hard time getting introduced to Ruth Lee at Stanford, once he had laid eyes on her at the football rally, was that her sorority, the Thetas, believed that his fraternity brothers, the Kappa Sigs, were "pretty rough characters."[39] Ruth Lee had her own comment: "Yes, pretty questionable to go out with," a bunch of machos who drank too much.[40] Phil wasn't a drinker — he had joined the fraternity against his inclination because it was his brother's fraternity and his brother insisted he join, too.[41] Phil wasn't interested in parties or even in athletics, but he did want to meet the pretty blond Spilman girl. He got his chance when he happened to notice a photograph of Ruth Lee on the bureau of his classmate and tennis partner, Jack Field. By then, Phil was a junior. He'd let two good years go by without meeting Ruth Lee Spilman. She later chalked this up to his shyness. He now asked Jack to fix him up with a blind date. Jack had no claims on Ruth Lee. She was merely a tennis partner, so he agreed.

Jack arranged a blind date of sorts. Phil and Ruth Lee drove to Pacific City, a resort on San Francisco Bay near San Mateo, and danced the night away. Since Jack was in love with a different girl, there were wonderful opportunities for double-dating. Soon after, Ruth Lee and Phil began taking hikes on weekends.[42] Their favorite place to go was the wilds of the Santa Cruz Mountains. The courtship picked up speed and both of their families got involved. Phil considered himself very lucky. "She was a vision of loveliness and it was love at first sight," he wrote. "I was a callow youth ... with little social skills and almost no contact with girls."[43] Phil somehow managed to have a Model T, which pleased Ruth Lee because he drove her around in it all the time. One day the Model T broke down. Ruth Lee's mother had gone along to chaperone. What was Phil to do? He asked Elizabeth if he could use her hat pin. He fixed the car with it, and off they drove.[44]

Both future mothers-in-law approved of the courtship, though Sylvie didn't like the fact that Ruth Lee was working as a stenographer to help support her studies and her family. As Ruth Lee told it, Sylvie considered stenographers to be a bit too "fast" for her taste. This was both amusing and ironic, as Sylvie had been a stenographer in her youth as well.

6. Courtship, a Wedding, and Victorian Values

The courtship may have been quick in terms of the calendar — Ruth Lee and Phil were married about a year after they first began dating seriously — but it wasn't fast in any other way. In fact, in a wonderfully old-fashioned moment, their intention to marry each other was sealed by a simple squeeze of the hand. Ruth Lee told the story of being with Phil and having him wordlessly take her hand and squeeze it. They both knew what it meant — that he had chosen her for his partner in life. She squeezed back and accepted.

There is little information about their wedding except that it was in what Ruth Lee called an "adorable little church," All Saints' Church, in Palo Alto.[1] They married in 1925, the year Phil graduated from Stanford and Ruth Lee would have graduated had she finished her studies. They went camping on their honeymoon, which was a very unusual way to spend a honeymoon in the 1920s, but a clear reflection of the man Ruth Lee married. In the middle of their first night together, there was a torrential rainstorm. Ruth Lee remembered Phil going out naked to build a fire in the rain.[2] She loved his practical, earthy side, and his gallantry. They had received $200 as a wedding gift, so they loaded up what Phil called "our $60 Model T touring car" and headed for Sproat Lake, British Columbia. "Ruth Lee had never been out of the Bay Area," Phil wrote, "so all the sights in Northern California, Oregon and Washington were new to her.... Ruth Lee, who had never been a camper or an outdoors girl, now became a real camper. She loved sleeping on the ground."[3] She also loved paddling with Phil in the birch bark canoe they borrowed to use on Sproat Lake. Before their marriage, Phil claimed, Ruth Lee had never seen snow. He loved the pleasure she took in discovering new aspects of nature.[4]

They were married in the so-called Roaring Twenties and Ruth Lee was very much of an early feminist in her belief in the equality of the sexes. It is said that Ruth Lee convinced Phil to vote for the Progressive Party candidate for president in 1924, Robert La Follette.[5] The left-leaning populist was not elected and Phil probably voted more conservatively for the next several decades. The newly married couple also exemplified an older set of values, that of Victorian England. When Ruth Lee and Lib were growing up, displayed prominently on the wall was a fine etching of Queen Victoria and Prince Albert in regal attire, attended by a hunting hound, lap dogs, a cherub, and several dead geese laid out on the divan and the floor. Dedicated to "Her Most Gracious Majesty, Victoria, Queen of Great Britain," its title was "Windsor Castle in the Present Time."

Ruth Lee and Phil's particular brand of Victorianism was characterized by a strong belief in right and wrong. They didn't see as many shades of gray or ambiguity in moral questions as most people did once the twentieth century was well launched.[6] At the same time, they were pragmatists and would do what they needed to do to accomplish their goals. Ruth Lee and Phil believed in hard work without complaint — or, at least, no complaining in public. They were firm believers in the Protestant work ethic. As described by Wayne E. Oates in his *Confessions of a Workaholic*, the ethic is quasi-religious in its vigor: "a universal taboo is placed on idleness, and industriousness is considered a religious ideal; waste is a vice, and frugality a virtue; complacency and failure are outlawed...."[7] Ruth Lee was in fact the less idle of the two. There were no real days off, except for illness, and no desire to have days off. Work itself gave meaning to life. However, they were not austere, except in their household spending habits. Nor was Phil particularly humble or tranquil.

There was no question in their minds that lack of temperance or chastity was unpardonable. There were things, after all, that one just did not do. Phil loved to hold Ruth Lee's hand in public, but he believed that not controlling one's sexual behavior was a sign of cultural and moral degeneracy. Sexually transmitted diseases were likewise freighted with moral taint, though Phil was careful not to express that view to his patients. As for sincerity, Ruth Lee was not publicly honest to the point of committing social faux pas in the name of candor. She had her company manners and her private views. She would greet a neighbor she did not particularly care for with tremendous politeness or stop to have tea with an unexpected visitor even though the visit was ill-timed. This could have been considered dishonest, but no one felt it ungracious. Phil knew how to be professionally diplomatic and then speak his truth behind closed doors, though sometimes he let his emotions spill over. He let Ruth Lee answer the phone because for the most part he didn't like to talk on the phone. Ruth Lee insisted on good phone manners, which she learned

6. Courtship, a Wedding, and Victorian Values

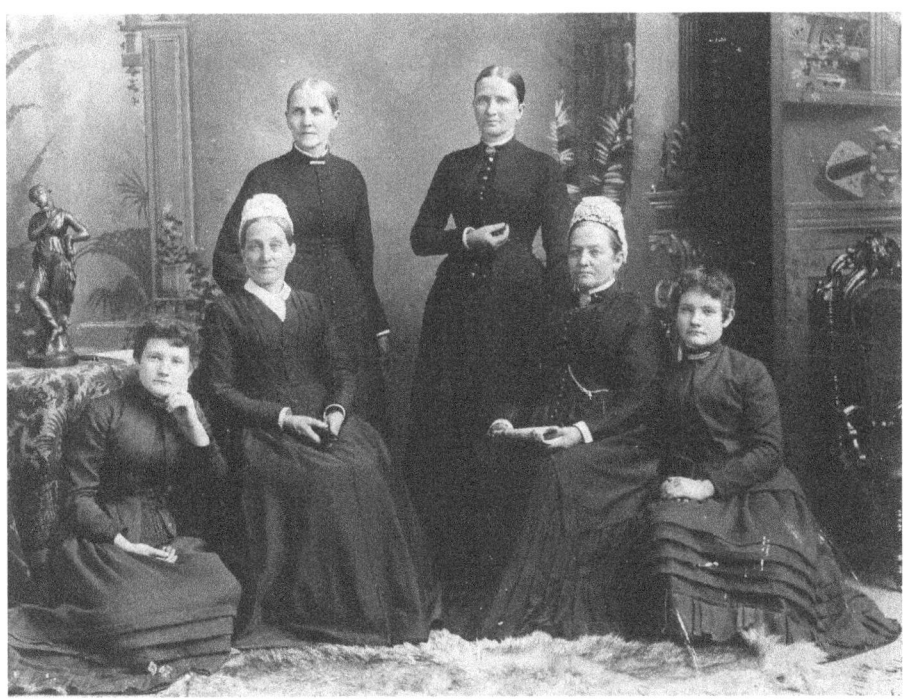

Ruth Lee Thygeson's Victorian ancestors, in Ontario, Canada.

from her father. If James Spilman answered the phone and the caller said, "Who is this?" James would reply, "I haven't the slightest idea." Ruth Lee insisted that everyone in her household initiate calls with, "This is so-and-so. May I please speak to so-and-so?"[8]

Ruth Lee and Phil believed in what many people would call Christian values, though they left God and Christ by the wayside.[9] Phil read a bit of the Bible, but his interest was archaeology, not religion.[10] A potential pitfall of Phil's values was the risk of rigidity and dogmatism. For him, change was not progress unless it was in the realm of science. Scientific progress meant the eradication of disease and human suffering, and it was the great hope of the future. Some scholars have referred to this belief system, writ large, as positivism. In *Pursuit of a Scientific Culture*, Peter Allan Dale defines positivism as "a considered philosophical position adopted by a wide variety of intellectuals who have in common simply the conviction that science offers the only viable way of thinking correctly about human affairs."[11]

Whereas for Victorianism there were clearly delineated areas of right and wrong, in science it was important to be skeptical and questioning. Thomas Henry Huxley captured this in an epigram: "The man of science has learned to believe in justification, not by faith, but by verification."[12] The issue of scientism is important, as Ruth Lee and Phil did not believe or participate in organized religion. Phil once told his son Fritjof that when he was in high school or a freshman at Stanford, he attended a church service with a neighbor girl. According to the story, "the minister spent the entire sermon criticizing people who didn't go to church." Phil told Fritjof, "That's the last time I ever went to church, and I never intend to go again."[13] In contrast, Fritjof believed Ruth Lee might have enjoyed being a churchgoer. She loved singing and would have enjoyed being in a choir. She also would have loved being a member of an organized community devoted to doing good works.[14]

Fritjof considered his mother a very spiritual person though she was also very scientific in her thinking. Members of their family have said that for Ruth Lee and Phil, science and nature, in the form of the American wilderness, occupied the place that most people reserve for religion. She was more interested in and influenced by the Bible than Phil was. In papers she kept in a special folder most of her adult life are quotations from the Bible she copied by hand. One of them, Isaiah 5:8, reads, "Woe unto them that join house to house, that lay field to field, till there be no place that they may be placed alone in the midst of the earth." In terms of Ruth Lee's life and values, this expresses her need for wild, open spaces and for preserving the earth's natural environment. The Thygesons saw science as the one rational and logical way to understand the world. The wilderness, in contrast, was their spiritual home, the place where they felt most connected to the beauty of the land and of living creatures. Ruth Lee loved wildflowers and birds; Phil loved bodies of water. Both loved mountain-climbing, canoeing, and animals.

7. Married and in Medical School

Phil and Ruth Lee entered their marriage facing tragedy and adversity. They were twenty-one and twenty years old, respectively. Phil's father was long gone and Phil did not have a close relationship with his mother. During the year Phil and Ruth Lee were courting, her father committed suicide. It was a private tragedy whose nature the family kept secret, even to other family members and for decades after the event. Ruth Lee did not discuss her father's death with her children or grandchildren except to say that he had suddenly developed a severe pneumonia and died quickly. In fact, as Ruth Lee's sister Lib eventually disclosed, James Spilman gassed himself with the family oven while despondent over what he saw as his failure to financially support his family.

The family secrecy was probably related to Victorianism and a perception of social shame and general condemnation of suicide. James had had a life insurance policy, and it may be that he thought that taking his own life would provide significant benefit to his wife and daughters. The life insurance policy did in fact pay a death benefit to James Spilman's widow, but it was not enough to support her. The myth of his having died of illness — rather than by his own hand — was perpetuated even by Phil. He wrote, "Ruth Lee, at age fifteen, was helping in the support of her family due to the ill health of her father. She was unable for this reason to finish Stanford University after her junior year."[1] But he was not ill in the usual way. He was depressed, and then he was dead. Ruth Lee began to earn money as a teenager by typing theses for graduate students at Stanford.

Ruth Lee always spoke of her father with love, compassion, and a tinge of sorrow. She referred to him sometimes as "my poor papa." Lib was less forgiving — she felt that his suicide caused great suffering and that he ought not to have done it. However, he was in the grip of deep depression, for which there was little help in his day. With their father gone, the need to help their mother financially grew more acute. Ruth Lee, so close to graduating from Stanford, withdrew from the university during her senior year. "I had to quit because my mother needed money desperately, and there wasn't anyone to get it; my father was gone. So I quit school after three and one quarter years. I was always going to go back just to tidy it up, but I never did."[2]

Phil did not graduate on time either because he chose to quit school for six months in order to work in commercial radio. He would have graduated in 1924, but instead graduated in 1925, after a quick make-up effort during the summer. Amateur radio had become more and more exciting, and obtaining a commercial radio license was an irresistible next step for him. He loved using ham radio to communicate with ever more distant and exotic destinations. It was "extending its range all the time. Why, when I got from St. Paul to Milwaukee to Cleveland, I was really getting somewhere." Before long, they had gotten all the way around the world and even to South Africa the "long way."[3] For ham operators like Phil, this was worth staying up all night!

The other reason Ruth Lee gave up her university education was to help support Phil and herself during his medical school years. As a newlywed, Ruth Lee earned $125 a month as a stenographer, and sent $80 of that salary to her mother for food, clothing, and medical care.[4] Ruth Lee and Phil supplemented the remaining $45 with $75 a month from Phil's mother, her contribution to his medical school expenses. Sylvie Thygeson continued to help the young couple financially even during the lean years after Phil became a doctor. The family lived frugally, and Ruth Lee kept a notebook in which she wrote down every penny they spent. She was so busy and so efficient that she would iron only the collars, cuffs, and front panel of Phil's shirts. He would look presentable with his lab coat on, but not an ounce of Ruth Lee's energy was wasted.

They rented a studio apartment on Sacramento Street just across from Lane Hospital in San Francisco, where Stanford's medical school was housed. Ruth Lee worked as a secretary downtown, riding the cable car to work. A bounteous Italian dinner at a San Francisco restaurant cost fifty cents. A steak from the butcher cost thirteen cents.[5] They were able to get gallery seats for operas and plays for a dollar apiece. "It was paradise on earth," Phil wrote. He did not even mind that he had to moonlight to earn extra money. He worked as a chauffeur for a "wealthy fur merchant from Alaska."[6]

When Phil graduated from Stanford in 1925, he was an engineering major. He decided, however, that his math deficits doomed him to failure in the field. He had done well in physiology and other science courses. Medicine seemed like a good choice. It didn't occur to him that he might not be admitted to the medical school, though he had a moment of doubt when eighty candidates showed up to register for what turned out to be only thirty slots. Stanford solved the problem by letting all eighty register, with the intention of whittling the field down to thirty by the end of eighteen months of preclinical studies. Phil was not good at anatomy and osteology. It has been said that if Ruth Lee hadn't drilled Phil over and over again on the bones in the human body, he never would have passed the course.[7] That may be an exaggeration, but it's hard to know. Ruth Lee definitely learned a lot of medicine alongside her husband. By his own account, Phil was bad at anatomy and called himself "clumsy at dissection."[8] He decided early on that he did not want to be a surgeon and went out of his way to avoid doing surgery.

Another unfortunate bit of luck was that Phil's rakish, reckless older brother, Elling, had preceded him into Stanford's medical school. Elling was "a gambler, a fraternity man, and a playboy." He liked to sleep late in the mornings and committed the unpardonable sin of letting his medical school cadaver dry out. "And so," Phil said, "Professors Danforth and Myers looked upon me with jaundiced eyes." During the period of Phil's preclinical coursework, Ruth Lee, who was employed as a secretary in the anatomy department, overheard a professor say, "Thygeson will never make it as a doctor!" Ruth Lee thought that was very funny and enjoyed teasing him about it years later.[9] Phil, who often enjoyed laughing at his own expense, thought it was funny, too, especially after it was proved wrong. He didn't consider himself a particularly good medical student at first; he was a "B average student."[10] Nonetheless, he went from being a B student to being an A student once he got married. The exception was pharmacology, where he received a B because a certain amount of math was required.[11]

Phil thought of Stanford's School of Medicine as a uniquely wonderful school for two reasons. First, it was research-oriented rather than clinically oriented. Second, it had fabulous staff, many of whom had trained at Johns Hopkins in Baltimore.[12] Johns Hopkins University was where the great physician and humanist William Osler had spent much of his career, and it was admired as a model for teaching, research, and patient care. Phil liked to point out that the University of California at Berkeley was much less research-oriented and didn't have illustrious faculty such as Thomas Addis, an expert in endocrinology and experimental medicine. Addis was a brilliant Scottish-born nephrologist and hematologist who became interested in the genetics of hemophilia. Addis invited all sorts of fellow luminaries, such as Walter Lilly and K. F. Meyer, to lecture to his medical students.[13] There were local stars as well. A. W. Hewlett, the father of Bill Hewlett of Hewlett-Packard fame, "wrote a wonderful book on pathophysiology in medicine."[14] The medical students were so excited about research that, of Phil's class of thirty students, twenty-seven went on to affiliate with universities as researchers or teaching faculty or both.[15] In fact, his training at Stanford set the tone for Phil's medical career. He always preferred research to clinical medicine, and he was disappointed when any protégé of his gave up the former for an exclusively clinical practice.

Phil was susceptible to the influence of mentors. A single exceptionally good teacher was enough to make him change his plans for the future. In his pre-medical coursework, Professor Heath was the greatest influence. In medical school, it was most likely Professor Edwin Schultz, who taught bacteriology. Phil judged Professor Schultz to be a "poor lecturer but an absolutely marvelous seminar man."[16] A preclinical thesis was one of the requirements for medical students, and Phil decided to survey sanitation and public health in Palo Alto. To that end, he "checked all the dairies and restaurants," which gave him a life-long aversion to restaurants.[17] He always preferred to eat at home and especially to eat Ruth Lee's simple but good cooking. "After I saw how dishes were washed in the restaurants of Palo Alto, I could no longer enjoy eating in a restaurant. This phobia about restaurants and restaurant dishes has continued all my life. I don't like to go out to eat!"[18]

In the course of his studies, Phil continued to be interested in public health. In addition to his preclinical thesis, he had to write a clinical thesis and chose for his subject a problem that plagued Ruth Lee—hay fever and other forms of allergy. It was a new field of study and there were various experimental treatments to explore, among them injections of minute amounts of pollen in an effort to desensitize the patient.[19] Phil had a rough time defending his thesis. The professor who questioned him didn't think much of this newfangled area of medicine. According to Phil, he considered it to be "verg-

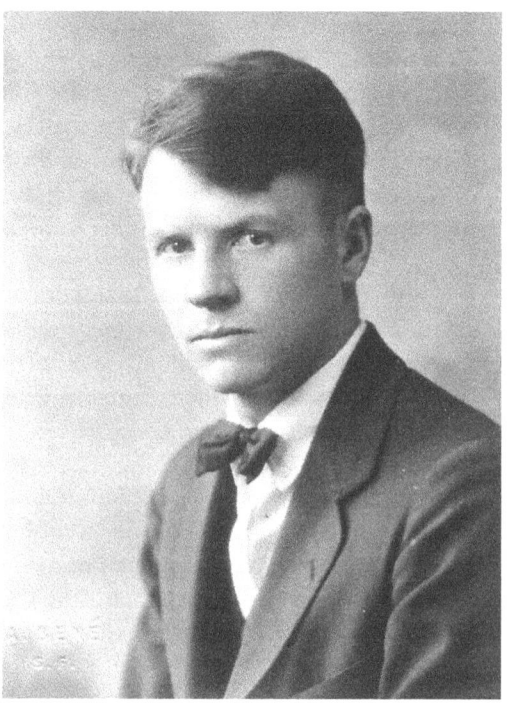

Phillips Thygeson as a young married medical student in San Francisco, mid–1920s.

ing on charlatanism."[20] Phil didn't consider the study of allergy a possible career path. However, he was briefly interested in pursuing internal medicine, the specialty of his sister Ruth's husband Dwight Shepardson, who invited Phil to join his internal medicine practice after graduation. However, Phil was much more interested in microbiology and infectious agents too small to see with the naked eye. He was also very interested in immunology.

While all of this medical training was going on, the Thygesons were learning how it felt to be married. They loved setting up house together and Phil was thrilled to have his bride by his side. Still, there were rocky moments. Ruth Lee had grown up in a very gentle, polite family and had a terrible shock when she learned that her in-laws were quite unlike her own family of origin. A story has been passed through the family — some say it happened before they married, but most family members recall it as happening when they were newlyweds — that Ruth Lee joined the Thygeson family at a small resort town on the Northern California coast one weekend, arriving under her own steam by way of public transportation. Sylvie was there with all four of her children, and as Ruth Lee walked down the road to the house where they were staying, she heard a terrific uproar of a fight, with yelling and harsh language. Ruth Lee arrived in time to see Sylvie hurl a can of tomato soup at Elling. Everyone was in a rage, including Phil. This was the first of many times Ruth Lee would deal with Phil in a rage.

It was a great shock to Ruth Lee because her parents and sister didn't raise their voices no matter what. She was stunned and horrified, and was especially disturbed by her discovery that Phil could behave this way.[21] She reflected long and hard about whether she could be happily married to someone who

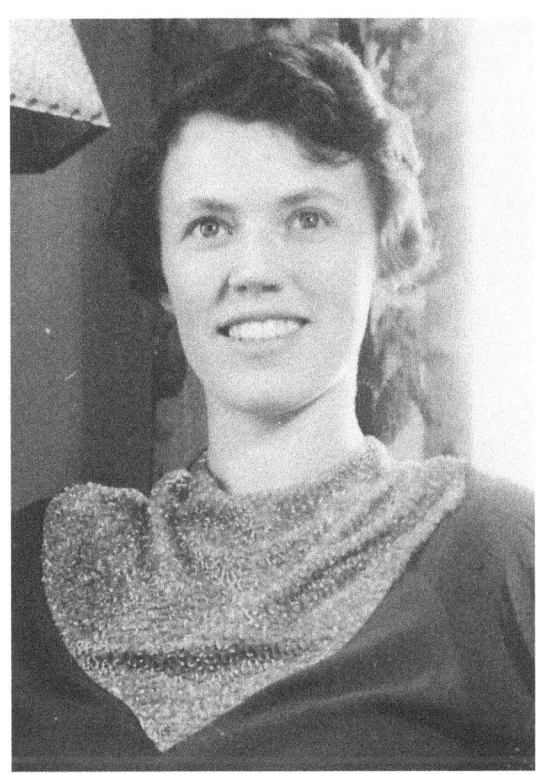

Ruth Lee Thygeson as a young married woman.

behaved like that. It was the greatest crisis of confidence in her first year of marriage and she later confided to her daughter that she had considered backing out of the marriage. She did go on, and occasionally had the Thygeson wrath directed at her. She was skilled at keeping the peace with Phil, which had the unfortunate side effect of his becoming used to having things his way. To outsiders, it looked like a harmonious, happy marriage; to intimate family, it was a happy marriage, but one that demanded compromises by Ruth Lee.

8. Frontier Medicine in Colorado

Stanford did not issue medical degrees after four years of coursework and clinical work. It required an additional year in the form of an internship. Phil decided he wanted to do his internship year in Colorado. His choice is revealing because it wasn't really motivated by the medical training opportunities presented by Colorado. He had passed through Colorado Springs on his return from a trip to the East and had been so attracted to the high Rocky Mountains he couldn't resist finding an excuse to live there. "The weather and the mountains and everything were so ideal that I thought I would have to intern in Colorado and then go back to San Francisco."[1] He signed up for a year at the University of Colorado in Denver, and in 1927 he and Ruth Lee made the fateful drive in their Model T, with Phil hemorrhaging from his incomplete operation. They camped along the way. "It was June and the Nevada deserts were in bloom with snow-capped mountains on all sides," Phil wrote. "It took us ten hours to cross the 60-mile Carson sink. The crust was so thin and we fell through so often that our progress was slow. Often we had to wait for someone to pull us out. At Salt Lake we felt so dirty that we checked into a cheap-looking hotel for a bath." After Salt Lake City, they chose a brand new road to Denver, the Victory Highway. "It rained every afternoon, which made the dirt road slippery. We frequently slipped off into the side ditch. On some hills we had to wait until the sun dried the road.... At Rabbit Ears Pass, we had to wait for snow removal.... Ruth Lee saw snow lilies for the first time and was enthralled."[2]

At that time, Phil and Ruth Lee were very interested in the history of the West, especially as it pertained to the pioneer era. The days of the open frontier were over, but the ways of the West were slow to die. Around 1800, the average American lifespan was only about forty years. A century later, with many medical innovations either established or about to come into being, it was still only fifty years.[3] The Rocky Mountains contributed its fair share to the short lifespan of Americans, as tuberculosis, typhoid, smallpox, malaria, cholera, and the vaguely defined Rocky Mountain fever were common.[4] People were allowed to call themselves doctors and behave as if they were doctors with little or no training.[5] They hung out their shingles and dispensed laudanum and other concoctions. A mining town resident observed, "Signs of 'Dr.' stick out from cabins, shanties, tents, and wagons, and the title is heard in almost every company in the diggings. A wag at Cherry Creek called out 'doc' in the street, and eighteen men turned around in response."[6] By the time Phil graduated from medical school, sanitation and science were rapidly improving the health and longevity of Americans. Helping effect the improvement was the sort of thing that interested him a great deal, as his undergraduate thesis showed. The intersection of sanitation and public health became central to his future research work on trachoma.

The first thing the Thygesons did when they got to Denver was to whisk Phil off to see Dr. William C. Finnoff about the hemorrhage he had while driving east through the Sierra Nevada. Meanwhile, Ruth Lee decided she wanted to continue her studies and work toward her college degree. She enrolled in summer school at CU Boulder and had to live in the dormitory there, while Phil was several hours away in Denver. They saw each other on Phil's day off, which was Sunday. Phil came every Sunday to pick her up and they headed for the high Rockies together.

Once he got to know Phil, Finnoff began a prolonged campaign to persuade him to become an ophthalmologist. Finnoff was considered the best ophthalmologist in the region, along with Edward Jackson, who was a professor emeritus at the University of Colorado. This was the era of preceptorships, when the most important aspect of advanced medical training was to be taken under the wing of a great teacher. Before long, Phil was working for Finnoff in Finnoff's office. He especially admired Finnoff's expertise in ocular pathology. "I had the world's best luck to have Dr. W. C. Finnoff as my mentor," Phil wrote. "He taught me to look on ophthalmology as a science and not as a clinical specialty. He taught me to be very proud of ophthalmology and its accomplishments."[7]

Though Phil admired his mentor, whom he considered the best ophthalmologist in the region, he didn't idolize him. In fact, he said that Finnoff had a "little man's complex." Finnoff "always had a great big car, and he drove it at high speed just the way all the little fellows do."[8] In a photo of University of Colorado interns, Phil is distinctly taller than all of the others. Finnoff knew he was the best of the best and would tell his patients as much. He had been trained by Edward Jackson under the preceptorship system, and had then gone to Vienna and learned ocular pathology from Ernst Fuchs. Phil reported that Finnoff had the first slit lamp microscope and did the first intracapsular cataract extraction "in the whole western United States."[9] Finnoff had grown up in Colorado, and Phil, a fellow westerner, loved that about him. Apparently, Finnoff had a personality problem, however — he could be blunt and abrasive. He was never made chairman of the department at the University of Colorado.

While at the University of Colorado, Phil had the benefit of studying under another great ophthalmologist, Edward Jackson. "Whenever Finnoff was away and I was faced with a rough case, I went to Dr. Jackson for advice. Jackson was never too busy to help me out."[10] In fact, the two great ophthalmologists had offices almost across the street from each other. In the late 1920s, Jackson was in his seventies and had officially retired from the University of Colorado, but Phil reported that he was "the principal teacher in the two-year course on ophthalmology" at the university. He was also editor of the *American Journal of Ophthalmology* and president of the esteemed Colorado Ophthalmology Society.[11] Phil credited Jackson with making "Colorado kind of a Vienna of ophthalmology,"[12] Vienna being the place where budding ophthalmologists from Europe and the United States practically felt they had to go for training. According to Phil, Jackson developed the first graduate course in ophthalmology in the United States and the first advanced degree in the specialty, a doctor of ophthalmology. Phil was one of the first to earn the doctor of ophthalmology degree. Jackson taught Phil one of the key concepts of what became Phil's philosophy of clinical practice. It was "that every ophthalmologist should know the natural history of disease and that treatment of disease had to be better than the natural history."[13] Phil taught this precept to his grandson Marcus in the course of time. As Marcus explained, Phil's commitment was "to know the natural history of the disease and ... manage what was really sort of a natural process. As a consequence, he had a much better sense of what was really likely to have a bad outcome, and a better sense of whether the treatment was worse than the disease."[14] Phil was in a unique position to have learned the natural history of eye diseases before medication altered the course of treatment. The lesson of avoiding overtreatment of infection was one he would preach and teach until his dying day.

Recognizing fresh talent, Jackson pressed Phil into service on behalf of his projects. "While I was still an intern," Phil wrote, "Dr. Jackson corralled me for his journal. He needed help with the abstract section of the journal."[15] With Ruth Lee's help, Phil began to read French medical journals and write abstracts of relevant articles in English. Dr. Jackson and Ruth Lee became very fond of each other and before long, she was doing secretarial work for him. It's unclear whether or not he paid her, but he certainly appreciated her. "We both were very fond of Dr. Jackson," Phil wrote. "He was a kindly, warm, very lovable man. And he was a very good friend."[16] Phil expressed his gratitude by driving Dr. Jackson's visitors around in their new Ford. Ruth Lee helped host social events for Jackson, as his wife had died and his daughter no longer lived nearby. More than Finnoff, Jackson made the crucial difference in Phil's decision to become an ophthalmologist. "It was really Dr. Jackson who persuaded me that my future lay in ophthalmology, with a subspecialty in microbiology," Phil wrote. "I was meant to be a microbe hunter and trachoma gave me my big chance."[17]

Phil liked physiology and thought of Jackson as the great innovator in physiological optics.[18] He also admired Jackson's seminal cross-cylinder refraction method. Jackson's cylinder was a lens that was powerful in only one direction. As Phil explained, if you held two of these cross cylinders at a ninety-degree angle to each other, it was easy to figure out the axis of a person's astigmatism or uneven shape of the cornea.[19] In its day, it was a breakthrough technique. Phil had never been exposed to cross-cylinder refraction before learning it directly from Jackson in Denver.

In contrast to William Finnoff, Edward Jackson had a gentle, diplomatic approach. Finnoff would tell a patient how the referring doctor had made a mess of his or her treatment. This led to Finnoff's being unpopular among his peers. In terms of role models, Phil had the opportunity to decide which man to emulate. He chose Jackson's model of not tattling on fellow physicians who made mistakes in diagnosis or treatment. He also followed Jackson's lead in working to eradicate fee-splitting, where "an optometrist would refer a cataract case to an ophthalmologist and then expect a kickback."[20] It can't be said, however, that Phil was an Edward Jackson by nature. He was more of a Finnoff sometimes in his leadership style.

Phil loved his internship year in the beautiful new University Hospital building, which had been financed by the Rockefeller Foundation. Ruth Lee and he lived in modest interns' quarters. Phil took the licensing exam to qualify for his M.D. at the beginning of his internship year rather than at the end, which was not the way it worked for the other interns. It's unclear whether he talked his way into being allowed to take the exam or how this unusual turn of events came to be, but he passed with flying colors and was a licensed physician in Colorado in spite of Stanford's rules. "Perhaps that was illegal but no one seemed concerned about that," Phil wrote.[21] The interns were given a shocking amount of responsibility given how inexperienced they were. Nine of them ran the hospital, where there "were no residents, no full-time staff. The interns gave all the anesthetics, did much of the routine laboratory work."[22] When he was a "green intern," Phil wrote, the "experienced ward nurses kept me from making serious mistakes and helped me learn the art of medicine."[23] They helped him do urinalysis and blood counts. Phil greatly admired the nurses, whom he felt were underappreciated and undervalued, and did his best to show them gratitude and respect.

Phil continued to help Finnoff with his surgeries and work in his laboratory on eye pathology issues. Their different areas of research expertise complemented each other. Phil was the stronger in microbiology and Finnoff knew more about ocular pathology. In addition, they shared a love of research. Phil felt that Colorado was a clinician's school and facility, not a research place, as Stanford was. He and Finnoff at least had each other. Phil enrolled in the University of Colorado's ophthalmological training program and by the early 1930s had earned a Master of Science degree in microbiology and a doctoral degree in ophthalmology. Phil's very first published papers had Finnoff as lead author. In 1929, they published "The finding of *Bacterium granulosis* (Noguchi) in trachoma" in the *American Journal of Ophthalmology*, an attempt to confirm Hideyo Noguchi's theory that *B. granulosis* caused trachoma. In fact, it didn't, but that discovery helped move Phil's research along. Two years later, they published "*Bacterium granulosis* in trachoma" in the *Archives of Ophthalmology*. By 1933, the precocious Phillips Thygeson was publishing seminal papers in English and in French on trachoma where he was sole author. Ruth Lee served as his editor.

Phil's academic talent was not overlooked. Professor Ivan C. Hall offered him a position as instructor of bacteriology at the University of Colorado. It paid $2,400 a year, a great fortune to Phil and Ruth Lee.[24] In spite of Phil's new duties, Finnoff and Jackson kept after him to become an ophthalmologist. He ended up combining his interests in bacteriology and ophthalmology, with their enthusiastic support. Because Phil often needed to work at night at Dr. Finnoff's house, Ruth Lee had a choice of staying home alone or joining them. She chose to join them, and soon became involved in the work. Her part-time day job gave her flexibility. Over time, she became quite a thinker in ophthalmology and helped Phil plan his research papers. "She was my catalyst. She was full of ideas for my research papers," he wrote. "I would not have had much of a career without her."[25]

The clinical side of things in Denver in the late 1920s was anything but dull. Phil wrote, "I recall seeing diseases now extinct. For example, I saw smallpox up close. I saw hemorrhagic smallpox. I saw smallpox of the eye." He also saw lupus, vaccinia, polio, "rabies of the dog and of the man," rheumatic and scarlet fever, "and almost all of the infectious diseases of man, except tropical diseases."[26] Not long before, Colorado medicine had included bloodletting, purging, all sorts of homemade, addictive remedies, and a pronounced lack of hygiene, antisepsis, good plumbing, or even clean water.[27]

The more benign of the home remedies included "arnica, powdered rhubarb, castor oil, camphor, horehound, sassafras bark, wild safe and chokecherry teas, oil of wintergreen, baking soda and Epsom salts."[28] More malignant options were popular as well. The *Denver Quaker Cook Book* touted a diarrhea-curing tincture that contained opium and was to be taken four times per hour. In case anyone was in doubt, the book promised readers, "This [recipe] alone is well worth the price of the book."[29]

In their early days in Colorado, settlers had to contend with scurvy, for there was a severe shortage of vitamin C-rich foods and they didn't know what local Native Americans knew, which is that they could have found vitamin C in berries, wild onions, and cactus.[30] Table salt and herbs were used to sterilize and stop bleeding.[31] There was also the problem of safely extracting arrowheads from people. One enterprising doctor sold specially designed arrowhead-extraction forceps in 1876, the year Colorado became a state.[32]

Mountain fever had probably been wiped out by the time Phil arrived as an intern in Colorado. It had baffled the doctors of its day, with some thinking that perhaps it was due to lead poisoning from water being drunk downstream from toxic gold mine tailings. Others thought it was most likely a kind of typhoid fever.[33] Poisons such as mercury were frequently used to treat venereal conditions,[34] and mountain doctors, who often doubled as gold miners, were considered extortionists of the first order. Pioneer-era physicians were paid in gold, venison, animal hides, and bear meat.[35] Lawrence N. Greenleaf, a Colorado poet of sorts, wrote a ditty to damn the "doctors" of 1868:

> A myriad shams, on every hand we see;
> Doctors grow rich although they disagree.
> While one prescribes a liberal dose for all,
> That of another is minutely small....
> Betwixt the doctors, doses large and small
> The wonder is, that we survive at all![36]

Over-the-counter remedies were full of alcohol, cocaine, and heroin. Cocaine-based remedies were pedaled to women for uterine complaints and Foster's Terp-Heroin was said to be good for respiratory ailments. Morphine was a mere ten cents an ounce in places and its sale was completely unregulated.[37] Even babies were given teething and "soothing" concoctions laced with opium derivatives. As late as 1914, the Denver Department of Health was still trying to alert the public to what it termed "baby killers," products such as Dr. Fahrney's Teething Syrup, which contained morphine and chloroform, and Dr. James's Soothing Syrup, which was full of heroin.[38] When Ruth Lee gave birth to a son, Fritjof, on February 24, 1930, in Denver, she may have heard the siren song of Mrs. Winslow's Soothing Syrup: "And so can all mothers with tuneful refrain/Delight in their infants, whose health they maintain."

The product was said to have been in use for over fifty years and used by "millions of mothers."[39]

Phil had to contend with the fact that doctors in Colorado were not held in high esteem. In 1923, *Colorado Medicine* published the following assessment: "[The doctor] is looked upon more or less as a member of an unfair and prejudiced class."[40] This was partly because of a prolonged period of price-gouging. Colorado doctors charged between $50 and $200 for the "complicated delivery" of a baby in 1860 and prices remained the same fifty years later.[41] Laborers earned so little that having a modest wound sutured could cost three days wages.[42]

Phil also had to deal with a prodigious number of sick people.[43] Tuberculosis was the disease most frequently diagnosed in the decades before his arrival, though pneumonia, typhoid, "insanity," and alcoholism were also common.[44] In the era of horse-drawn ambulances, hospitalization at the local County Hospital cost one dollar a day, and there was an alarming lack of sanitation. As Colorado medical historian Robert H. Shikes wrote, "An outbreak of typhoid in the hospital was traced to the contamination of refrigerated food by a misdirected hospital sewer line—but not before a doctor and a head nurse had died."[45] Conditions for hospital patients were considered "deplorable"[46] very shortly before Phil and Ruth Lee arrived. In a publication entitled "Municipal Facts, November—December 1925," the hospital was upbraided for its "rat-infested kitchen, beds without clean sheets, blankets too thin for warmth, confusion, dirt and poor food!"[47] A local newspaper described the place as being a "scandalous death trap ... so crowded that beds are placed in the aisles."[48]

Denver was a locus of typhoid, mainly due to contaminated drinking water and poor sanitation. Dr. James McDonald wrote to the *Rocky Mountain News*, "Our water is not only filthy, but it is damned filthy; not only opaque, but it stinks."[49] By 1922, five years before the Thygesons' arrival, the death rates from typhoid had fallen considerably, though Colorado was still one of the most typhoid-ridden states in the country.[50] In 1928, Denver's water was still deemed unsafe, intestinal disease was prevalent, and the city dumped raw sewage into local rivers that ran unchecked to downstream urban communities.[51]

Fortunately, Phil's internship didn't lead him to the infamous County Hospital but rather to the new Colorado General Hospital building, established in 1921. The University of Colorado had combined the old (classrooms in Boulder and County/Denver General Hospital for clinical training of medical students) with the new, the Colorado General Hospital building.[52] This hospital, also known as University Hospital, was where Phil did most of his clinical work.[53]

Colorado's best medical school, at the University of Colorado at Boulder, opened in 1883. As during the early days at Stanford, tuition at CU Boulder was free. Women were admitted, but they were encouraged to remain unmarried if they wanted to practice medicine. Faculty were often part-time and volunteer; they would cancel class when they had emergencies with their patients.[54] The Denver and Gross College of Medicine, which predated the University of Colorado program, did not fare well when Abraham Flexner made his famous 1909 inspection tour of every medical school in the country. The College of Medicine was accused of "a total absence of scientific activity," and criticized for its dearth of medical books. One dean was characterized by Flexner as being afflicted by "unadulterated cussedness, ... raw malice, ... and percolated venom."[55] In contrast, Flexner approved of the University of Colorado's medical school, which caused the Denver and Gross program to disappear.[56] Early CU medical faculty did not have time for research. The Regent's Report for 1919–1920 included the blunt assessment that the medical school was "seriously hampered by insufficient personnel and equipment."[57] It was in the 1920s that this situation finally changed, and Phil Thygeson's early research work was part of the change. As an intern, however, he first had to contend with healing Colorado's sick.

During the 1920s, one of every ten Coloradans died from tuberculosis, a mortality rate double that of the other forty-seven states.[58] Colorado was a tuberculosis hub, in large measure because many consumptives from the East were told they might save their lives if they moved to the dryer climates in the West. The tuberculosis bacillus thrives in conditions of high oxygen concentration. In the Mile High City of Denver, the air was thin enough to kill off at least some of the ubiquitous bug. With this particular form of suffering came a certain kind of tourist propaganda. Eastern medical journals published articles on the salubrious effects of Colorado's climate and the Denver & Rio Grande Railroad advertised that "Invalids and Pleasure Seekers" would find "health and pleasure" in Colorado.[59] The situation for many years was less than healthy and uplifting. For a long time, "as many as one out of every three Coloradans had active tuberculosis, one out of every four Coloradans died of the disease, and the state was known as much for the 'white plague' as for its mountains and mines."[60] Not long before Ruth Lee and Phil's arrival, tuberculosis was still the single highest recorded cause of death, with infectious diseases such as scarlet fever and diphtheria a close second.[61] Ruth Lee was exposed to tuberculosis there, had a spot on her lungs, and had positive skin tests for the rest of her life.

Up until 1882, when German microbiologist Robert Koch proved that a bacterium was the cause of tuberculosis, the prevailing notion was that it was caused by everything from heredity to what you ate. A Colorado doctor suggested that tuberculosis be treated with mercury and the *Denver Medical Times* published the more memorable proposal of a concoction of copious amounts of kerosene, whiskey, and creosote.[62] Even Robert Koch had a treatment to peddle, a drug he called "lymph," and he made a good deal of money selling it, though it was of no use.[63]

Naturally, there was a great fear of tuberculosis. The Colorado legislature actually debated a bill that would have required a "lunger" to wear a bell around his or her neck to warn the public.[64] Surprisingly, it wasn't until 1913 that a law was passed requiring doctors to report cases of tuberculosis to public health authorities.[65] The *Journal of the American Medical Association* published what turned out to be a rumor that Colorado might close its borders to consumptives.[66] A public campaign against spitting on the streets and in other public places was undertaken, and spittoons, sputum cups, and flasks became popular.

Phil had several harrowing experiences while doing his internship at University Hospital. One of them would haunt him all his life. A young woman was admitted with internal bleeding. According to Marcus Thygeson, she most likely had an ectopic pregnancy that had ruptured her fallopian tube. "She basically bled to death and he was not able to get control of the bleeding or give her enough transfusions. Her death greatly upset him. He felt responsible somehow, that if he'd been able to do something differently, he might have been able to save her."[67] Another case had a less dire outcome, but was nonetheless memorable and unsettling. Phil helped treat a farmer diagnosed with acute appendicitis. He scrubbed in alongside the surgeon and when they opened up the man's abdomen, they could not find his appendix. They called in a second surgical team and they, too, could not find an appendix. The chief surgeon turned to Phil in the operating room and said, "'Listen, Phil, close up here and then you explain to the patient what happened.' And then he left." So there was Phil, wondering what he could possibly say to the patient. He thought about it for a while, went to visit him, and said, "Mr. So-and-so, you have a rare disorder. You have obliterative appendicitis.... Your appendicitis is gone and you should be fine." No such disease existed. The story ended, "A few months later he got a card from the guy saying, 'Thank you so much for all the good care. I want you to know my belly pain is gone. I'm back on my tractor and doing fine.'"[68]

Patients loved Phil. He had a natural talent for expressing gentleness and care, to which they responded. The incident of "obliterative appendicitis" speaks to one of Phil's beliefs as a physician, which was that the placebo effect should never be underestimated. The story is really a case of placebo surgery. "He was very big on bedside manner," Marcus Thygeson said. Phil recognized that "there was still something he could do as a person to relieve discomfort or allay concerns and anxieties ... or just basically commiserate with them as they dealt with oftentimes devastating illnesses that led to blindness." A grateful patient once said to Ruth Lee, "Your husband, he is such a good doctor and such a good man." Phil confided in Marcus, "The patients of mine who are most grateful are often the ones for whom I could do the least."[69]

Denver was not the safest place to practice medicine and have a baby, but Ruth Lee and Phil were willing to take the risk. Shockingly, at that time Denver's infant mortality was the highest of any major city in the United States.[70] Fritjof Peder Thygeson was born on February 24, 1930. He later told his own birth story: "I was born three weeks premature. According to my mother I was bright yellow, I had yellow jaundice. I was very long, very skinny, no chin, and my mother says that of all the people in the world, the person she appreciates most in one sense is the nurse who came in and said to her, 'Oh, Mrs. Thygeson, you have such a beautiful baby!'"[71] Ruth Lee was thrilled with her baby. She had, after all, been married for several years before he was born, and he was a planned baby. She worked full-time until Fritjof's birth. Her mother still needed support, though as a widow she was now living with her other daughter, Lib, and Lib's husband Milton. Ruth Lee was a secretary/stenographer at a Denver mental hospital known as Mt. Airy.[72]

Ruth Lee was committed to providing her mother with $75 in monthly support.[73] According to Phil, she became "manager, secretary, hostess and general factotum for the little hospital." At the time, she earned $150 a month and Phil earned only $20 a month. Ruth Lee's job provided her with room and board, and once more they found themselves living apart, seeing each other just once a day and spending all day Sunday together. It was Ruth Lee's salary that permitted them to buy a Model A Ford convertible, which they both loved.

After she gave birth, Ruth Lee was cared for by her dear friend Jessie Wilson. "In those days a new mother stayed in bed for two weeks, so everything needed to be done" for her.[74] In the era when Fritjof and his sister Kristin were born, it was thought to be harmful to handle a baby too much. "I was not held," Kristin said. "Probably Fritjof wasn't either." Feeding was on a "rigorous four-hour schedule.... No matter how much the baby cried, you didn't go in and pick up the baby...."[75] Neither baby was breastfed, though that was not Ruth Lee's wish. She "always wanted to breastfeed but wasn't able to, probably because they had the view, well, if you can't do it right away, you can't do it. So you give up and feed the baby canned milk, canned cows' milk, which is what I was raised on.... My mother always kind of grieved that."[76]

9. Building a Real Log Cabin

Remarkably, Phil and Ruth Lee had barely crossed the threshold into parenthood when they took on a new challenge, which was to build themselves a summer cabin high in the front range of the Colorado Rocky Mountains. The Rockies had undergone a tourism boom when the railroad arrived in the 1870s. Colorado was touted as the "Switzerland of America," and tourists were drawn to newly built resorts in the front range of the Rockies.[1] There was a gold rush in 1859, and the boomtowns that followed eventually turned into another sort of tourist attraction — Colorado ghost towns.[2] In the meantime, people like Ruth Lee and Phil came to the Rockies in automobiles. People visited by the thousands in cars powered by everything from gas to steam. F. O. Stanley, a pioneer in the establishment of Estes Park, a town at the main entrance to Rocky Mountain National Park, arrived there in 1903 in his own special invention, the Stanley Steamer. By 1909, he had built an elegant hotel there with 105 rooms with private bathrooms.[3] Henry Ford had just made the Model T affordable. Weekend trips to the high country were possible.

In 1915, Rocky Mountain National Park became the country's thirteenth national park.[4] The park's supervisor, Charles R. Trowbridge, had very little money to work with — something like $10,000, with no office space, automobiles, trucks, or employees.[5] In 1920, the famous Fall River Road, one of the highest in the nation, was completed. Convicts from the state penitentiary in Canon City did much of the work, which was a product of brute labor, picks and shovels, and dynamite.[6] The road was so steep, narrow, and full of switchbacks that some drivers drove up it in reverse, the strongest gear. The grade in places climbed as much as 15 percent on the way to the summit at 11,796 feet. Park rangers helped drivers manage the hairpin turns and a strict speed limit of twelve miles an hour was assigned to the steeper grades. This is the sort of adventure Phil and Ruth Lee adored, and they visited the Park before they built what became known as the Paiute cabin. In the end, they got their very own wilderness, for there was dramatic hiking, with peaks of over 13,000 feet, only a few miles from their cabin's doorstep. There were also many fewer tourists where they built their summer cabin, about thirty-five miles from Rocky Mountain National Park.

While the building of the Thygeson cabin by hand with simple, traditional tools was a pioneering effort in the best sense, it was also part of an important American tradition. In the 1930s, the Civilian Conservation Corps (CCC) collaborated with the Forest Service and National Park Service to build national park and forest cabins as part of a national recreational infrastructure and to provide jobs to those who desperately needed them.[7] The classic Rocky Mountain "rustic style," exemplified by the Fall River Ranger Station in the national park to come, was exactly what Phil and Ruth Lee built. It featured a simple "fieldstone foundation, log walls with saddle-notched corners, small multi-paned windows and an overhanging wood-shingle roof."[8]

The Park Service later wrote about its famous rustic style: "Successfully handled, it is a style which, through the use of native materials in proper scale ... gives the feeling of having been executed by pioneer craftsmen with limited hand tools. It thus achieves sympathy with natural surroundings and with the past."[9] Perhaps the renaissance in log cabin building was a sign of nostalgia for the frontier days. Phil Thygeson had been born too late for certain endeavors, such as being a Lewis and Clark figure.

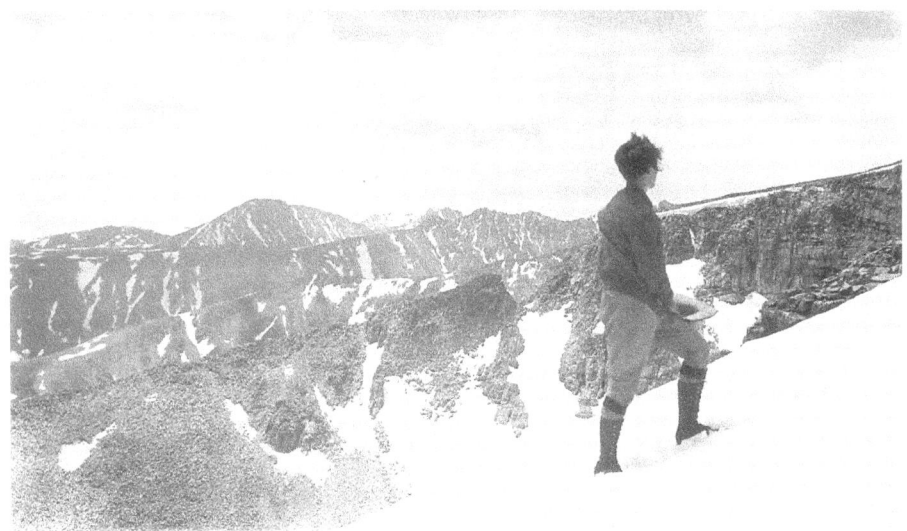

Ruth Lee Thygeson on the flank of Mount Audubon, a 13,200-foot peak near where she and her husband built their log cabin.

Phil and Ruth Lee first laid eyes on the site where they would build the cabin in the summer of 1929. In their "little flivver, a little Ford,"[10] they drove up to the mountains to camp and then go hiking the next morning with Fritjof, a babe in arms. Because Phil had to work all day, they weren't able to leave Denver until nearly dusk. It was a long, slow drive, much of it over single-lane dirt roads. The weekend began with their driving to the little mining town of Ward, established in 1860 after gold was discovered in nearby Gold Hill. Named for Calvin Ward, who mined a claim known as Miser's Dream, the little town built on a steep hillside was soon a boomtown. At one point Ward had several thousand residents and a number of productive silver and gold mines. In 1898, a narrow gauge railroad reached Ward. The train had to climb nearly 4,000 vertical feet up steep canyons on the "Switzerland Trail" to reach a shingle-roofed depot. The town's steep hills were dotted with little miners' shacks, and there was a church with a steeple, an old-fashioned schoolhouse with a bell mounted on its roof, a five-sided hotel, and a primitive, two-cell jail with pine platforms for sleeping and sand pits for the inmates' latrines. The town faded to almost nothing after a catastrophic fire in 1900.

In the 1920s, the town of Ward, located at around 9,000 feet, was still nearly deserted. There were only half a dozen people living there, the mines were abandoned, and dangerous open shafts and mine tailings could be found right in town. There was a tiny store run by Mr. and Mrs. Miller. Mr. Miller doubled as the postmaster and would drive to Boulder to pick up the town's mail. Phil and Ruth Lee and baby Fritjof passed right on through Ward and began to climb the steeply winding one-lane dirt road to Brainard Lake, at 10,300 feet.

Arriving not long before midnight, they set up camp a mile shy of Brainard Lake. They pitched a heavy canvas tent and spread out their bedroll of wool blankets held together by large blanket pins. When they awoke early the next morning, they were stunned by the beauty of the snow-capped peaks jutting up only a couple of miles away. The peaks loomed three thousand feet above them in the near distance. They had a revelation — they should build a log cabin on that very site. They were not daunted by the fact that they had no experience with log cabins or that the land belonged to the U.S. Forest Service. They set out to explore the area on foot. Over time, they climbed all of the peaks in the group known as the Indian Peaks. The peaks had names such as Paiute Horn, Arikaree, Pawnee, and Navajo. Alpine lakes at 11,000 and 12,000 feet were frozen until well into June each year, and they hiked the barely visible trails to reach them. There were a couple of cabins already in this area, but the nearest neighbor was half a mile away. When Phil first approached the local Forest Service ranger to ask for permission to build,

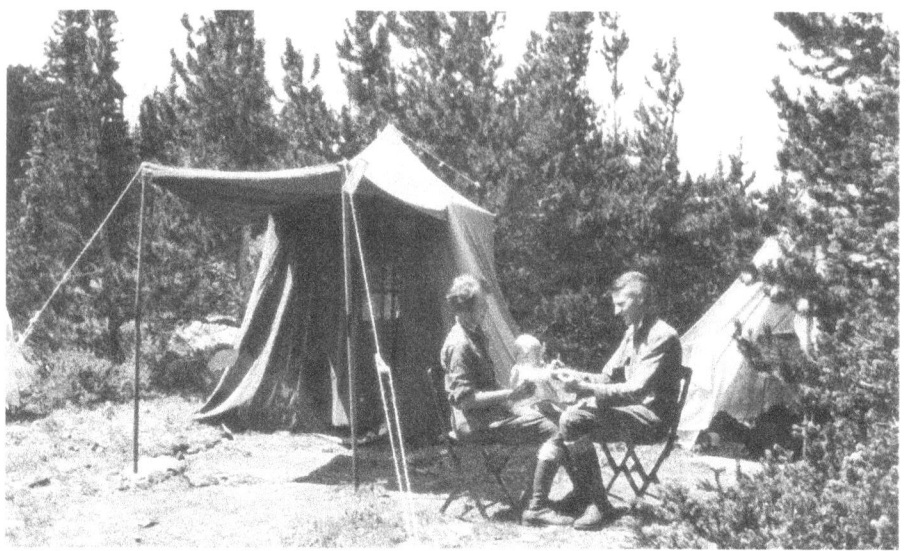

Ruth Lee, Fritjof, and Phillips Thygeson at the cabin-building site, 1930.

he was told that the site was unsuitable, as it had no source of water. Somehow, though, they talked him into it.[11]

It was not easy to work full-time, care for a baby, and build a log cabin on almost no money and their own physical labor, but that's what they did. They borrowed a thousand dollars to pay for cash expenses. Phil never minded borrowing money; he had supreme confidence that he could repay it. After what had happened to Ruth Lee's father, she was much more nervous about debt. Aside from store-bought windows and wrought iron hinges and hardware for windows and doors, Phil and Ruth Lee made just about everything by hand. Phil had learned a lot from his own father and from his years as an avid Boy Scout. He firmly believed in his own ability to accomplish just about anything if he had a good set of instructions. It was a family joke that he was the original consumer of the popular genre, the how-to manual. For the Paiute cabin, which stands to this day, Ruth Lee and Phil bought a book, now lost, entitled something like, *How to Build a Real Log Cabin*.

The tradition of log cabins appears to go back thousands of years to northern Europe, especially to Scandinavia. Softwood forests, such as those filled with pines, were perfect. Originally, cabins were crude and simple, with round logs piled high and a hole in the roof for smoke to escape. Phil and Ruth Lee's cabin was simple but elegant — round logs carefully notched at the corners with log ends extending beyond them, doors and windows cut from the logs, a beautiful hand-laid stone hearth and chimney, and a not very steeply peaked shingle roof. In the book they were using, flat roofs were discouraged on the grounds that only a peaked roof would keep dangerous amounts of winter snow from accumulating. But Phil and Ruth Lee didn't like the look of a peaked roof.

Building the cabin was an enormous effort. First, Ruth Lee and Phil had to ask the U.S. Forest Service for permission to lease a plot of land. Permission was granted in exchange for a small annual fee and an understanding that the lease would need to be renewed regularly. The next step was to get permission to cut down healthy, straight, tall pines in the nearby forest. A Forest Service ranger chose the trees they were allowed to cut and marked them with ribbons. Phil swapped call nights with fellow residents in order to get summer weekends off and rush to the mountains to work on the cabin.[12] With a cross-cut saw with handles on each end and long teeth, Phil and Ruth Lee together sawed down each tree. The trees were then "limbed," their branches removed with an ax. The logs had to be smooth, without knots sticking out where limbs had been, so bulges were pared away. Slash had to be burned and the site kept clean. Horses dragged the downed logs one by one to the cabin site. The logs then had to dry, a process of some months. Although they could have spared themselves a great deal of trouble by leaving the bark on the logs, they didn't like how that looked. It was Ruth Lee's job to skin the logs, which she managed while keeping an eye on young Fritjof. She straddled each log and used a two-handled draw knife to slip under the pine bark and drag toward herself over and over.

They chose a simple design, with three rooms in a rectangular cabin only 25

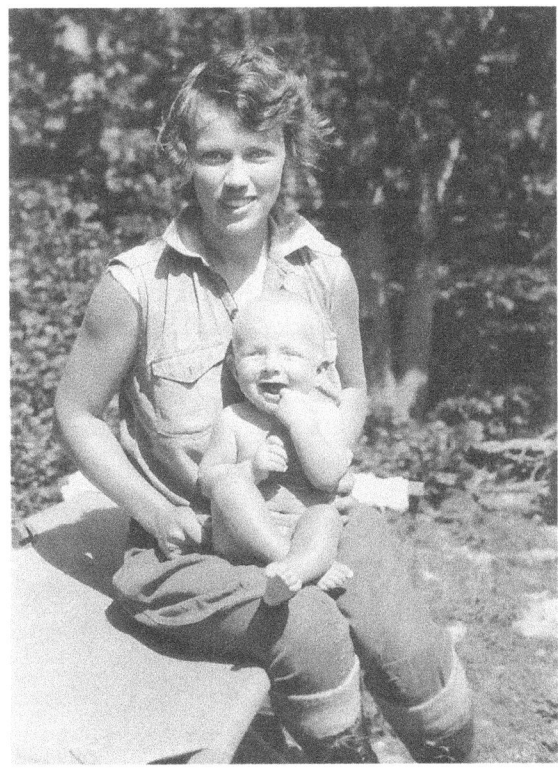

Ruth Lee Thygeson and son Fritjof in the Colorado Rockies, 1930.

by 40 feet, including log ends. Actual living space was modest, perhaps 600 square feet. A small bedroom was separated from an even smaller kitchen by a partial wall of vertical, peeled logs. The tools they used are still at the cabin today — a two-man crosscut saw, a carpenter's saw, an ax, an adz, a drawknife, a mallet, a chisel, and various tools to create good plumb lines and right angles.[13] The cabin's foundation was made of carefully chosen stones and the floor was a few feet above the bare ground. In Rocky Mountain National Park, where similar cabin building was going on, "rounded glacial rock and weathered granite — often with lichen growing on the surface — were placed around the base of these buildings and used to build chimneys."[14] From the kitchen door and the front door, the one that was rarely used, steps of rough granite and mortar that led to the rocky ground were laid by hand. The cabin was oriented so that its one large window — an unusual window in the days of small, divided-light windows that opened like shutters — faced the peaks to the west.

    Constructing the cabin walls was a considerable challenge. The sill logs, which were the longest and straightest, had to be on the bottom of the cabin's long axis, running north-south, with their butt ends opposite to each other. After each pair of sill logs was laid on, a pair of end logs was notched to fit into them. The log-end notches, known as "saddle notches," were scooped carefully out of each log as it was prepared for the log to be laid on top of it. Great care was needed as each new pair of logs were selected, to try to keep the walls as level as possible.[15] Phil and Ruth Lee used an ax to trim the cabin's log ends to an exposed line, another esthetic touch that required extra work but made their cabin more beautiful to them. Two strong young people could maneuver the lower logs into place with a great deal of effort. Ruth Lee and Phil began this process themselves, notching each log carefully just before rolling it into place. They used skids, strong planks placed at an angle, on which they could roll and drag logs up to the top of the cabin wall. Sometimes ropes or metal staffs were used to help get the logs into place. As the walls rose higher, it became impossible for them to roll the logs onto the growing stack without help. They hired a pair of local men.

    For the chinking, they bought large quantities of oakum, hemp dipped in creosote. Oakum was traditionally used in shipbuilding, to caulk or stabilize joints and seams where timbers came together. Oakum was at one point made of old rope, yet was so effective plumbers used it to seal pipes. It had the added benefit of repelling rodents and insects.[16] Ruth Lee and Phil stuffed it carefully and copiously between the logs so that no daylight came through to the inside of the cabin. On the outside, they added wire mesh in the curved space between two logs, attaching it with long nails and covering it with mortar. On the inside, they took aspen saplings, cut them into quarter rounds, and nailed them with very small, almost headless nails into the spaces between the log rounds.

There was a lot to learn from the book they used. It was essential, for example, that the fireplace chimney be lined on the inside with firebrick or similar material, because rocks could explode when exposed to extreme heat.[17] They mixed concrete in a wheelbarrow, one part cement to three parts clean sand. The fireplace, built with rocks hand-picked and hauled to the site, was designed with an internal damper and smoke shelf that caused it to draw well and throw out heat. The fireplace dominated the north end of the cabin and exposed stone ran all the way from the ground up to three feet above the eaves on the cabin's exterior. A soot-blackened kettle hung from a forged iron arm at the left side of the fireplace to heat the family's wash water. The hearth was flat and jutted out into the room to keep cinders off the oak floor. It also had a stone sitting bench built into it so that the fire tender or cook had a place to sit. That was Ruth Lee and Phil's special design.

The cabin was Phil and Ruth Lee's first and in some ways greatest creative work. Though it took several summers of hard labor to build it, they took pleasure in the artistry and the physical labor involved. They bought windows and heavy, two-inch-thick doors. The custom-designed black wrought iron hardware for the massive wooden front and back doors of the cabin was one of the few luxuries they allowed themselves. It was Ruth Lee's project to design the hardware and commission a blacksmith. The kitchen door was a windowless Dutch door that could be left half-open to let the sunlight into the kitchen but keep a young child inside. Both of the cabin doors could be closed and locked from the inside with heavy sliding iron pieces, which turned out to be very helpful when black bears occasionally sought entry.

When the cabin was finished, the logs were covered in coats of boiled linseed oil, which turned them a beautiful golden color that was warm and welcoming in the kerosene lamplight. After a number of years, the cabin was encased in a sort of protective resin — the rain and snow were repelled, and even the lumbering black carpenter ants had a hard time getting a meal. Phil constructed the bed frames from skinned aspen poles, and he made by hand the couch, the chairs, and even the little coffee table. He managed to do it with a minimum of hardware and store-bought materials. "My father would make a peg at one end of a small aspen log and a hole in another piece that he was going to join it to," Kristin explained. "By this method, he could build a ninety degree angle in a bed frame or the couch."[18] He broke down and bought pine planks, however, and varnished them to create table tops. He also bought single layers of hard wire webbing, the kind used in military cots, to support mattresses.

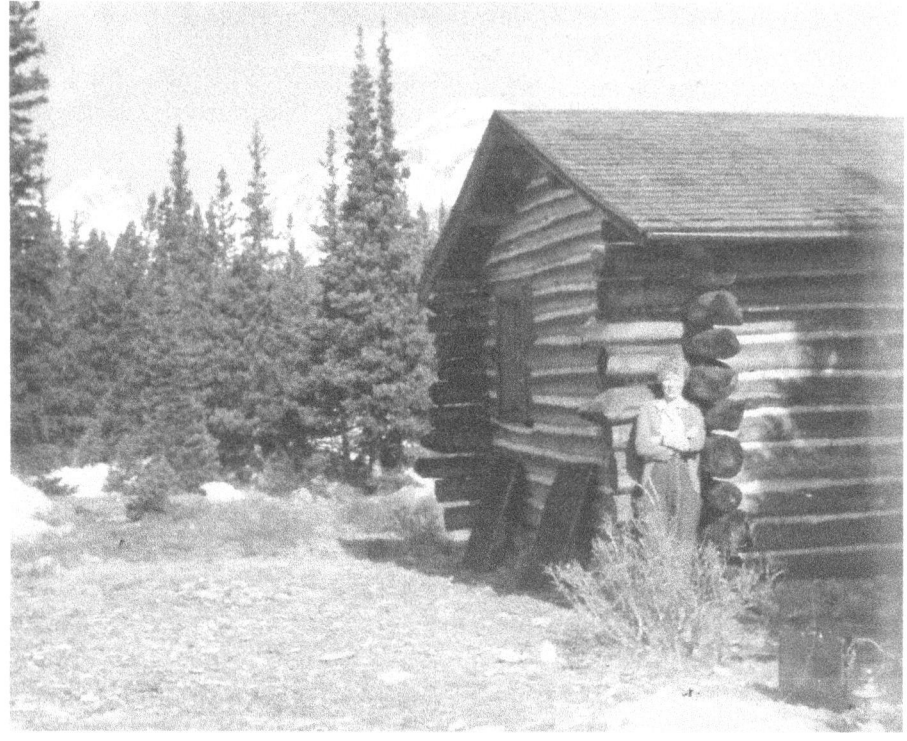

Ruth Lee Thygeson outside the cabin she helped build, with the Indian Peaks in the background.

The kitchen sink was made of zinc set in a linoleum-covered counter with a short length of pipe draining into a slop bucket. This sink and bucket system endures to this day, and the cabin still has no electricity and no running water, not even a well. In the early years, cooking was done over the fireplace, with meat laid into a two-sided metal grill that could be propped over the coals. They left ears of corn in the husk to steam and cooked potatoes wrapped in tinfoil. Phil always loved making and tending fires. The fireplace had a set of fire irons and a bellows, though Phil liked to blow on his coals. In time, a simple two-burner Coleman stove that used white gas supplemented the fireplace cooking. It had to be pumped by hand to give pressure to the gas and would often send up a funnel of flames when lighted. Pots and pans were hung on the wall. Food that needed to remain cold was stored in metal cylinders with lids and nestled inside snow drifts under the firs and spruce outside the cabin during the early weeks of summer. Later in summer, a hole was dug for the can to be inserted into the cool earth.

In the early days of the cabin, the latrine was a hole Phil dug in the ground with a raised pine board with a hole for sitting. It was out in the woods among the trees, and nothing but the forest gave it privacy. Phil was enough of a creature of civilization to buy a toilet seat for it. It came from the Montgomery Ward catalogue, which Ruth Lee affectionately called "Monkey Ward." After World War II, the Forest Service banned open pit toilets. When they were able to visit Colorado after the war, Phil built a small pine building divided into two tiny rooms — a tool shed on one side and an outhouse on the other. The chemical pit toilet, which used a foul-smelling concoction made of creosote, tar, and pine oil, ran into a hand-dug drain field.[19]

In the cabin, bath water was heated in the black cast iron kettle hanging over the open fire. It was ladled out into a zinc bathing tub and baths consisted of four or five inches of warm water, a bar of soap, and a wash cloth. The Thygesons shared bath water, starting with the youngest member of the family going first. The family washed their hair on warm days outside in the sun, using tubs balanced on the sawhorse. Ruth Lee washed clothes and diapers by hand with a small scrubbing board and a tub of rain water. Wash water drained off the roof into gutters that in turn drained into a 50-gallon wooden pickle barrel by the back door. Delicious drinking water came from a natural spring about a mile down the road toward Ward. Water-loving blue-purple wildflowers known as Tall Chiming Bells grew in abundance right where water spilled out of the hillside. Phil hauled drinking water in five-gallon metal cans.

For recreation, the family went hiking. The more developed trails had single, ax-flattened logs to serve as bridges over swollen streams, with the white water of early summer snowmelt roaring below. How they got baby Fritjof across those streams is an intriguing question. Where did they draw the line in terms of taking risks with their lives? Ruth Lee and Phil were both very strong and fit, so they were able to climb the 13,000 foot peaks in the area. One of the harder summits is Paiute Peak, a Matterhorn-shaped peak in back of Mt. Audubon, which reaches 13,200 feet. First they had to climb Audubon, which takes several hours, and then travel out a knife-ridge about half a mile toward the Continental Divide. There is no other way up Paiute Peak because its face is too sheer. In a glacial bowl below the peak is a frozen tarn that rarely thaws. There are no trees or windbreaks above the tarn, just a rock promontory exposed to wind. Ruth Lee made it part of the way to Paiute Peak along that knife ridge, thought better of the risk, sat down with one leg straddling each side of the ridge, and slowly made her way back to safety.[20] Phil, who was, in essence, an intrepid mountain goat, went on without her.

10. To Egypt in Search of Trachoma

In medicine, Phil was beginning to be a research pioneer. His interest in infectious ocular disease meant he would probably need to do research overseas. Opportunities came to him through a remarkable stroke of good fortune. He became the chosen protégé of Dr. Francis I. Proctor, a wealthy ophthalmologist who developed a strong interest in trachoma, the most common and devastating cause of preventable blindness in the world. Proctor had graduated from Harvard Medical School in 1892 and was a highly respected cataract surgeon in Boston. He became interested in trachoma late in life. He was led to the interest through his hobby of photography, a hobby Phil also shared. Proctor enjoyed stereoscopic photography and when he was retired, he read about the Carnegie archaeological excavation begun in 1924 at the Chichén Itzá ruins in Mexico. He decided to photograph the ruins and became a volunteer on the excavation team. While there, he discovered that the indigenous people of the region, who were primarily of Maya descent, were suffering terribly from trachoma.[1]

Following his retirement from practice in Boston, Proctor and his wife Elizabeth built a pueblo-style home on a hundred acres of land just outside of Santa Fe, New Mexico. Proctor became, as Phil put it, "obsessed with trachoma and its cause and cure" upon meeting Native Americans who also suffered terribly from the disease.[2] At the peak of Proctor's involvement with the disease, he became a consultant on trachoma to the Bureau of Indian Affairs. Since he lacked the research skills to do specialized laboratory work himself, he supported others in that effort, including the Japanese bacteriologist and immunologist Hideyo Noguchi. Noguchi graduated from Tokyo Medical College in 1897 and emigrated to the United States soon thereafter. He spent over two decades doing research at the Rockefeller Institute.

10. To Egypt in Search of Trachoma

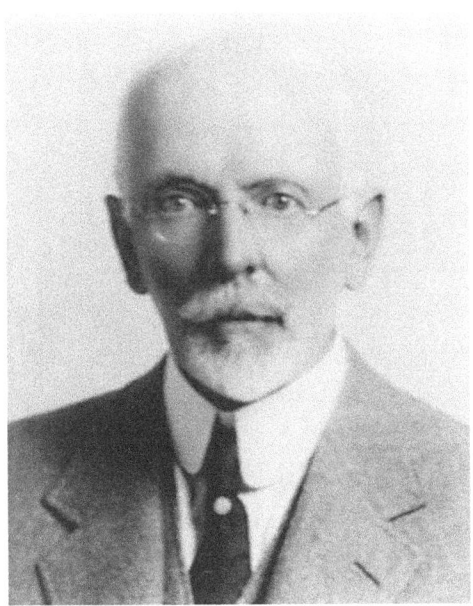

Francis I. Proctor, Phillips Thygeson's benefactor and mentor who encouraged his work on trachoma and after whom the Francis I. Proctor Foundation for Research in Ophthalmology was named.

In 1929, Phil and Dr. Finnoff published an article on Noguchi's finding of *Bacterium granulosis* in trachoma in the *American Journal of Ophthalmology*. The article caught Dr. Proctor's eye, as he had persuaded Noguchi to do trachoma-related research. Noguchi had joined the staff of the Rockefeller Institute in 1904, and did seminal studies on snake venom and on smallpox and yellow fever vaccines. He also identified the cause of syphilis and developed a skin test to diagnose it. Tragically, he died in 1928 in Accra, Gold Coast (now Ghana), of yellow fever. His death, Phil wrote, was devastating to Proctor, who "had a deep personal and scientific relationship with him."[3] Sadly, Noguchi died an unhappy man. Based on research he did in Latin America, he believed that yellow fever was caused by a leptospiral infection. When research results coming out of Africa revealed, instead, that the cause was a filterable virus, Noguchi went to Africa to try to figure it out for himself and, he hoped, confirm his own research. Before his death, he discovered that he had indeed been wrong.[4] After his death, Phil Thygeson was to prove him wrong once again, this time in relation to the cause of trachoma. Nonetheless, Noguchi's work stands as a brilliant contribution to microbiological research.

Proctor lacked the expertise to confirm Noguchi's work on trachoma, but he wanted this work done quickly. After Noguchi died, and Finnoff and Thygeson's paper on *Bacterium granulosis* was published, Proctor made a special trip to Denver to meet the two of them. According to Phil, Finnoff was "especially interested in trachoma because trachoma was rampant in Colorado and [was] the world's leading cause of blindness."[5] With their shared excitement about trying to find both a cause of and a cure for trachoma, they quickly agreed to collaborate. Though the University of Colorado simply did not have the money to support this kind of research, Phil chose trachoma research as the subject of his graduate thesis at CU.

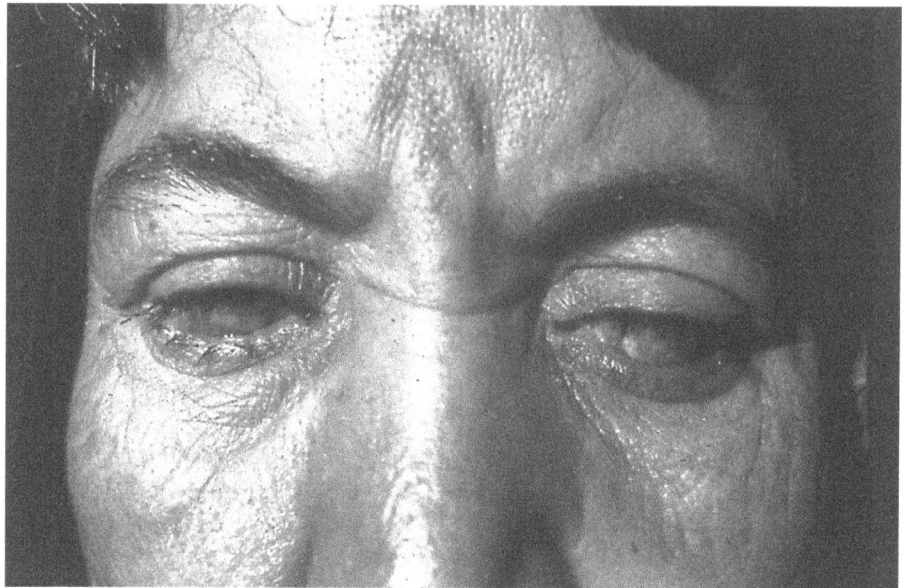

Native American with severe trachoma. From Phillips Thygeson's collection.

The collaboration among the three physicians was soon settled: Proctor would provide the funds, Finnoff the pathology expertise, and Thygeson the microbiology. There were other great doctors in the background. Finnoff, for example, had been trained by Karl Lindner in Vienna. Proctor recommended that the newly formed trachoma team collaborate with Polk Richards, head of the Indian Health Service trachoma unit. Very early in their relationship with Dr. Proctor, Phil and Ruth Lee got to know Dr. Proctor's wife, Elizabeth. Phil found her beautiful and elegant and, in the idiom of the day, "a wonderful hostess." "She was a tall blond woman in her forties who radiated charm and good will," he wrote, and she was just as interested in trachoma as was Francis Proctor.[6]

In 1929, Proctor recommended that he, his wife Elizabeth, and Phil take a research trip to the Giza Memorial Institute in Egypt, as Egypt had the highest rate of blindness in the world.[7] The institute had been established in Cairo as "a memorial to the camel drivers of Egypt in World War I."[8] All of the war materiel that supported Edmund H. H. Allenby's conquering army had been transported on camels at great risk to the camel drivers. Allenby was a British viscount who led the Egyptian Expeditionary Force to conquer Syria and Palestine in 1917–1918. So many camel drivers were killed that the British government built a memorial to their memory. Phil believed the institute was made possible by Dr. H. F. MacCallan, who helped create a hospital-based

10. To Egypt in Search of Trachoma

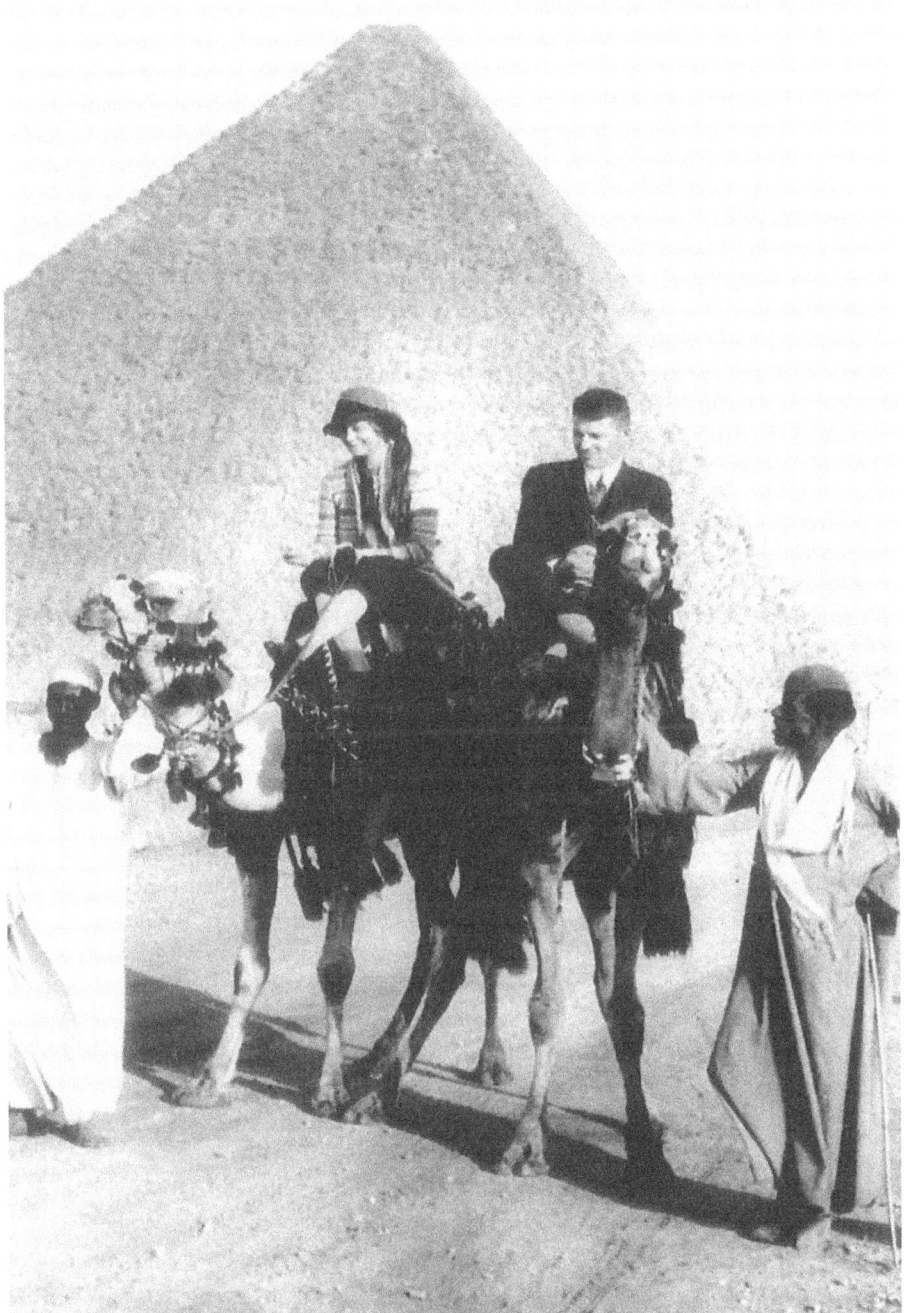

Elizabeth C. Proctor and Phillips Thygeson in Egypt in 1930.

ophthalmic service in Egypt. Phil admired MacCallan's book on trachoma and the "MacCallan classification" system for trachoma.[9] The Giza Institute was remarkable in that it had four full-time researchers, an almost unparalleled luxury. The staff was Egyptian and British, led by director Roland P. Wilson, a researcher whose achievements Phil felt "were largely unrecognized, except for a few like me."[10] Wilson didn't like MacCallan, but Phil was able to distinguish between personality shortcomings and research prowess, and he was willing to overlook the one in his admiration for the other.

Travel to the Giza Memorial Institute was a memorable adventure. Phil went with Dr. and Mrs. Proctor aboard the deluxe S. S. *Augustus*. "Mrs. Proctor was a real Maryland belle," Phil wrote. "She was a real beauty and used to all the best things in life. She wouldn't accept anything other than first class."[11] After a crossing of nine days, they arrived in Naples, where they were greeted by the chief of police, escorted without incident through customs, and taken to the Hotel Excelsior, where they were given, in Phil's words, "the big treatment." They were offered an opportunity to meet with Mussolini, which Dr. Proctor declined.[12] Ruth Lee was not invited on this trip, probably because of her new baby, and Phil missed her greatly.

From there they traveled by boat to Egypt, via Alexandria. Elizabeth Proctor was something of an expert on the Nile valley and ancient Egypt, so she served as the group's host and tour guide.[13] "The interesting thing on that voyage, which took two days, was that our two rhesus monkeys, that we had brought with us and that supposedly had *Bacterium granulosis* conjunctivitis, got loose and went all over the boat," Phil wrote. "They scared all the passengers."[14] From Alexandria, they traveled to Cairo by train. While at the Giza Institute, a lovely two-story building with modern facilities, they were put up in a fancy boarding house.[15] The Proctors, who had spent a winter learning bacteriology in a laboratory in Tucson,[16] worked in the Giza laboratory alongside Phil and Wilson for several months until they concluded that their usefulness had ended. Before the Proctors left, they showed Phil a number of ancient sites around Cairo and took him on an unforgettable ride on the back of a camel from Giza to the pyramids of Sakara, the "dead city of Memphis," a tailbone-bruising distance of over ten miles.[17] The Proctors went on to tour the Nile River by boat, leaving Phil to his lab work. They then went back to Sicily and enjoyed the rest of the mild winter there.

Phil admired and learned from Wilson. He appreciated the well-equipped laboratory and the supply of monkeys they used for trachoma and other ocular research. He credited Wilson with understanding the crucial role of flies in transmitting trachoma from one human eye to another. He was also impressed by Wilson's study of pathology and his fabulous collection of biopsies of eyes at all stages of trachoma, including the very early stages. "His study of the cytology of the incipient [trachomatous] follicle was outstanding.... It was the stimulus for my work on the cytology of expressed follicular material.... He pointed out that there is a world of difference between trachoma, follicular conjunctivitis, and folliculosis."[18] Phil also was inspired by Wilson and Egyptian researcher El Tobgy's work on vernal catarrh, a sort of seasonal allergic conjunctivitis. As Phil was fond of acknowledging, other people's work gave him "many ideas for my own studies."[19] What fascinated him most was Wilson's view that the inclusion body of trachoma was all-important and could be found in the incubation period of the disease process. It was the first detectable sign of the disease.[20] Wilson drew this conclusion from studying Egyptian newborns. Phil noticed that this crucial observation about the early role of the inclusion body "never seemed to get into the literature."[21] Phil would eventually remedy that omission, but the credit never really went to Wilson. During this time, Phil did the work for a paper on bacterial flora of the eye in patients with trachoma.[22]

After Finnoff's rigorous work schedule for interns back in Colorado, Phil was a bit wide-eyed at how things were done in Cairo. "I was amazed to see how so much work was being done, despite the short work hours." Work began at 9:00 A.M., with Turkish coffee and conversation. At 11:30, there was a break for tea and more conversation. "The work day ended at 1 P.M." This was followed by a big lunch and time for a nap, exercise, bathing, and "a high tea with crumpets." Then they dressed for dinner and a night on the town.[23] All the same, Wilson was able to study the spring and fall epidemics of Koch-Weeks and gonococcal conjunctivitis, and link them to the Egyptian fly-hatching seasons. It was excellent training in epidemiology for Phil.[24] After Phil's trip to Egypt, an even more profound set of lessons lay directly ahead.

11. Learning from a Nobel Laureate in Tunisia

This time, Phil was to go to the Pasteur Institute in Tunis, North Africa. At Dr. Proctor's urging, Phil had applied for a National Research Council Fellowship almost immediately after his return from Egypt in 1930. His goal was to study trachoma in Tunis with the Nobel Prize winner, Charles Nicolle. Nicolle and Charles Le Bailly (or Lebailly) had done important research on influenza. The two French researchers determined that influenza was a filter-passing or filterable virus and proposed that a new category of microbes be added to the nomenclature. In 1919, the two embarked on a study of microscopic infectious agents in rodents, and in 1928, Nicolle received the Nobel Prize in Medicine for his typhus research, which helped advance his work in the microbiology of trachoma.[1] He had reported the filtration of the trachoma-causing agent with Berkefeld B filters. These were the first filtrations of the trachoma agent and were done using Algerian mangeby monkeys.[2] Nicolle became cofounder and president of the International Organization Against Trachoma.

In 1931, Phil was awarded a National Research Council Fellowship to go to Tunis to study the microbiology of trachoma with Nicolle. It was a great help because it paid $200 a month plus $150 for crossing the Atlantic by ship. A year was too long for the young family to be separated and the Proctors provided the crucial financial assistance — a thousand dollars — that permitted Ruth Lee and Fritjof to go along for the research year. Dr. Proctor had associates connected with the American Export Line, a transatlantic freighter operation, and so the Thygeson family got to ship out for free on S.S. *Exermont*, a freighter that normally took no passengers at all. They spent twenty-six days in the crossing and had a wonderful adventure. Because they were the only passengers, they got to eat with the ship captain at his table,[3] which

II. Learning from a Nobel Laureate in Tunisia

Ruth Lee particularly enjoyed. The captain took a shine to the newly toddling Fritjof and set up a net so that he could safely run around part of the bridge. Fritjof loved the captain's Victrola playing the folk song, "Yes, We Have No Bananas Today."[4] There was a mutiny aboard ship near Gibraltar, provoked by a fight between a steward and an oiler. The steward took a heavy

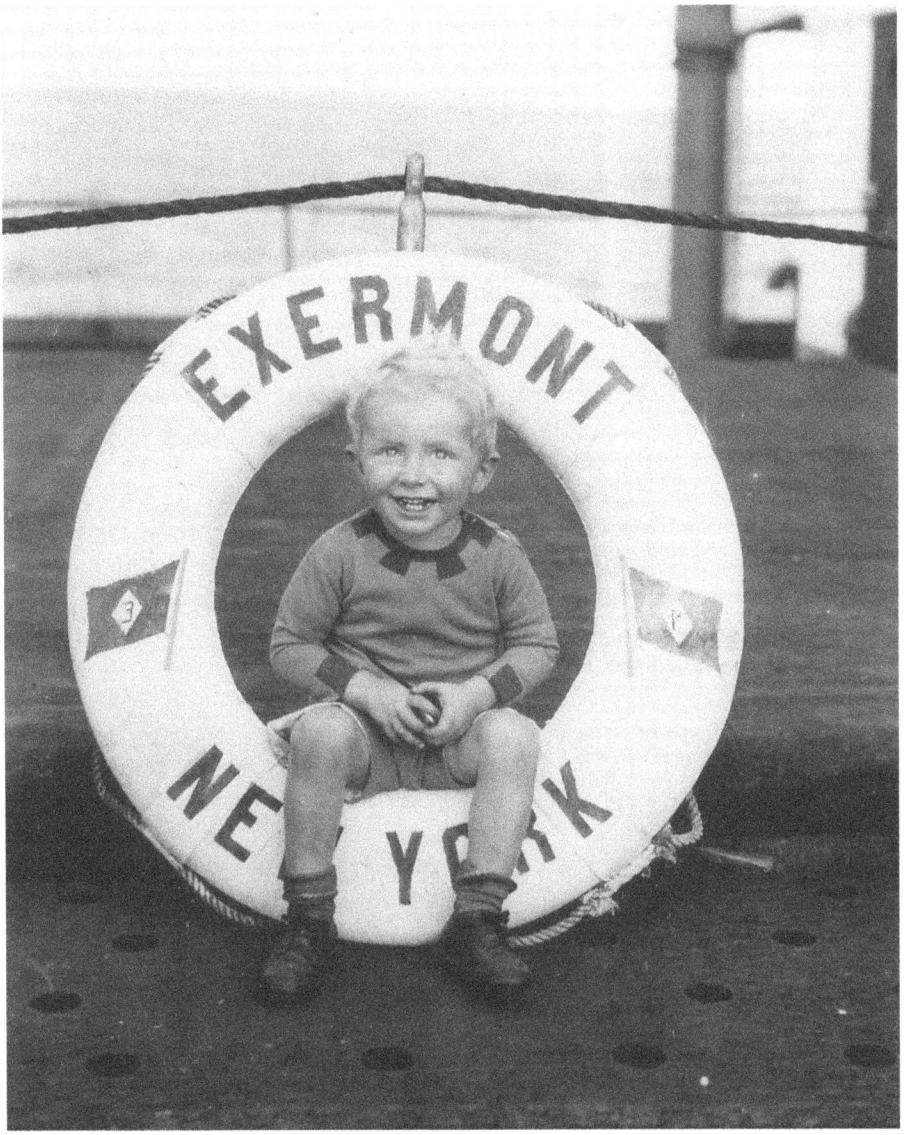

Fritjof Thygeson aboard the S. S. *Exermont*, en route to Tunisia, 1931.

wrench down to the engine room and knocked the oiler unconscious. "This was high seas mutiny because it put the engines in jeopardy," Phil said.[5] The captain locked the steward in the brig and turned him over to authorities somewhere along the coast of Africa. The mutiny was also memorable because of the enraged reactions of the oiler's friends and shipmates.

Phil, Ruth Lee, and little Fritjof moved into a villa in Carthage with a French family, the Déchenaux. Monsieur Déchenaux was a retired teacher, so they hired him to tutor them in French. They learned a lot and spoke fondly of the warm, friendly couple all of their lives. Ruth Lee was much more linguistically adept than Phil, though she had her own struggles getting started with French. According to Fritjof, she didn't understand what the French in Tunisia were saying to her until she practiced conversing with an Arab shopkeeper who had learned French as a second language. After a few weeks of that, she was able to converse with anyone.[6] For his part, Phil reported that he "couldn't speak it worth anything at all," though he had chosen it as his medical school language and was able to understand medical literature in French.[7] Charles Nicolle, Phil's French-born mentor at the Pasteur Institute, was profoundly deaf. He was a wonderful lip reader but, of course, it was essential that the person with whom he was conversing be speaking French.[8] Phil became conversational in French.

Phil and Ruth Lee loved the ruins of ancient Carthage, an archeological site with pre–Byzantine-era tombs. They spent their weekends exploring the ruins and collecting ancient artifacts. Phil photographed and they enjoyed hunting for Roman, Punic, and Byzantine coins. Phil's favorite discovery was a silver Louis Philippe five-franc coin from 1830 that he found while sifting beach sand at Carthage. Ruth Lee and Phil also collected pieces of Carthaginian marble. Little Fritjof had a wonderful year. He later remembered watching a camel drawing water from a well and young women turning grapes into wine.[9]

Phil believed that Nicolle took a liking to him partly because of his Norwegian name and heritage. Nicolle liked to vacation in Norway. He honored the "fellows" who came to work in his laboratory by permanently noting their names on the marble wall of his personal library. As a young doctor being trained mainly through a series of preceptorships, Phil was excited to learn what he could from a famous new mentor. Nicolle taught him something invaluable — how to run a laboratory. "He had a wonderful system," Phil said. "He had Charles Anderson, who was the associate director, and Anderson did all the leg work, all the scut work, as they call it. He left Nicolle free to do his laboratory studies. Nicolle made the policies, but Anderson settled all the disputes and everything like that...."[10] With the extra time this arrangement gave him, Nicolle became a prolific novelist. Phil was learning the valuable

11. Learning from a Nobel Laureate in Tunisia

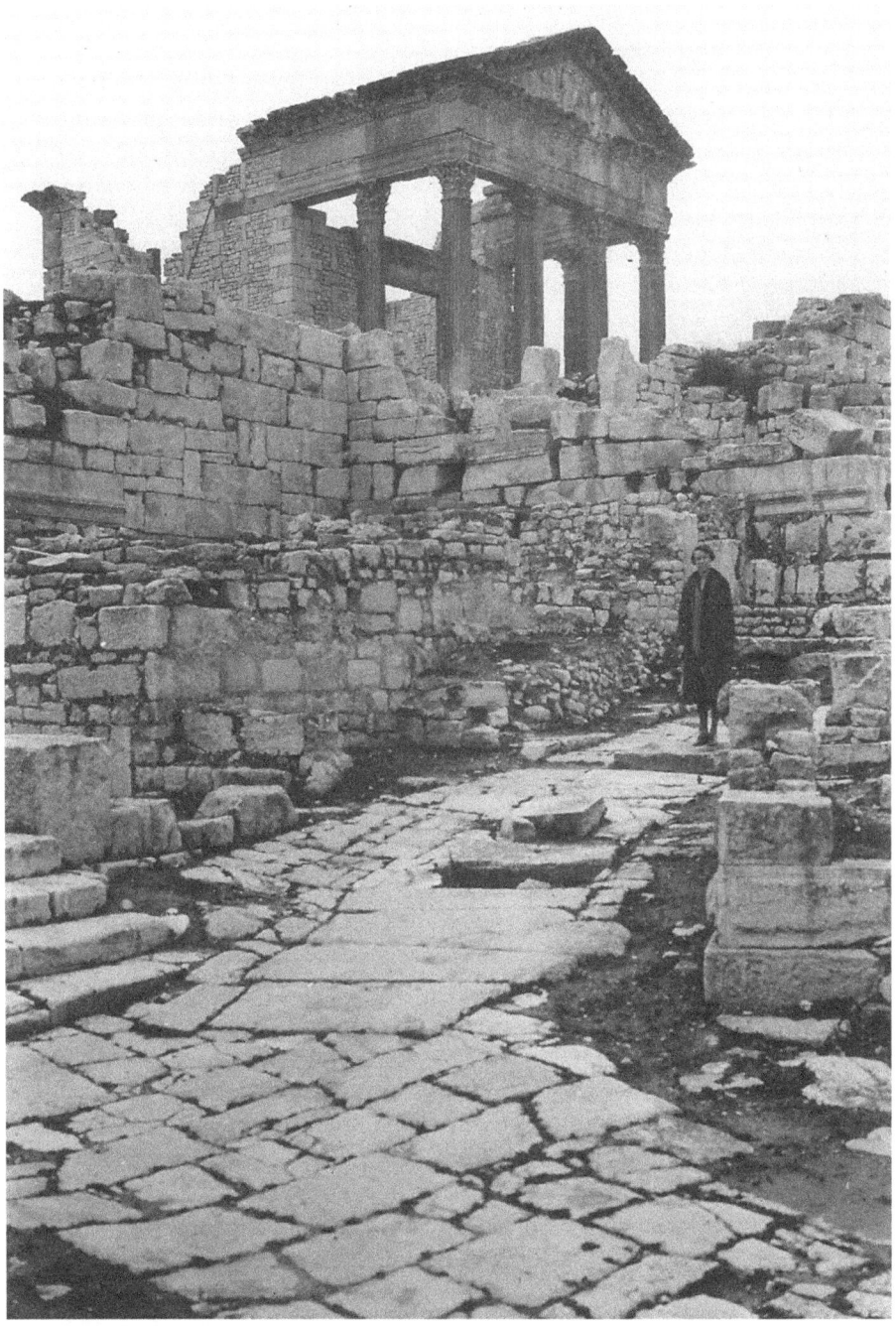

Ruth Lee Thygeson in the ruins of Carthage, near Tunis, Tunisia, 1931.

lesson that a good researcher supported by a good administrator could have more than one passion.

The Pasteur Institute of Tunis was "number two in the so-called jewels of Pasteur Institutes all around the Mediterranean," Phil said. "They were in Algiers, Casablanca, Istanbul, Athens. They had one in Indo-China, too."[11] The one in Asia was located in what was then Saigon and is now Ho Chi Minh City, Vietnam. It was established in response to a great need for public health support around rabies and other diseases. According to Phil, it was because of Nicolle's international status as a Nobel Prize winner that Tunis was considered number two. Phil was treated very handsomely there and given his own laboratory and technician. Nicolle also gave him advice and shared his view that the cause of trachoma, which was that the infectious agent would be found in the follicle. Phil believed the answer lay in the inclusion bodies and the epithelium.[12]

At the time, there were three predominant theories of the cause or etiology of trachoma. One was Noguchi's *Bacterium granulosis* theory, which was proved wrong. The second was the Halberstaedter-Prowazek (H.P.) inclusion body theory. Dr. Proctor was interested in this theory and Phil was interested in the story behind the theory. Max Neisser, the researcher who identified the agent that causes gonorrhea, was in Java doing research and had his assistants Ludwig von Halberstaedter and Stanislaus J. V. von Prowazek with him. They asked to be allowed to do trachoma research, but Neisser didn't want them to be distracted from his work on gonorrhea, so he refused their request. "[O]n the side they surreptitiously started studying trachoma," Phil said. "What they did was to inoculate orangutans with trachoma scrapings."[13] They were able to produce experimental trachoma infections this way, but they mistakenly thought that tiny intracellular bodies they saw in the epithelia of their orangutans were the cause of trachoma. They called the bodies "chlamydozoa." Because these bodies were also found in inclusion blennorrhea, microbiologists believed that they couldn't be the cause of trachoma.[14] Prowazek and others thought a virus was at work, but eventually the virus turned out to be a small bacterium, *Chlamydia trachomatis*.

In Tunis, Phil was able to show that inclusion bodies could consistently be found in active trachoma, but that sometimes they were very few in number. Nicolle supported this work as due diligence in research, but he did not believe it was the answer to the mystery of what caused trachoma. Nicolle thought the Halberstaedter-Prowazek inclusion bodies were merely "artifacts" of the disease, not its cause. Phil summed up Nicolle's view as "Le virus, c'est dans le follicule" ("The virus is in the follicle.").[15] Nicolle arranged for Phil to work with Roger Nataf, a French scientist deeply committed to trachoma research. Phil and Nataf repeatedly tried to replicate Nicolle's trachoma filtration experiments, in which he had "produced experimental trachoma in an Algerian Magat monkey ... with a Berkefeld V filtrate of trachomatous material." The attempt to reproduce the experiment failed repeatedly. "It was clear to me that follicular material was clogging the filters," Phil wrote, "and later I was to prove that this was so when I switched to graded collodion (Elford) filters."[16] When someone was proved incorrect, Phil was never one to mince words. Of Nicolle, he remarked, "He wrote and spoke as a world authority. But he happened to be all wrong on trachoma."[17]

At some point during their year in Tunis, Phil took a solo trip to Paris to visit the number one Pasteur Institute and learn from Victor Morax, a Swiss doctor of French nationality whom Dr. Proctor knew. Phil thought of Morax as "an early pioneer in ocular microbiology" and as a marvel of a doctor because he could do so many things well, including invent surgical techniques.[18] A group of bacteria known as Moraxella was named after Morax, who discovered them.[19] Thanks to Morax, Phil got to see Louis Pasteur's rooftop laboratory. What stayed with Phil all his life was how the great Pasteur had been memorialized by having his laboratory kept intact. "It had been left with an experiment half completed, just as Pasteur had left it before his death," Phil later wrote.[20]

Morax introduced Phil to the Pasteur Institute's concierge, who was the first person to receive Pasteur's experimental rabies vaccine. The story of the vaccine experiment was later documented in Paul de Kruif's *Microbe Hunters*, a book Phil loved. Phil often referred to himself as a "microbe hunter," which suited his swashbuckling, pioneer self-image. Meeting Morax and the concierge also made Phil feel he had a "direct link" back to Pasteur, one of his all-time heroes.[21] Phil and Morax spent hours together looking at Morax's research, which included studies of what was then known as "swimming pool conjunctivitis" because it could be passed among people swimming in the same pool.[22] Some researchers confused this disease with trachoma, but neither Morax nor Phil made that mistake. Though follicular conjunctivitis was shared by both diseases, they were actually quite different, and monkey experiments were a good way to prove it.

Phil returned to Morax's laboratory again the following year and took a one-week intensive course in ocular microbiology, perhaps the first ever offered in the subject.[23] Ruth Lee and Fritjof accompanied Phil on one of these trips. Phil had little experience taking care of Fritjof single-handedly, but Ruth Lee desperately wanted to see the Louvre, so he volunteered to take care of him for an entire day. "I think it was probably one of the hardest, most awful days my father ever had," Fritjof said. They stayed in a small hotel with an elevator. "What I wanted to do was to go up and down that elevator, up and down, all day long. My father would try to get me to stop and I'd start crying." Phil didn't know how to cope with that, so together they rode the elevator all day long.[24]

Phil enjoyed Morax's laboratory monkeys. One of the monkeys could spit all the way across a room and would spit at everyone except for Morax. "Morax sent a keeper ahead to draw off the spit before our examination. Morax seemed to have a way with chimps. They sat on his lap and let him evert their lids — something my apes would not let me do."[25] Morax was also a good host; he took Phil out to an elegant French restaurant and then to a show similar to the Folies Bergère. Phil admired him because he was insightful about trachoma and the inclusion bodies and because he was a "Renaissance man," which is what Phil aspired to be. "He was an innovative surgeon, pathologist, microbiologist, and historian."[26]

Phil often talked about the other paths in life he could have taken — the farmer, forester, or public health epidemiologist he could have been — and what he considered himself to be, a medical researcher. "I am interested in the plagues that affect mankind," he wrote, not just the plagues themselves but the history of the plagues.[27] To this end, he read with great interest about the first microscope in the hands of Antonie van Leeuwenhoek, born in 1632 in Delft, the Netherlands. In the hands of Paul de Kruif, author of *Microbe Hunters*, every significant scientific discovery was a rollicking adventure. In the historical lineage of microbe hunters who deeply influenced Phil and other research scientists, we must count Antonie van Leeuwenhoek, Louis Pasteur, Joseph Lister, and Robert Koch. Leeuwenhoek was a great role model for Phil because he made his own tools. He could have been satisfied with using microscope lenses ground by expert lens grinders of the Netherlands, but he wanted to make them himself.[28] Remarkably, when Phil managed to isolate the *Chlamydia* bacterium that causes trachoma, the discovery was possible because he had made some of his own laboratory materials by hand.

Leeuwenhoek was deeply fascinated by the newly discovered world of microorganisms. He looked at samples of all kinds of water, rainwater, canal water, and well water.

> Everywhere he found those beasts. He gaped at their enormous littleness... he compared them to a cheese-mite and they were to this filthy little creature as a bee is to a horse. He was never tired of watching them "swim about among one another gently like a swarm of mosquitoes in the air...."[29]

When Leeuwenhoek finally wrote to the Royal Society of England to announce his discoveries, he was not believed.[30] Phil admired scientists who were ahead of their time and were not believed, but who were eventually redeemed for posterity. He could see how scientific discovery and belief might not be in sync.

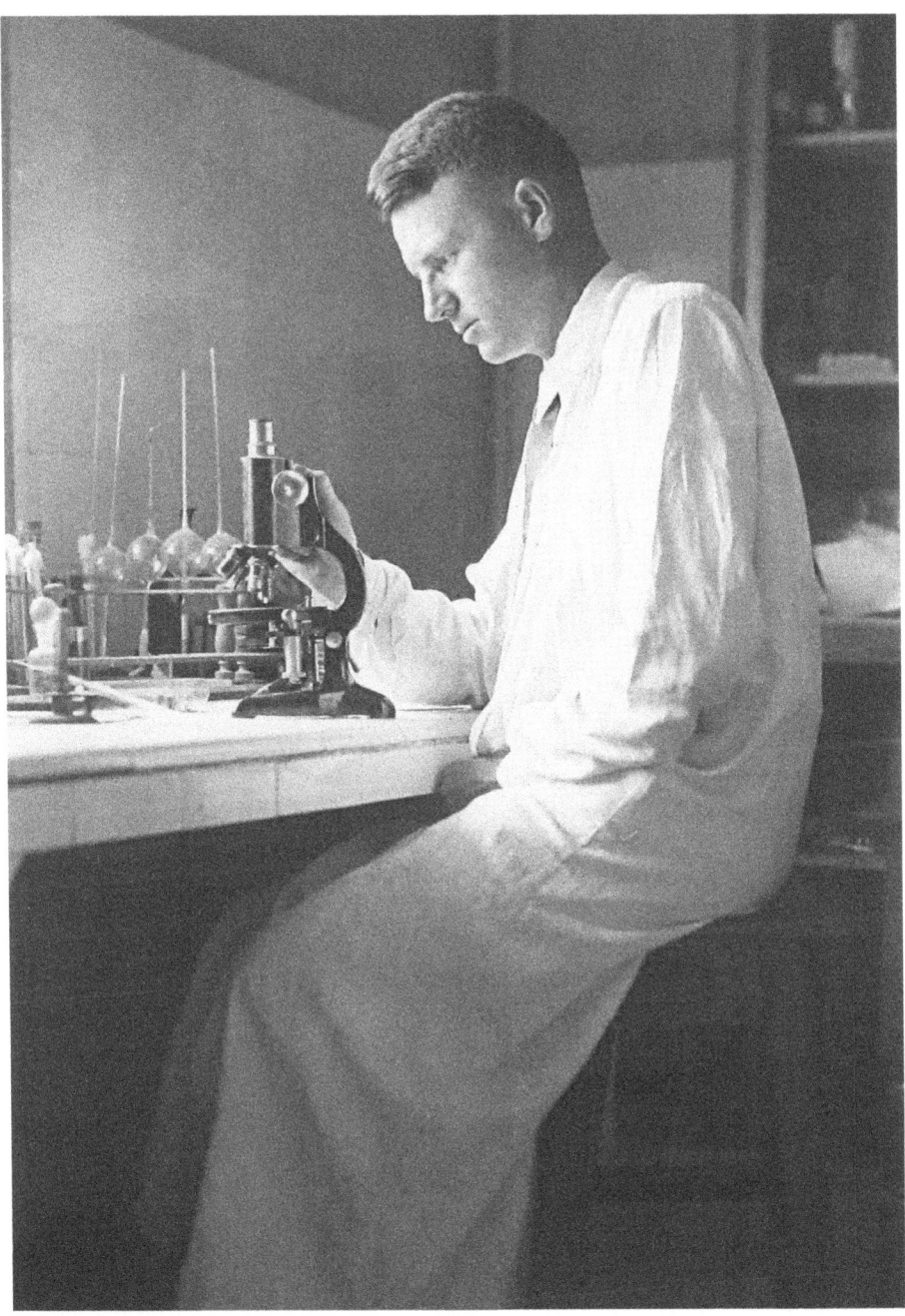

Phillips Thygeson doing trachoma research in his laboratory at the Pasteur Institute in Tunis, 1931.

Of the microbe hunters who preceded him, Phil admired Pasteur most of all, as the father of microbiology and as the one who revolutionized scientific belief and made the "germ theory" of disease common knowledge. Pasteur was born in 1822, two thousand years into a belief system dominated by the theory of "spontaneous generation," which held that organisms arose spontaneously in organic materials. "The idea," one historian wrote, "that beetles, eels, maggots and now microbes could arise spontaneously from putrefying matter was speculated on from Greek and Roman times. And in the 1860's spontaneous generation was still a subject of debate in the exalted French Academy of Sciences."[31] With the help of a colleague whose clever vision resulted in a swan-neck flask that didn't let dust from the air contaminate the sterilized contents, Pasteur was able to show that air often carries contaminating organisms but that it's possible to prevent air from becoming contaminated. For the public, this became a new awareness that life forms beget life forms. As Pasteur said, "There is now no circumstance known in which it can be affirmed that microscopic beings came into the world without germs, without parents similar to themselves."[32]

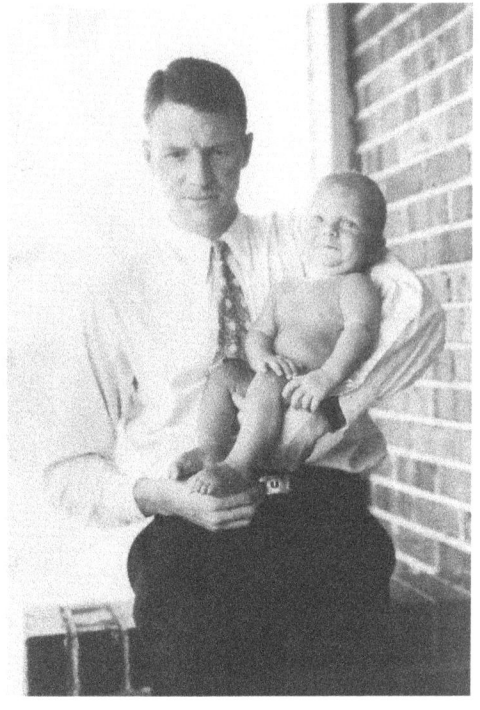

Phillips Thygeson and baby son Fritjof, late 1930.

Pasteur modeled the scientific method and urged scientists not to make claims they couldn't back up with replicable experiments. Pasteur's own achievements in scientific research were said to be "enchaînée," linked together in a logically evolving way. He began with understanding the structure of crystals and the molecular structure of living things. From there, and with the help of the swan-neck flask, he learned about the process of fermenting alcohol and all of the ways that process could go awry and doom a batch of wine or beer. Microorganisms were the key to understanding the processes. Sterilization — which in the realm of food and beverage became known as "pasteurization" — was the remedy. From silk worm disease, Pasteur came to an understanding of the communicable nature of infectious disease in humans. He understood the horrendous number of casualties of surgery and childbirth due to lack of antiseptic habits by physicians and nurses in hospitals. This led him to create vaccines. The problem for women giving birth was so severe, according to Pasteur's son-in-law and biographer René Vallery-Radot, that in a span of six weeks in 1856 in the Paris Maternity Hospital, 64 of the 347 women giving birth died of "childbirth fever."[33]

Pasteur's discovery soon gained a reputation as an avoidable nosocomial or hospital-acquired infection. Passionately committed to preventing more deaths, Pasteur lectured to the French Academy of Medicine about how easy it was to introduce pathogenic germs into a patient's wound and how if he "had the honor of being a surgeon" he would sterilize his instruments and bandages and wash his hands with the greatest of care.[34] Pasteur also introduced many fellow scientists to the notion of anaerobic bacteria and explained how septicemia and gangrene were made possible. Phil was in total agreement with Pasteur and worked hard during the course of his career to avoid physician-induced infections and counsel fellow ophthalmologists who discovered they were having a problem with infections in their offices.

A difference between Pasteur and Phil Thygeson was that Pasteur's work played out very publicly. Pasteur accidentally discovered a cholera vaccine for birds. He left his cholera cultures stored on a shelf in Arbois during the heat of summer. His laboratory assistant didn't pay close attention, and when Pasteur returned, the homegrown cholera bacillus no longer killed chickens. Thinking the experiments ruined, the assistant proposed throwing out the useless cultures, but Pasteur had an inkling that perhaps the cultures had another use. Indeed, they did — chickens exposed to the killed cultures were immune to cholera and those that hadn't been dosed with the cultures died quickly when injected with the cholera bacillus. The elated Pasteur worked to replicate and retest his vaccine, with great success. Before long, however, he was challenged to publicly demonstrate that he could protect sheep from anthrax with a new, barely tested vaccine. Twenty-five sheep were vaccinated, twenty-five others were used as controls, and all were injected with a fatal dose of anthrax. It worked! "The publicity was intense. A reporter from the London *Times* sent back daily dispatches. Newspapers in France followed the events with daily bulletins. There were crowds of onlookers, farmers, engineers, veterinarians, physicians, scientists and a carnival atmosphere."[35] This sort of attention is what Phil Thygeson did not get, at least not outside ophthalmologic circles. He lived in a different era, after the key tenets of microbiological research had been established.

Phil also relied on the work of Joseph Lister and Heinrich Hermann

Robert Koch. Lister was born soon after Pasteur and aided in the effort to encourage surgeons to use sterile technique. He argued against the prevailing notion that the bad-smelling air in surgical wards and sickrooms was due to "miasma," a vague foulness of air that arose spontaneously. He pointed out what should have been obvious, that the bad smell was due to rotting, infected wounds and illness. Pasteur had three ideas about how to get rid of infection—filter out the organisms, kill them by superheating them, or kill them with chemicals. Since only the third idea could easily be applied to human wounds, Lister focused his experiments on that idea.[36] He tried carbolic acid on wounds and discovered that it reduced gangrene. He talked surgeons into sterilizing their hands and wearing gloves. It is said that he saved Edward VII's life by making sure his appendectomy was done right.[37]

Koch was able to further Pasteur's work by more definitively proving how a single organism caused a specific disease. Using a concoction of gelatin and potatoes, he created a nutrient medium on which any number of pathogenic bacteria could be cultured. This helped other scientists with their lab work. By the time Phil was born, disease agents were being isolated and identified one after another. As Koch expressed it, "As soon as the right method was found, discoveries came as easily as ripe apples from a tree." Koch's most famous contribution to fellow scientists was his four criteria to establish a causal relationship between an organism and the disease it caused. "Koch's Postulates," laid out in 1882, remain the definitive way experimentally to prove disease agency. The organism in question has to be found in all cases of the disease, isolated and maintained in a culture medium, capable of producing the same disease even after several generations as a laboratory culture, and retrieved from an experimentally infected animal or person and successfully cultured in the lab again.[38] Koch's use of this nutrient medium in Petri dishes is still standard today. His most famous work in this vein was on cholera, anthrax, and tuberculosis. In 1905, he was awarded the Nobel Prize in Physiology or Medicine.

Koch's refinement of microbiological laboratory technique enabled Phil to produce publishable research results and to have confidence in his laboratory technique. After his time at the Giza Institute, Phil was able to publish on his own and, in 1931, "Bacterial flora in Egyptian trachoma" appeared in the *American Journal of Ophthalmology*. His experiences at the Pasteur Institute of Tunis and Paris led him in 1933 to publish several articles on trachoma in French as well, both in the *Archives de l'Institut Pasteur de Tunis* and the *Revue Internationale du Trachome*. His method for writing article drafts was to dictate them aloud to Ruth Lee, who was expert at shorthand. He was known to wake her up in the middle of the night to take dictation. For many years, she kept a stenography pad by their bed for just those moments. It is possible that Ruth Lee did the initial translation of the articles published in French and someone at the Pasteur Institute in Tunis corrected the French.[39]

Phil's career progressed at an incredibly rapid pace through the late 1920s and 1930s, largely thanks to Dr. Proctor's support and Phil's obvious talent as a researcher. Even before he left for Tunis, Dr. C. S. O'Brien, chairman of the Department of Ophthalmology at the University of Iowa, was trying to recruit Phil to join his teaching staff. Again, Phil was drawn by the appeal of star faculty. He later said that the Iowa department had the best ophthalmological residency program in the country because of C. S. O'Brien himself. He knew O'Brien was a star, much like Finnoff, Jackson, Morax, and Nicolle, and he wanted to learn from the very best and to become a star himself. Phil was excited by O'Brien's passionate commitment to ocular pathology and research. When invited to join the Iowa department as an assistant professor, Phil quickly accepted the offer. The salary was to have been $4,000,[40] but because of the Great Depression it was reduced to $3,150 a year.[41] The Thygesons returned from Tunis in 1931 and began to pack their things for a move to Iowa City.

12. Research Idyll in Iowa City

Cecil Starling O'Brien, Phil's mentor and supervisor at the University of Iowa, came on board in 1925 as head of the "newly autonomous" Department of Ophthalmology. Before 1925, ophthalmology was served through an eye, ear, nose, and throat clinic at the university.[1] One of O'Brien's goals was to attract the best faculty to the new eye department, which is why he recruited Phil, an up and coming ocular microbiologist. O'Brien, who went on to become a director of the American Board of Ophthalmology in 1937, was not afraid to surround himself with fellow rising stars. O'Brien "was the ideal boss." He embodied a "combination of very high standards ... expected very high performance and [expressed] great appreciation for the performance."[2] In Iowa, Phil made a wonderful life-long friend in Alson E. Braley, who began as a resident in Phil's training program in external disease and took over O'Brien's role as department chairman in 1950. Braley and Phil had ham radio and many other interests in common. During the Thygesons' years in Iowa City, O'Brien worked his staff very hard and made them observe the traditions of good patient care. Not only did his staff work six days a week, but he had them accompany him from bed to bed on daily morning rounds at the hospital.[3] O'Brien also worked Sunday mornings and presented special courses two nights a week.[4] Through all of this, he became friends with Phil.

For Phil, moving to Iowa was faintly reminiscent of growing up in the midwestern state of Minnesota. Both regions had had thriving Native-American populations that were pushed aside by white settlers, and both became agrarian and industrial centers. Both became home to major medical research centers. There was plenty to interest Ruth Lee and Phil about the history of Iowa. By the early nineteenth century, Native Americans known as Meskwakis had begun to earn substantial sums mining lead.[5] Not surprisingly, there was strife between them and white speculators arriving from the East.[6] In 1839, Iowa City was chosen to be the capital of Iowa Territory. The name "Iowa" derived from the Ioway Indians who lived in the Des Moines River valley. The year 1833 marked a sad turning point for the Native Americans of Iowa. In that year, under the terms of the Black Hawk Purchase, it became legal for white settlers to claim Indian lands. Before long, a massive land rush pushed the Ioway Indians far to the West. By 1851, it was all over, as "all Indian lands in Iowa had been ceded to the U.S. government."[7] Statehood had been announced five years earlier, and Iowa City lost its prominence as a seat of government. What followed was a fairly standard tale of midwestern agricultural development. Wheat was an early crop; Iowa later became famous for its hogs, cattle, soybeans, and corn. Herbert Hoover, John Wayne, and John Ringling (of circus fame) were all born there. Mennonites and Mormons arrived early, and the Mormons pushed farther West. A railroad line from Chicago connected to Iowa City in 1856.

A progressive streak manifested itself in the University of Iowa, founded in 1847, two months after Iowa declared statehood. In 1860, the university admitted women and men "on an equal basis."[8] In 1870, what was to develop into the College of Medicine offered its first courses. The eight women admitted to the first class marked the University of Iowa as the first coeducational medical school in the country.[9] During Phil and Ruth Lee's time there, from 1931 to 1936, the University of Iowa Hospitals established the nation's "first and only statewide hospital ambulance service for patients unable to pay for their own transportation."[10] Many years later, the Ophthalmology Department at the university became the first in the nation to train morticians to remove eyes with the intention of preserving corneas for transplantation.[11]

The several years Ruth Lee and Phil spent in Iowa City were by all accounts Phil's happiest years as a researcher. He had the most freedom he would ever have to devote himself to his greatest love, pure laboratory research. In Denver, he had had many clinical duties. In many ways the time at Iowa was also his most productive as a basic researcher. "In the long discussions I had with him in the last year of his life," Fritjof said, "it was clear that that's when he, as a scientist, was his happiest, most creative, and when it was most exciting for him. Their boss [at Iowa] was a real task master. They worked four hours on Saturday, they worked eight to five during the week. My father loved the work he was doing."[12]

Iowa City in 1931 was still essentially a farm town. A student who arrived a few years before Phil and Ruth Lee was not dazzled by the glamour of the place. "If there was beauty in the Iowa landscape in September 1923, I scarcely noticed it," Philip D. Jordan wrote. "Corn stalks, withered to brown, stood like scarecrows in fields, hogs rooted in pens, and, now and again, neat houses and dilapidated, unpainted barns flashed by. We were traveling in an old Dodge at 30 miles an hours, a speed which fretted my mother so that she kept nagging my father to slow down on 'these awful dirt roads.'"[13] At the time, the elegant University Hospital was a prominent feature on the east bank of the Iowa River. Its beautiful Gothic tower was completed in 1928. However, there wasn't a single decent bookstore in town. "Farmers came to town to trade, and the Amish, in crowned hats and black suits, tied horse drawn buggies to hitching posts."[14] For Ruth Lee, with her unquenchable curiosity, Iowa City was a wonderful place to live.

The same Abraham Flexner who gave scathing reports of many medical schools around the country stopped by Iowa City on his famous 1909 tour. He arrived by train at four P.M. one April afternoon and left again, for Nebraska, at the toll of the midnight bell. What could he learn in eight hours? Whatever he gleaned, he had a profound impact and his recommendations on how to correct a spate of deficiencies at Iowa were the blueprint for change.[15] They were based to some degree on what was working well at Flexner's undergraduate alma mater, Johns Hopkins, which William Osler had worked so hard to help make into a model center of medical education.

Flexner thought the admissions standards at Iowa were not rigorous enough, that laboratory sciences and clinical instruction were deficient, that part-time faculty needed to be turned into full-time faculty, and that the record-keeping system was atrocious.[16] He wrote that University of Iowa president George E. MacLean "witnessed my unavailing efforts to find anyone — nurse or physician — who could describe the system on which bedside teaching was conducted. There are, for example, no hospital records worthy [of] the name."[17] Flexner recommended that the Rockefeller Foundation help fund Iowa's efforts to fix itself. In contrast, he recommended that the doors of other medical schools be shut for good.

Iowa specialized in disorders of the head. Half of its teaching cases were related to cases involving EENT disorders, including ophthalmology issues.[18] Flexner urged Iowa's hospital administration to get a strong dean of medicine to provide new leadership. To James Trewin, president of the Iowa State Board of Education, he wrote, "May I add that your attitude and that of your associates on the board leads me to believe that you are thoroughly alive to the needs of the situation and thoroughly equal to them?" He signed his letter: "I am, with best wishes, Very sincerely yours, Abraham Flexner."[19]

As Flexner's recommendations began to be implemented, enrollment in the medical school declined significantly, then rebounded to over 400 in the 1920s.[20] It wasn't until the 1930s, when Phil and Ruth Lee came to town, that the internship and residency system, now standard in medical education, were in place. During the Depression, the University of Iowa cut faculty salaries repeatedly.[21] By 1933, more than half of Iowa's banks closed or were taken over by other institutions, agricultural prices collapsed, and many farms were lost.[22] The mission of caring for Iowa's indigent population was proving a hardship for the state's coffers. Nearly 90 percent of "patient days" at the University Hospitals in 1931–1932 were considered indigent patient days.[23] Waiting lists for care ranged from "weeks to months" by 1930, and prospective patients began to die while waiting for treatment.[24] The wealthy had a distinct advantage, with good care available and private or semi-private rooms staffed by private-duty nurses in some cases.[25]

One of Phil's responsibilities was to "care for a ward of more than 40 newborns with neonatal ophthalmia" at a time when antibiotics had not yet been invented.[26] He became quite interested in inclusion conjunctivitis and experimented with inoculating his own eye and the unaffected eye of newborns with "unilateral inclusion conjunctivitis." He was thus able to determine how long it took for the Chlamydia to grow. He discovered the symptoms of clinical disease appeared six days after inoculation, at the end of the third cycle.[27]

In spite of the dire financial situation for Iowa's University Hospitals, Ruth Lee was finally getting a break from wage-earning. There is no record she worked outside the home during their years in Iowa. She needed a break from wage-earning to raise Fritjof, now a quickly growing toddler, and to give birth to Kristin, born October 25, 1934. It was the first time since her teenaged years that she was not earning money to support her mother, her husband or herself. Kristin, known to her family and friends as Krissy, was born when Fritjof was five years old. Both children were blonde, blue-eyed, and freckle-faced.

Phil was a sweet and affectionate father with very young children, but his aptitude for fathering children past babyhood was by all accounts severely limited. "As long as we were basically below three [years old]," Fritjof said, "he was just fine as a father. He'd be very affectionate and cuddle, do simple roughhousing and so on. I think the moment either one of us began to develop any kind of individuality, that became very difficult for him. I think my father's greatest failing was his lack of imagination and lack of empathy. He could not understand anything that he had not experienced himself, and this lasted his entire life.... If he hadn't experienced it, it either wasn't worth knowing or it was some total mystery that was beyond him."[28] Ruth Lee was the opposite. She was naturally empathetic and able to imagine being someone other than who she was. She was willing to suffer alongside those she loved. In a letter, she wrote, "It is a privilege of love to share the troubles and sorrows of those one loves as well as their good fortunes and happiness. Almost a right, I would say, if there are such things as 'rights' mixed up with so pure a thing as love."[29]

Although the hospital of the University of Iowa was grand by prevailing standards when Phil and Ruth Lee arrived — it was several stories tall, with two wings, two courtyards, and a grand Gothic tower as its centerpiece — an operating room was still a simple affair, with a gurney, a lamp, a sink, and a couple of metal carts to hold supplies. Facilities were modest for the ophthalmology department, too, though the staff performed nearly 500 surgeries in 1933–1934, including glaucoma surgeries.[30] Even in the late 1940s, the ophthalmology clinic was a room of less than 500 square feet. There was also a small dark room for the slit lamps, the keratometer, and an ophthalmoscope. Four refraction "lanes" were separated by plywood partitions that didn't reach to the ceiling. At the beginning of the new millennium, in contrast, there are now 60,000 square feet of clinical space for ophthalmology, and the faculty has grown from three to twenty-two.[31]

Medical technology was expanding rapidly in the early decades of the twentieth century. The X-ray machine came in relatively early in the century, followed by the EKG, higher-powered and better microscopes, microtomes for slicing tissue for pathological examination, and centrifuges for studying blood and urine.[32] Also helpful were electricity, telephones, power tools (which helped with surgery), and incubators (to save premature and sick babies).[33] In addition, there were intravenous fluids and sterilization. At the University Hospitals of Iowa, there was a broadening view of services in the form of new departments of housekeeping, nutrition, and social services.[34] By 1938–1939, the life-saving innovation of blood banking had arrived as well.[35]

Medical research had not been a priority at the University of Iowa in the 1920s, but that changed in the 1930s. Hiring Phil Thygeson was part of the change. Medical faculty began to participate actively in national organizations and symposia, and turn their attention to producing original research. Funding for research rose and fell with the university's fortunes during the Depression, but the Department of Ophthalmology forged ahead. Phil wasn't shy in his use of superlatives to describe Cecil S. O'Brien or in his description of the department at Iowa. Of O'Brien, he said, "He made a department, which I didn't know at the time but I knew later, by far the best in the country, much better than Harvard or Columbia or Hopkins or any other. It was by far the best."[36] Phil was delighted to have his own laboratory. "I was also in charge of refraction and external disease. Then the other field I had was neuro-ophthalmology."[37] He was assigned to the neurology ward to examine patients daily for eye-related issues, and was always on the lookout for teaching opportunities for medical students and residents.[38] One of Phil's achievements was to develop a training program in external disease for ophthalmology residents. He believed it to be the first such program in the United States. Two residents entered the program each year. After he taught them refraction and external disease, Phil assigned research projects that they were

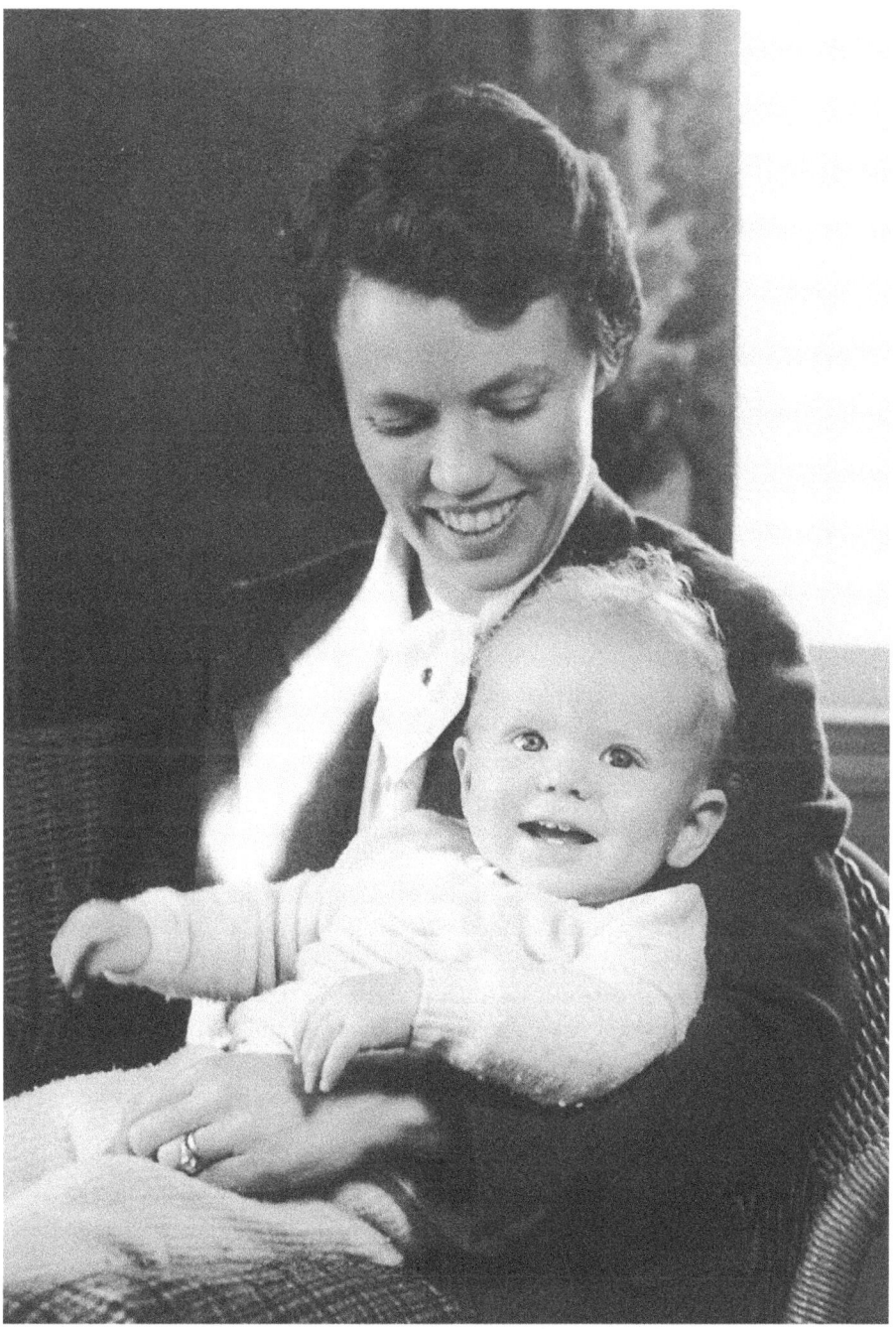

Ruth Lee with daughter Kristin, Iowa City, 1935.

to do in his laboratory. In this way, Phil met Al Braley, James Allen, and others who went on to become well-known academicians.[39]

Phil loved the interdisciplinary collaboration at Iowa. "We had a great time in Iowa," he said. "I learned more in those three and a half or four years than I have ever learned in a similar time later. It was such an intense study time. We had wonderful contacts with other departments, particularly pathology and biochemistry, so we got a lot of basic ophthalmology there that you don't get nowadays because they don't have the close contacts with the other disciplines now."[40] Phil loved his small team of colleagues, which consisted of Braley, Allen, and a woman medical artist. They were young, talented, and full of energy.

Just as Phil rode the wave of the pharmacological revolution that was to begin in earnest in the 1940s, he lived through the era of increasing specialization and compartmentalization of medical practice areas. When he started in medicine, many professors in the field were part-time academicians who volunteered their time and supported themselves with private practice. Over the course of Phil's career, they would become full-time, paid faculty.

A number of Phil's most important medical research papers were written during his years in Iowa. Ruth Lee was his invaluable collaborator. She took dictation on her shorthand pad and typed up draft after draft of Phil's "papers," as she always called them, on her manual typewriter. Over the years she had large upright typewriters and small portable typewriters. She would edit a typed draft with a pen, then type the revision. Ruth Lee's practice for many years was to type drafts on blue paper she referred to as "blue copy." Often the process was repeated several times. She used carbon paper when necessary and if there were too many mistakes on "clean copy," she would start whole pages over. She was expert at asking Phil questions about what he was trying to say and then expressing his points in the most economical, direct, and elegant way possible. Her sentences were short and wonderfully clear, yet a sense of personal style came through. "She had a philosophy of the writing of technical papers, which was that everything should be intelligible to the relatively uninitiated. It shouldn't be so full of jargon and so obscure and convoluted that anybody could possible wonder, 'Now what was the meaning of that sentence?'"[41]

Phil always said he didn't feel he could write without Ruth Lee's help and in fact might not have achieved nearly as much without her unending collaboration. "She could take a scratch copy of mine, study it, rearrange the paragraphs and produce a fine paper in perfect English." A professor at Iowa began using her papers "as teaching models for his students.... Soon my colleagues at Iowa began to consult her about their papers." Phil and Ruth Lee would go to American Ophthalmological Society (AOS) meetings together, and she would help anyone and everyone make last-minute changes to their presentations. "Her reputation spread. She was much more popular with the AOS boys," Phil noted, "than with the AOS girls."[42] By this, he meant that she got along well with the physicians, and she wasn't interested in the conversations of their wives. She preferred to work.

One of Phil's early published papers was on inclusion blennorrhea, also known as ophthalmia neonatorum, a conjunctivitis (or pus-characterized infection) affecting newborns. The disease was sometimes confused with trachoma, and was even called "genital trachoma" or "paratrachoma," but Phil distinguished between the two. Karl Lindner of Vienna showed that real trachoma usually caused long-term scarring and damage, which was not the case with inclusion blennorrhea. The confusion was a case of microbiologists thinking one thing and clinical ophthalmologists thinking another. It took experts skilled in both areas to clarify the question. In this particular research on inclusion blennorrhea, Phil did something he candidly admitted was later considered unethical. He wanted to demonstrate the role of the inclusions in the disease.

> We did a number of things you can't do nowadays. You would be sued right now.... [S]ince this was a harmless disease — it didn't cause any damage to the eye — I didn't hesitate to transfer a unilateral case into the other eye [of a patient]. That way I could tell when the inclusions started in the epithelium. About five or six days before the clinical disease started, I could find two or three cycles of development of the inclusion bodies all in the incubation period. So it was very clear that this agent was the cause of the disease.[43]

These were the "Wild West" days of ophthalmological research. In addition to filtering the elementary bodies and using the filtrate to infect the eyes of baboons, monkeys, and human volunteers, Phil inoculated himself! It took a week for his infection to appear. Another volunteer "had a much more severe disease than I did. She got over hers in three or four months while mine hung on for about seven months."[44] One wonders whether the other volunteer received any compensation. Phil and the volunteers suffered from acute conjunctivitis, but they had no scarring or long-term effects.

Trachoma was the subject of a great deal of confusion that lasted for much longer than that associated with inclusion blennorrhea. For a long time, it was thought that trachoma was caused by a virus. Phil's early published papers on the subject reflect this line of thinking. In 1934, he published "The Nature of the Elementary and Initial Bodies of Trachoma,"[45] which called the infectious agent a virus because its "filterability and the presence of inclusion bodies and ... the intracellular nature of the organisms ... at that time were considered to be viral characteristics."[46] That year, he also published one of his most important papers, "The Etiology of Trachoma." Phil was not the one to prove that trachoma was not a virus. It was James W. Moulder who years later showed that the agent conformed to the life cycle of bacteria — in this case, Chlamydia. As Phil explained after Moulder's discovery was made public, "There's RNA in the cycle of the Chlamydia which is not present in the usual viral molecule. So it became obvious that we were dealing with a completely distinct group of organisms, Chlamydia, which resemble the rickettsiae on one side, and have some resemblances to the viruses on the other side...."[47]

Phil was a pioneer in the United States in seeing that the Chlamydia behaved differently from viruses and rickettsiae. He arrived at his insights by using Elford collodion filters to filter trachoma materials. These filters were so thin that the pore size was measurable. William J. Elford of London, who created them, had worked out a way to let researchers choose the size of the pores. To make the filters, Phil recounted, "We poured the collodion by a special technique. I had to learn all this, and we had to make our own filter holders and everything.... It was a tricky thing to measure the pore size."[48]

Phil believed the Berkefeld filters used by Nicolle and others adsorbed too much material and confused the question of the infectious agent.[49] Nicolle was thirty-six years older than Phil, and was using older and, to some extent, outmoded technology. Phil had the advantage of the brashness and energy of youth. If he had to make his own filters, so be it. He used Poiseuille's Law, a law of physics, to calculate the average pore size of his filters. Phil's lab made by hand Elford filters with a pore size Phil said in his oral history was three to six millimicrons. (Phil's colleague G. Richard O'Connor believes the term "millimicron" to be in error — Phil should have said .3 to .6 microns.) The goal was to stop all bacteria from passing through the filters, but to let the viruses through. Using monkeys, Phil learned that a bacteria-free filtrate would still induce an infection with trachoma. Before long, he would need to test his theory on people, in the form of a famous experiment on a human volunteer. Before that could happen, however, he had other work to do.

In 1935, Phil published "Acute Follicular Conjunctivitis, Beal's Type," which was a further discussion of a fever- and pharyngitis-related illness illuminated by R. Beal, who worked for Victor Morax in Paris. The following year, Phil published "The Virus of Inclusion Conjunctivitis" with a gynecologist at Iowa named W. F. Mengert. The article was the result of studying the genital epithelial tissues of mothers who gave birth to babies who developed ocular inclusion blennorrhea, which could cause very serious disease in newborns. As with many of Phil's research innovations, a memorable story was attached to the work. A young gynecologist, Dr. Randall, whom Mengert knew, was doing a dilation and curettage on a young woman and got hit in the eye with genital material from the D & C. He developed full-blown inclusion conjunctivitis, which led the team to reexamine the woman for inclusion bodies in her cervical epithelium, and to Mengert and Thygeson collaborating on their paper.[50] The disease that infected Dr. Randall and his patient was known for decades as "swimming pool conjunctivitis" because it could be passed around in public swimming pools, that is, until the age of chlorination, which wiped out the problem. For that particular disease, in

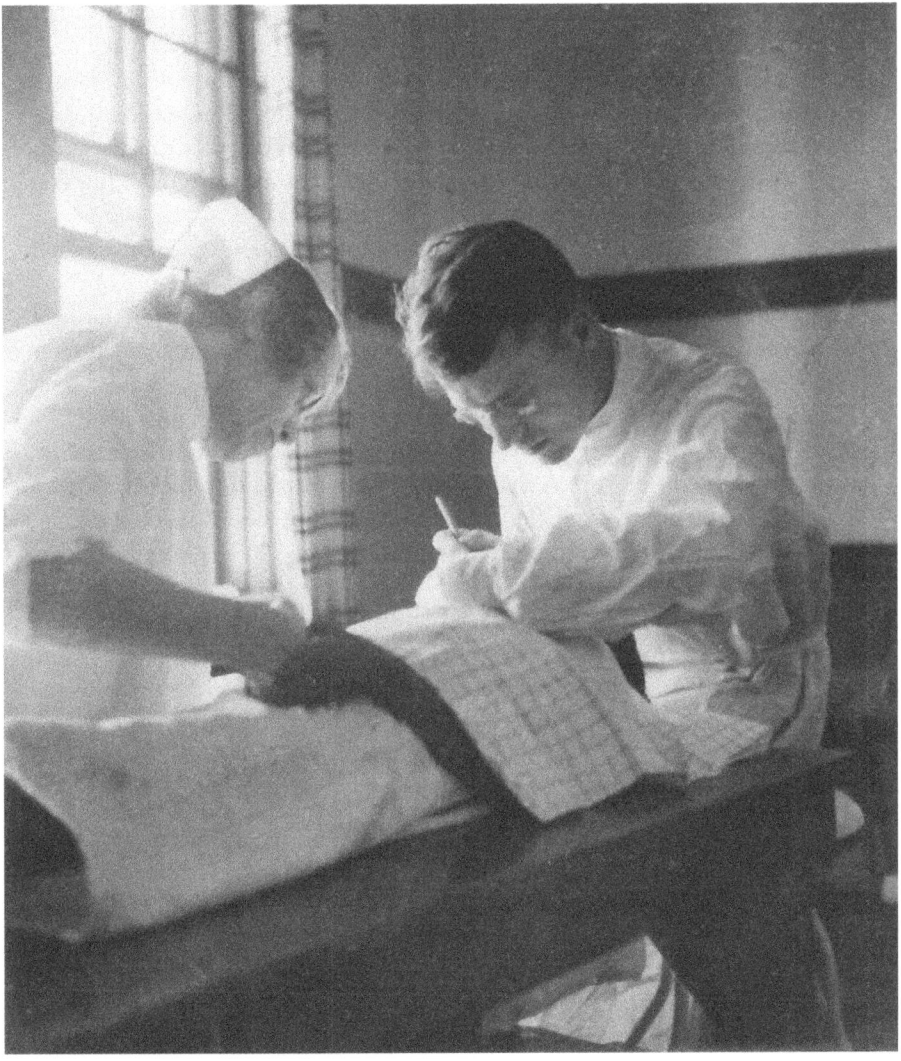

A nurse assists Phillips Thygeson as he does a procedure on a monkey.

the days before chlorine, a little urination or discharge of fluids was enough for pool water to become infected. There was a great deal of relief when the problem was eliminated.

In the course of his Chlamydia research with Mengert, Phil and his fellow researcher discovered that Chlamydia prefer the cervix over the uterus and fallopian tubes. This discovery led them to experiments on humans. "[W]e made a couple of experimental inoculations of the cervix of volunteers. We felt it wasn't dangerous," Phil said. He and Mengert got their volunteers with the help of Everett Plass, head of gynecology at Iowa, and they introduced venereal disease in nonpregnant women. It would have been dangerous for a pregnant woman, but they chose those who, theoretically at least, wouldn't suffer long-term damage from an experimentally induced, self-limited disease. Phil reported that it took three to five months for the disease to clear up on its own. "We couldn't do that type of experiment on volunteers any more! That's all completely off," he later said.[51]

Phil tried to be aware of the ways in which researchers could close their minds to ideas that conflicted with the prevailing notion of the cause of a disease. For example, inclusions were found in so few ocular diseases in the early days that many researchers decided — through faulty logic — that inclusions did not play a role in the cause of trachoma. Phil took mental notes about keeping an open scientific mind. He also learned from his own mistakes. One of his mistakes, a laboratory error, involved a monkey — a sooty mangabee, a type new to Phil. He didn't know that this monkey had needle-sharp teeth rather than the flat teeth of the baboons with which he had been working. He grabbed the monkey and it bit him right through this thick leather glove. He got a severe infection in his finger. In a classic bit of storytelling, he later spoke of the death of a young researcher who had been bitten by a monkey and had died of *Herpes simiae* encephalitis. This death occurred right before Phil was bitten by his monkey. He laughed when he told the story of waiting to come down with his own encephalitis and die.[52]

13. Fort Apache and the Great Experiment

Though Phil was interested in a number of diseases, his chief passion remained trachoma. The trachoma puzzle intrigued Phil. Treatment involved anesthetizing the conjunctiva and squeezing exudates out of the conjunctival follicles. Why this worked was something of a mystery. Phil's best guess was that it brought blood and its healing lymphocytes into closer contact with the trachoma agent. In the course of his early work, he concluded that trachoma was the world's "number one" worst eye problem.[1] He estimated that "in the United States about fifty percent of the Indians had active trachoma."[2] There were frequent reinfections and many people ended up with severe scarring and blindness.

Phil became interested in trachoma in Appalachia. The disease was carried into the region by the colonists of Virginia and West Virginia, most of them Scots and Irish who decided to keep moving west from the Virginias. The region has long had a reputation for being a "trachoma belt" with the nickname of the trachoma-endemic region being the Daniel Boone Trail. The mountain people of Appalachia, often poor and with limited access to running water and sanitation, had many of the same challenges as North Africans in combating trachoma. It is quite possible that Ruth Lee and Phil empathized with these impoverished Americans. Frugality was a very strong trait in them. Having lived through the Depression and having known lean times, they were both quite conservative in their spending habits and acquisition of worldly goods.[3]

Trachoma had been a problem of great national concern not long before. The Public Health Service (PHS) had rejected all prospective immigrants arriving at Ellis Island if they showed signs of infection. At this time, small temporary hospitals were opened in Appalachian areas, with a single trained physician working with nurses. In 1913, President Woodrow Wilson authorized the Public Health Service to devote money from its special fund for "epidemics" to trachoma prevention and control.[4] Six hospitals in Appalachia treated trachoma and attempted to correct "lid deformities" that occurred when trachoma produced so much scarring that lids turned inward, causing eyelashes to scratch the corneas.[5]

The Public Health Service (PHS) grew out of a need in the eighteenth century to provide care for seamen. Infectious diseases of the nineteenth century — cholera, smallpox, and yellow fever — merely increased the need for Congress to take steps to finance and support public health.[6] According to Phil, the involvement of the PHS was a great asset to trachoma diagnosis and treatment, especially for Native Americans. Although the Indian Service was charged with providing health care, Phil reported that it just didn't have the necessary specialists and thus couldn't provide the care. This was true for tuberculosis as well. "There wasn't any money, and it was under the Department of the Interior, not the Public Health Service,"[7] he recalled.

Dr. Proctor, who was head of the Indian Service trachoma program, helped set up a trachoma research laboratory at a boarding school at Fort Apache, located on the White River Reservation in Arizona. Fort Apache was how Phil got actively involved in rural public health in the United States. The fort itself was a cavalry headquarters during the tragic wars between the U.S. government and the Apache.[8] Nearby were prehistoric ruins and petroglyphs. After the unfortunate incursion of the U.S. Army, a military cemetery sheltered the dead. At Dr. Proctor's instigation, old army barracks were used to house children with trachoma, who often received the conventional treatment of the time, copper sulfate.[9] This treatment dated to ancient Egyptian times. At Fort Apache, they also used silver nitrate and chaulmoogra oil. Phil and his staff set up a laboratory that included research primates.[10] They did a sort of clinical trial where they took three groups of children, gave each one of the three treatments daily, and compared the outcomes. They had an annual cure rate of approximately 20 percent in each group, which led them to conclude that none of the treatments was particularly effective. Phil's analysis was that because the infectious agent lives in the surface epithelium, anything that got rid of that layer was of some benefit.

Phil's connection to Dr. Polk Richards, an Indian Service doctor, was a great help to him professionally. Richards had been put in charge of the Indian Service trachoma program by Dr. Proctor. In 1935, Phil, Richards, and Proctor coauthored a paper published in the *American Journal of Ophthalmology* entitled "Etiologic Significance of the Elementary Body in Trachoma." Phil called Richards a jack-of-all-trades. Richards could do cataract extractions, lid surgery, and gall bladder removal. He could even pull teeth. "He was just a natural, all-purpose doctor. He was the first man I ran into in the Indian Service," Phil wrote. Richards had spent twenty-five years working with the Navajo at Fort Defiance. There, he had done everything from "pulling leeches to delivering babies."[11] He was very likeable, a great story teller, and a favorite among the nurses. Ruth Lee suggested doing a tape-recorded oral history of Richards, but he wanted his stories to be for personal amusement only, not for posterity. For his part, Phil liked to make fun of Richards, referring to him as roly-poly and teasing him for driving his government car at 25 mph no matter what the posted speed limit. Richards had an idea that this was the most efficient, best way to treat a car, and he refused to do otherwise.[12] Phil nicknamed him Polk-a-dot.

Phil noted that Richards accidentally infected himself with trachoma while expressing a patient's infected follicles. "Some of the material went into his eyes. Five days later he came down with a violent trachoma."[13] Richards treated himself with copper sulfate and recovered with only minimal scarring. His and Phil's collaboration lasted for years. A highlight was when they were invited to attend the International Congress of Ophthalmology in Cairo, to report on trachoma. They crossed the Atlantic together on the *Queen Elizabeth I* and spent a week in Italy waiting for the boat to Egypt.[14]

Phil loved learning about the Apache Indian culture and the historical conflict between the U.S. Army and the Apache. When he and Ruth Lee arrived at Fort Apache to do research, it was not long after the army had decamped. Fort Apache had been established in 1870 in order to make it easier to control and subjugate the Apache population. The army initially got the upper hand. Much misery-inducing dislocation ensued. In 1875, 800 Apache were forced to leave Fort Apache and move to the San Carlos Reservation. Many other forced marches followed. Their leader, Geronimo, who earlier had escaped from the army's clutches altogether, was transported in chains. Some of the resettlement sites were cramped and malarious, and there was unrest and resistance.[15]

For parts of three summers in the 1930s, Phil and his family lived in General Crook's cabin, whose walls formed one corner of the actual fort of Fort Apache. The canvas-floored log cabin, built in the 1870s, while not as handsome as and even smaller than the cabin Phil and Ruth Lee built, was just as interesting. In its original form, the kitchen was a shed in the yard. Old cooking kettles were still there, and Ruth Lee used one of them to pasteurize milk she bought raw from local farmers for her children. She used a thermometer to monitor the process. In an adjutant's house on the grounds of Fort Apache, Phil discovered reams of old army records and documentation of the Cibecue Massacre of 1881 in which Apache killed several soldiers who had arrested their medicine man. Noch-ay-del-klinne, the medicine man, had proclaimed that two beloved, dead leaders would come back to life and chase the white man from Apache lands. The medicine man died in the battle.

In 1876, Geronimo took some of his people and fled to Mexico, only to return to Arizona, settle in, and flee to Mexico again in 1885. Remarkably, the second time he fled, five thousand soldiers were used to hunt down Geronimo's "tiny band of 35 warriors and 80 women and children."[16] When they were finally caught, they and other tribal members who had not fled were forcibly moved to Florida. Geronimo died in 1909 in Oklahoma, far from his homeland. Phil was fascinated by the fact that several of Geronimo's wives still lived at Fort Apache and that some of the Apache scouts who had helped the army track the Apache were living there too. The scouts had been awarded medals by the army, which they wore with pride even in the 1930s. "Some of them could speak English," Phil said, "and so I would talk to them and get the history of where they had been."[17] Phil found the Apache friendly on the whole and did his best to treat the medicine men with respect. "We were very careful with the medicine men, who were very important in the tribal life.... The medicine men accepted us, too, as fellow doctors. They were psychiatrists. So we made sure always to consult with the medicine men."[18]

When Dr. Proctor and Phil felt they had done enough research, Phil wrote, we "would make side trips to the Grand Canyon, the petrified forest and the Canyon de Chelly and the painted desert."[19] The relationship with

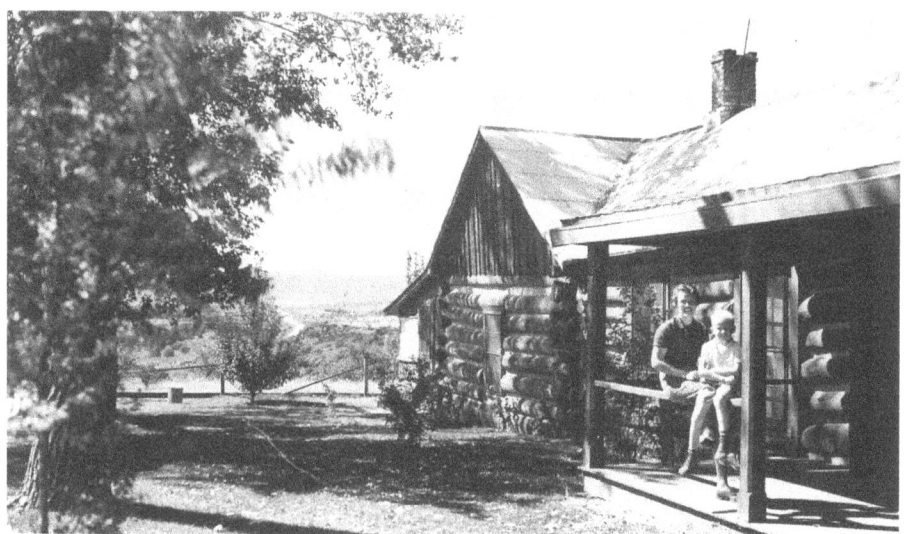

Ruth Lee and Fritjof Thygeson on the porch of General Crook's quarters at Fort Apache, Arizona, where Phillips Thygeson was doing trachoma research related to the local Apache people.

Fort Apache endured for years, and Phil and Ruth Lee's children vividly remember their visits there. It was located on the White River Reservation. Kristin remembered her father criticizing her for not being like the Native-American children. He claimed they didn't protest when he took scrapings of their epithelia, whereas his own children protested when he asked the same of them.[20] "The Indians were wonderful patients," he said. "They never complained. The children very seldom cried. White children would have gone crazy."[21]

The Proctors had both a cultural and a medical interest in Native Americans. They collected Navajo rugs, Navajo and Hopi jewelry, and pueblo-style pottery. Soon, Ruth Lee and Phil were doing the same.[22] The Proctors also cultivated good relationships with Native Americans who, like them, lived near Santa Fe. Phil observed their success and tried to emulate them in his relationships with patients and staff in his trachoma research in Arizona.

Phil performed arguably his most important experiment at Fort Apache. He inoculated a human volunteer with virulent trachoma. Clarence Brown was a patient in the clinic at Iowa "who had lost an eye through neglect." Phil always hated to see an eye lost, especially if the loss could have been avoided. "This was a sad story," Phil said. Brown had a virulent tumor on his eye. In medical terms, he had an "epidermoid carcinoma ... on his bulbar conjunctiva."[23] Due to an unfortunate error, he was never told the results of his biopsy. The cancer grew and when Brown finally sought treatment, his eye had to be removed. The cancer in his olfactory tract couldn't be removed, which gave him the sensation of terrible odors, and he was told he would soon die. "[W]e figured he didn't have long to live but that he might live long enough for the experiment. So we gave him the story of what we wanted [to accomplish with the experiment], and it interested him. He knew he was going to die, and so he volunteered."[24] Dr. Proctor gave him a thousand dollars in compensation, good money in those days, and Brown accompanied Phil to Fort Apache, where there was an abundance of active trachoma material.

"I thought he was going to die on the way down there. He scared me all the way," said Phil. The experiment consisted of scraping active trachoma from the fifteen worst child cases known to the medical staff at Fort Apache. With the help of Francis Proctor and Polk Richards, Phil ground up the scrapings, filtered them to get rid of irrelevant bacteria, and then filtered the "small stuff" through an Elford collodion filter. They hoped to be able to isolate the elementary bodies of trachoma and then to measure them using the highly calibrated pore size of their Elford filters, which had been an incredible help in detecting and measuring the polio virus.[25] They took the filtrate and divided it into three batches — one for Brown's remaining eye, one put through the ultracentrifuge to check for the presence of elementary bodies, and one to culture for the presence of bacteria. Five days later, Brown had a "violent acute trachoma loaded with inclusion bodies" in his one eye.[26] Within a week, pannus — the beginning of the scarring process — had begun. Pannus comes from the Latin and means "a piece of cloth." In the eye, it means a vascularization of the cornea with granulomatous tissue — blood vessels, opacity, and possible eventual blindness.

The goal was not to leave Brown blind in both eyes for the short remainder of his life. He had completed a noble act of volunteerism by allowing Phil and his colleagues to prove definitively in a human being what agent caused trachoma. Their experiment was a huge success because they believed no other bacteria had contaminated the filtrate with which they infected Brown's eye. The disease they caused was limited to trachoma, a disease which in turn was caused by *Chlamydia trachomatis*. Phil's great achievement was in isolating the trachoma agent — so that it was no longer confused with other infectious agents — and fulfilling Koch's postulates, definitively proving etiology of the disease.

Phil and his colleagues didn't yet know the disease agent belonged to the Chlamydia family, but they were close to that discovery as well. They immediately began treating Brown with copper sulfate. In a year, he was well. To

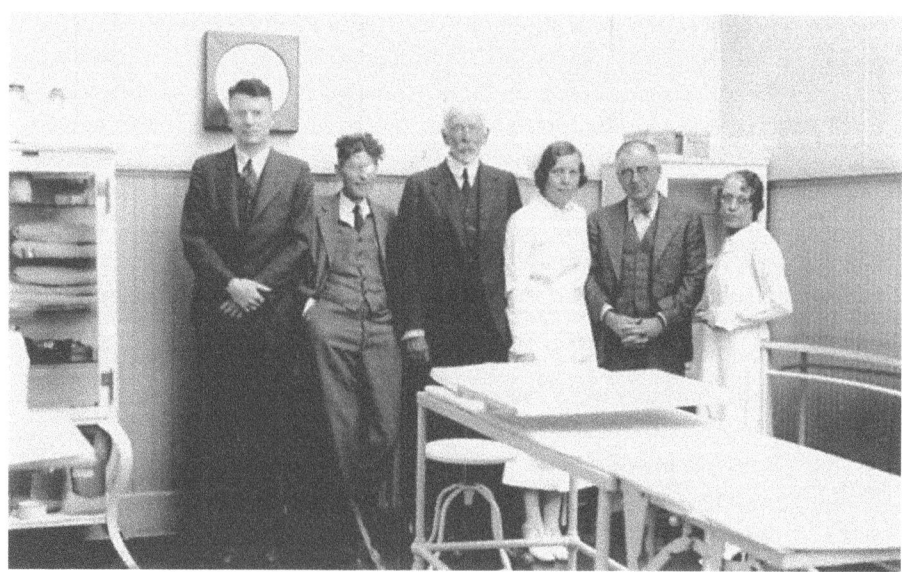

The great Clarence Brown experiment definitively proving the etiology or cause of trachoma, 1935. From left, Phillips Thygeson, Clarence Brown, Francis I. Proctor, and others.

everyone's surprise, he didn't die of his cancer, which went into remission. Instead, a year after the experiment, he and his wife died in a car accident.

As a result of this experiment, Phil was thrust into the limelight of international ophthalmology. He was now a research star. The research resulted in a medal from the AMA Section on Ophthalmology. He was also briefly and unhappily a star in the popular media. At Fort Apache, he was working with laboratory monkeys when a nurse dashed in and said, "You're on the air!" Phil was on the radio show "The March of Time," which was very popular in the 1930s. Its device was "dramatic retellings or re-imaginings of true events, much in the way Depression-era photographers sometimes posed their subjects — a poor family, or their pointedly meager belongings, for example...."[27] The program's research staff tried to get hold of credible source material and documentation, but imagination and poetic license often took over. In egregious cases, "writers were given the dramatic license to contrive and 're-create' such dialogue as seemed appropriate to the characters and situation."[28]

"The March of Time" was an interesting cultural phenomenon. "Broadcasts were taken so seriously by some that the White House regularly complained about its imitations of President Roosevelt, who was annoyed because he 'was getting calls and notes from political advisers regarding statements and remarks [made by the impersonator]. These statements reflected Roosevelt's policies, but, in fact, had never been uttered by the President.'"[29] For the trachoma story, the researchers found an article by Thygeson, Proctor, and Richards that appeared in 1935 in the *American Journal of Ophthalmology*, entitled "Etiologic Significance of the Elementary Body in Trachoma." The journalists distorted the facts for the sake of drama. As Phil told the story of the broadcast, "I got ... to hear myself say, 'Mr. Brown, the experiment is a success. You are blind.'"[30] It wasn't true, though, and the horrible thing was that Brown's mother was listening to the broadcast. When she heard that her son was blind, "she practically had a heart attack. She hadn't known about this experiment." The popular media then went wild trying to get Brown to participate in pulp journalism articles, which he found repulsive.[31]

Phil expected a lot of teasing from his colleagues in ophthalmology, but the show aired during the day when most of them were working and Phil was grateful few of them heard it. However, Paul de Kruif got hold of the Clarence Brown story. In 1940, he published a dramatic article entitled "They Wait for Light" in *The Country Gentleman*. De Kruif had a flair for making microbiological research sound like fabulously romantic adventure in addition to being essential to the betterment of the species. For him, trachoma was an "ages-old curse" that had "blinded countless millions." Its victims didn't just want sight; they waited for "the light." And in case readers had no idea what trachoma was like, his descriptions conveyed the deep physical misery of it:

> The disease is a years-long smoldering torment. It drives you wild with pain, unable to stand even the light of a dimmed room without tears. It makes you feel, for months, as if there were big cinders in both your eyes.... It makes you, if it's bad, hideous by turning your eyelids outward.[32]

He added, "In spite of modern science, trachoma is so widespread among the poverty-stricken millions of the Eastern Hemisphere that it taints the eyes of half the earth's population...."[33] This was not true, but it certainly got the point across. Other misinformation followed in the article. For example, de Kruif referred to trachoma as being caused by a virus and claimed that this fact had been proved by Charles Nicolle. This was a commonly held belief at the time. He also claimed that Hideyo Noguchi was "famed for his mistakes in science," a crushing misstatement of Noguchi's legacy. He further claimed that Phillips Thygeson provided the "finishing touches to the cleaning up of this phony science — disastrous to millions waiting for light!"[34]

In de Kruif's version of the story, Phil tried and failed three times to infect Brown with trachoma filtrate flown to Iowa City from Fort Apache.[35] Only after these failures did they decide to drive to Fort Apache together. De Kruif wrote that Brown nearly went blind before copper sulfate turned things around for him. He quoted Phil as having written, "At no time did Mr. Brown say he regretted the experiment. He was a good soldier throughout."[36] The rest of the article is dedicated to appreciating the other scientists involved in trachoma work — Fred Loe, Proctor, Richards, and others — and to discussing the fabulous new treatment drug, sulfanilamide. For that, he took readers to the "hill people" of Little Egypt, Illinois, whom he claimed were so poor as to have only one washbasin and towel per family. Sulfanilamide was available but — in a version of the story not told by Phil — it was "dangerous." "[T]he big doses needed to fight the trachoma virus should be given in a hospital or, to say the least, under the close watch of doctors." In Little Egypt, that was impossible, and when the pills were handed out and the hill people returned to their "hovels and cabins," de Kruif said they "began getting dizzy, nauseated, and their lips and nails turned blue" from the drug. However, they also reported dramatic relief from their trachoma.

In reality, Loe had been testing sulfanilamide among Native-American patients, reporting only eight serious drug-related complications in a thousand cases.[37] Why the difference between de Kruif's Little Egypt story and that of Loe's patients? De Kruif did not say, and we must take his story with a proverbial grain of salt. His affinity for hyperbole got the better of him at times in his excitement to tell the tale.

A number of other papers came out of Phil's years of intermittent work at Fort Apache. In 1937, he published "Trachomatous Keratitis: A Biomicroscopic Study of Two Hundred Eighty Indian School Children." The following year, with Richards, he published, "Nature of the Filtrable Agent of Trachoma," and, with W. G. Forster, "Observations of Trachoma of the White Mountain Apache Indians." Papers on treatment of trachoma with sulfanilamide followed in 1939, both solo and coauthored by his Fort Apache collaborators, Richards and Forster. Six months earlier, Fred Loe, an Indian Service ophthalmologist, had published the first treatment study results. Phil and his colleagues were able to confirm his results.[38]

The idea to use sulfanilamide, an early antimicrobial drug, for treatment of trachoma came about in an interesting way — by way of a dog sick with distemper. At one point, Proctor, Richards, and Loe were all visiting Phil and Ruth Lee in New Jersey. Together, they attended a lecture at Columbia by Alphonse Dochez in which Dochez reported that he had cured distemper in a dog by using sulfanilamide. Loe, who was then working on trachoma among the Sioux at the Pine Ridge Reservation in South Dakota, proposed that they try this drug on trachoma. Their logic was not quite right, as they thought both distemper and trachoma were viral in origin. Interestingly, it was known in the 1930s that trachoma was caused by Chlamydia. What wasn't known until well into the 1940s was that Chlamydia is a bacterium, not a virus. There's a large early body of literature on trachoma referring over and over again to the virus that actually isn't a virus at all.[39]

The outcome of the treatment experiments was the same — a high cure rate. Loe achieved ninety percent and Proctor, Richards and Thygeson reached eighty-five percent cure in their first Fort Apache-based study.[40] This was vastly better than the previous cure rate — with copper sulfate — of 20 percent. The article by Phil et al. appeared in 1939 in the *Archives of Ophthalmology*. Confirming studies were also conducted in Indonesia and France, and all of the news was good in regard to the efficacy of sulfanilamide in treating trachoma.[41]

At first, researchers thought the drug killed the trachoma agent, but it turned out not to be true. Instead, it stopped the "developmental cycle" of the bacteria so that they couldn't reproduce. Once the bacteria were knocked out, "natural desquamation of the conjunctival epithelium" would get rid of the bad tissue and the patient could be pronounced cured.[42] Ophthalmologists worked out the sulfanilamide dosage by trial and error and settled on a therapeutic level of "five milligram percent in the blood," which meant about four grams of medication a day per adult and less for children.[43] Children were the best subjects for treatment studies because they were more likely to have virulent trachoma. Adults tended to have milder trachoma but more scarring. Because of sulfanilamide and other antibiotics yet to be developed, the history of infectious blindness worldwide was about to change. Millions of people's sight would be saved due to the discoveries of the 1930s and 1940s.

14. The New York Chapter: Two Kinds of Politics

The unique era in Phil and Ruth Lee's life that Iowa represented came to an end. They loved their bucolic life in Iowa City, where Phil could ride a bicycle or walk to work. But Phil's career was in ascendancy and once he established a name for himself in the research world, it's not surprising that he was lured away. According to Fritjof, leaving Iowa was Phil's biggest professional regret. Never again would he have so few administrative duties and so much uninterrupted laboratory time. He was offered a prestigious position as assistant professor in the College of Physicians and Surgeons at Columbia University. Finnoff had given a dinner in Denver for speakers who came to present a special course. Dr. John Wheeler, head of ophthalmology at Columbia, was looking for the best possible people for a new eye institute at Columbia-Presbyterian Medical Center in New York, to be called the Edward S. Harkness Eye Institute. Finnoff was outspoken about Phil's achievements and promise in microbiology and external eye disease. Phil was offered the job of research director, which sounded glamorous and which he quickly accepted. He thought the facilities and the funding behind them would be better than at Iowa. It was also a rare, full-time academic position in ophthalmology at a time when most academic ophthalmologists were volunteer professors who supported themselves through part-time private practice. According to Phil, very few universities could afford full-time ophthalmologists at that time, among them Columbia, Iowa, Harvard, and Johns Hopkins.[1]

Because this was before the era of state and federal research grants, Phil's salary came from an endowment provided by Edward Harkness, founder of the eye institute. A grateful patient of Dr. Wheeler's, Harkness had made a magnificent gesture of gratitude. Phil's job title in 1936, when he accepted the job in New York, was research director of the Institute of Ophthalmology at Columbia University. With his endowed salary came salaries for a secretary and lab technician, and money for miscellaneous research expenses.[2] Though there was very little liability for physicians, the administration of the hospital decided to insure Phil. The policy cost eighty dollars per year.[3]

The university did not have much to offer, but the eye institute, which was part of Columbia-Presbyterian Medical Center, was well-funded. Though Phil had teaching duties, especially with medical students, he also had a wonderful amount of freedom at Columbia. "I had what I might call a roving appointment, because I could leave without any red tape for special work such as in Europe or with the Indians.... I could take my technician and secretary with me. So this was a very interesting and unusual appointment."[4]

His work was quite different now. In lieu of the close collaboration Phil had had with C. S. O'Brien in Iowa, where they would talk in Phil's laboratory every day, Wheeler visited only once, to show visitors the various laboratories. There was virtually no sense of collegiality. Wheeler was a surgeon, not a researcher. His and Phil's interactions were over money, management, and an occasional consultation on one of Wheeler's plastic surgery cases.[5] According to Phil, Wheeler performed cataract surgery on the king of Siam, charging him $25,000, a huge sum in those days.

Phil appreciated the talent pool at Columbia. "[T]he College of Physicians and Surgeons had a wonderful staff," he said, "so you could get consultations on every subject. It has a wonderful library with good librarians, and it had this marvelous outpatient clinic."[6] The outpatient clinic had been funded by the Vanderbilt family. Phil took advantage of opportunities to improve his knowledge base. "Columbia had the best mycologist of the time, a woman, Rhoda Williams Benham. She was by far the best mycologist in the country. She had a course every year, so I took her course. It lasted all winter, several hours a day.... This was the first time I got down to real nitty gritty on the fungi, so it did me a lot of good."[7] Phil also learned tissue culture techniques in Alexis Carrel's laboratory at the Rockefeller Foundation.[8] He was conscientious about his teaching responsibilities and, despite a lack of funding, established a basic course in science for residents in ophthalmology.

Phil had productive exchanges with a number of researchers while in New York, including Albert Sabin, who was interested in toxoplasmosis and herpes. Phil's interest in toxoplasmosis dated back to his work with Charles Nicolle in Tunis. Nicolle had discovered the *Toxoplasma* organism in a rodent indigenous to North Africa, the gondi. The *Toxoplasma* organism is relatively large and has an affinity for nervous tissue, such as the eye. "I was very fortunate to see the first human case," Phil said. A baby died in the hospital at

Columbia and an autopsy showed toxoplasma in both of its retinas.[9] Columbia was also the place where Phil and Ruth Lee met Ludvig von Sallmann, a Viennese ophthalmologist. Von Sallman had been a student of the famed Viennese ophthalmologist Ernst Fuchs, and specialized in radiation damage to eyes, including radiation-related cataract. Von Sallmann did a lot of work for the Lawrence Berkeley National Laboratory. He was also very interested in the toxic effects on the eye of metals such as lead and mercury. He and the Thygesons became lifelong friends.

Phil's role as an administrator during his years in New York meant he had to trade his white lab coat for a suit and tie a good deal of the time. This he didn't like. Left to his own devices, he preferred very informal clothes, and favored the colors red and green.[10] Moving to New York in 1936, however, and receiving a good salary opened up new possibilities for the family of four. They moved first to Harrington Park, living in rental housing, and then built an elegant, two-story, shingle-covered home near Tenafly, New Jersey, in a woody area known as the Palisades. The construction cost, Phil proudly recalled, was four dollars per square foot.[11] It was a modern house in a certain way; it had a more open floor plan than most houses of its day and its large rooms were full of light. Ruth Lee had the lead role in designing and building the house, and she was proud of her achievement.

For Phil, the commute to Manhattan was a real hardship. He found both the commute and the city dirty, noisy, and dangerous.[12] One of the difficulties was that Phil was trapped on buses with smokers. "It was real torture for him and it's one reason why almost every night he came home with a splitting headache ... from the smoke of the buses," Fritjof said.[13] The commute was not very long by today's standards, but it was grueling in the winter. "See, everybody smoked except me," Phil said, "and they had their windows closed because of the cold air, so I suffocated morning and night from this tobacco smoke.... It was terrible."[14] Phil also had inherited migraines, which could be provoked by smoke. He took aspirin much of his life and did his best to work when in pain. When he had to drive in the New York area, he was a stickler for the traffic laws. Phil was law abiding almost to a fault. During his years working at Columbia, he was stopped once by a police officer for speeding. Because he never drove over the speed limit, he was indignant enough to take the matter to court. The ticket was thrown out.[15] Phil also quite frankly disliked the northeastern climate. He did not like heavy, wet snow or humidity in the winter, nor did he like the hot, humid summers. He missed the West.

From all reports, Ruth Lee enjoyed New York City more than Phil. She would take one or both children on outings to the Radio City Music Hall in Rockefeller Center to see the Rockettes and other performers. She was long-legged and a fast walker, and she made her children keep up with her. Fritjof

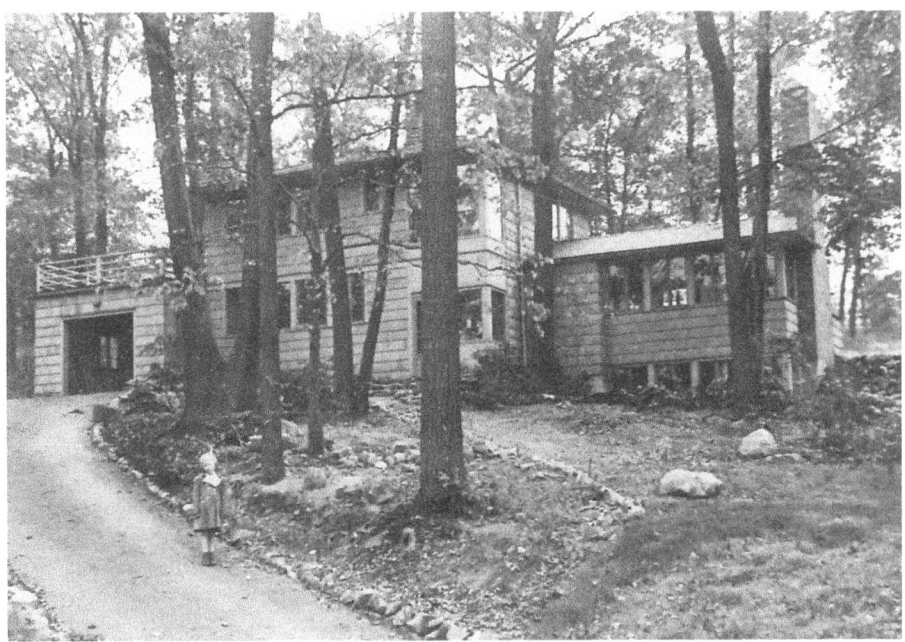

Kristin Thygeson standing in front of the Thygeson family home in Tenafly, New Jersey. The home was built by the Thygesons but sold at the end of World War II.

remembers her as having a great enthusiasm for life and for adventure, though she would temper that spontaneous joy with more sobering messages. She told Fritjof at one point, "You can't just expect life to always be happy."[16] She found her way to maximum personal fulfillment though reading copiously to her children and getting to know neighbors and other people in their community. She was an optimist by nature and had boundless energy.

In Tenafly, Ruth Lee's progressive political views, which had been formed by her challenging childhood, the tragic circumstances of her father's death, and the influence of Dr. Mosher, her proto-feminist mentor and employer at Stanford, became more central to her life. Now that her children were no longer infants and Fritjof was school-aged, she had more time for adult pursuits. Both of her children recall that she started going to political meetings in the evenings on behalf of her great passion, world federalism. "She felt so compelled to work for the good of humanity, for the saving of humanity, she just felt she had to do it," Kristin explained.[17] Ruth Lee paid close attention to world events during the 1930s, and she grew progressively more alarmed at the specter of another world war. World War I was with her daily because of her sister Lib's marriage to a veteran of trench warfare, Milton Snyder

Rosenfield. In the wake of a series of surgeries to get ahead of the gangrene that had crept inexorably up his leg after he was hit by a shell in no-man's-land in France, Milton lived with excruciating nerve pain, a sort of "phantom limb" syndrome. Lib lived with it too, of course, and referred to World War I as "that terrible war." Ruth Lee felt it was her duty to do what she could to create an international governance system where there could never be another world war.

Both children recalled how poorly Phil tolerated Ruth Lee's political passion and her absences. "She would just not be home in the evening," said Kristin, "and my father would be kind of pacing around and left with the children. I had a vague sense that he wasn't happy, but I just didn't know. She went to a meeting, that's all I knew." Over time, Phil became more and more unhappy, Kristin recalled:

> This just really rocked my father's boat.... This was ... one way in which [my mother] strayed from her early resolve to not upset my father because she couldn't take the consequences of his rage.... Eventually she stopped doing it at night. She would only go to meetings during the day when my father was away at work. Whether she told him about them or not, I have no idea. I rather doubt she told him but I don't know.[18]

Fritjof had his own, more dramatic version of this story to tell. "I was coming home. It was maybe ten, nine o'clock in the evening.... I heard all this noise, and there were only two houses on Dogwood Lane at that time — including the Parsons, who I thought were ancient.... I knew it wasn't the Parsons screaming, but I couldn't imagine what was going on. When I actually got to the house I could distinguish my father, just shouting at the top of his lungs, obviously in an absolute fury. The next morning my mother — I think it's probably the saddest I'd ever seen her — she said, 'We're not going to be able to do anything more at night for Union Now because your father just insists that I be home at night. Anything we're going to do we're going to have to do during the day.'"[19] This was disappointing for Frijtof, too.

> I was having the time of my life going to the meetings. I would take money at the door, I would handle the literature, and the people got a kick out of this little kid up to his eyeballs in the activity and obviously following the conversation and so on.... My mother ... was terrified of public speaking so she never spoke in a public meeting and she never chaired a meeting, but she was kind of the number one person behind the organizing, seeing that the literature got done, the arrangements were made, the publicity went out.... She was an extraordinary organizer.[20]

The primary goal of Ruth Lee's work was to recruit new members to the world federalism organization, which sought to unite the nations of the world in a federation of peaceful democracies. Kristin observed that her mother became more discreet — one could say almost clandestine — about her political activities "for her own protection because she couldn't deal with [Phil's] anger...."[21]

Ruth Lee believed that the more you loved someone, the more you should control destructive expressions of anger. She often told members of her family that one should treat one's family with the greatest care. She did not believe that relative strangers deserved greater politeness and consideration than one's most intimate relations. In the file she kept of special quotations and poems there is an excerpt of a hymn composed in 1867 by Horatio R. Palmer. Its refrain is overtly Christian and it is noteworthy that she did not copy the refrain into her files. However, what she did copy is a clear reflection of her values:

> Angry words! O let them never,
> From the tongue unbridled slip,
> May the heart's best impulse ever,
> Check them ere they soil the lip.
> Love is much too pure and holy,
> Friendship is too sacred far,
> For a moment's reckless folly,
> Thus to desolate and mar.

In the same file where she kept these verses is another echo of this sentiment, this time penned by the American poet Will Carleton:

> Thoughts unexpressed may
> sometimes fall back dead
> But God himself can't kill
> them once they're said.

Phil did not live by these words. Over the years, there was speculation about Phil's notorious temper. He could turn very red in the face when he was angry. He saved most of his outbursts for his family. "The story went through the family that my father had low blood pressure, just genetically low blood pressure, but that being in conflict got him charged and he felt better.... So the myth went around, true or false, ... that he just felt wonderful having a fight," Kristin said.[22] Perhaps because Ruth Lee's and Lib's mother had told her two daughters as children that Ruth Lee had a naturally sunny disposition and Lib's was cloudy and in need of improvement, Ruth Lee came to believe that Phil was of the dark and cloudy variety himself. She once said compassionately, "He has a very unhappy disposition. The poor boy is just unhappy."[23]

As a small child, Kristin wasn't very aware of conflict between her parents or the ways in which Ruth Lee stood up to Phil. "As a child, I saw their relationship as idyllic, as perfection, because my father would dote on my mother and she appeared to dote on him and she was always a ready recipient of his demonstrative affection. He was very demonstrative in front of his children," she said. Still, there was something unsettling about the balance of power in the relationship. "She ... never put him off. She always ... acquiesced to what he wanted."[24] Phil certainly had that impression as well, though he did not perceive Ruth Lee as acquiescing to him. Rather, he believed she agreed with him.

Growing up, the children were aware of Ruth Lee's passion for political activism. In their view, she wanted a peace-oriented world government and political leaders with "global vision." She believed in international law and hoped that if a few democracies came together to create a federation of nations, more and more nations would join until there was a universally accepted world government. The dream, of course, was that there would be a great deal less warfare, nationalism, and strife. Kristin thought that her mother's attraction to this vision was rooted in history. "She understood that historically we'd begun with warring tribes throughout the world. Then we'd gone to the nation state." With a federation of nations, there was the possibility of lowering the level of "tribal skirmishes" that characterized the world in the age of imperialism.[25] To this end, Ruth Lee supported Wendell Wilke for U.S. president, to no avail. Then she worked very hard to raise public awareness about the League of Nations. "She'd have meetings and groups and she'd pound the pavement." Phil and Ruth Lee often voted differently. "My father voted for John Dewey and my mother voted for Roosevelt," recalled Kristin. "She would vote Democratic and he would vote Republican."[26]

Phil did not discuss how he felt about Ruth Lee's political passions during their New Jersey years, or whether he knew what she did while he was away at work. Perhaps they had a 'don't ask, don't tell' understanding about her personal time. She was always available to her children when they needed her and for Phil when he needed her to help him write a medical paper. It was during their New Jersey years that Ruth Lee moved from editing for Phil only to being a professional, though unpaid, editor for other ophthalmologists. During the recording of Phil's oral history in the late 1980s, there was charming banter over her transition. "I don't know how you got started with those colleagues sending manuscripts home to me," Ruth Lee said, "but they sure as heck did. They advertised me." Phil's answer was, "They liked the way you worked on mine, so they wanted to get a part of it, I guess." "You must have told them," she said. Among what she called her "lovely clientele" were Ludvig von Sallmann and Algernon B. Reese. She particularly enjoyed working with Reese on his book on pathology. "He referred to himself as that illiterate southern boy from Georgia," she said with a laugh. "He was very generous in his praise. He sent me red roses."[27]

Ruth Lee became so busy she had to turn away work. Reese resorted to begging her for help. In a letter he wrote in 1949, after she returned a manuscript to him unedited, he wrote, "Won't you *PLEASE* reconsider and do this for us. If you will, I will promise you solemnly that I will not call on you again. We are very anxious to have this in fine shape ... and you are the only person who can do it as well as we would like to have it. Write your own price."[28] A mere year later, he was again begging her for help on a different paper he had written, with the words, "I shall appreciate immensely your smoothing it out."[29]

Being edited by Ruth Lee was not an easy experience. She required detailed author's meetings where she went over her editorial choices, asking questions about the author's intention and meaning at least every page and most likely every paragraph. Some doctors found it hard to sit patiently as she discussed the fine shades of meaning between different words or explained to them their grammatical errors. She quite enjoyed the work and said, "It entertained me to do it."

Asked how she learned how to edit, she credited her father. "He was in love with the English language," she said. "I got a great feeling for words and the use of words, and for rhythm in writing, a kind of rhythm, if you know what I mean."[30] Her father was a poetic writer and excellent stylist and her mother filled her childhood with classical music and her expert piano playing. Ruth Lee had an ear for language, whether English, French, or any other. She had an unusual ability to imitate what she heard and, to her chagrin, would find herself unconsciously (and impolitely) mimicking the accents of non-native speakers of English.

A good editor has to be able to take someone else's prose, decipher the meaning, and find a way to best express the meaning while still preserving the writer's voice and style. Ruth Lee's sister Lib also became an editor, who later in life specialized in turning doctoral dissertations by Stanford history students into publishable books. Ruth Lee and Lib subscribed to the same philosophy, articulated by E. Colin Cherry: "The rules we call grammar and syntax are not inviolate, but the more we break them, the lower are our chances of successful communication."[31]

Ruth Lee's editing work required both great talent with English and an ability to work closely with writers, some of whom had prickly egos and did not like to have their work covered in ink marks or have long conferences addressing each correction or query. "I wouldn't say I had ever had any formal training," Ruth Lee acknowledged. She had an English course at Stanford that she found very stimulating. Her professor didn't just toss a few comments onto her work. She *corrected* it, Ruth Lee reported. That professor was her role model. Ruth Lee appreciated that Phil always accepted her editorial suggestions, unlike other physicians. As for Phil, he was both humble and profusely grateful to his wife. He had been told in high school that his significantly younger sister Mary could write a better composition than he could.[32] He decided at that moment that he was not a good writer and never would be.

Ruth Lee saw her editorial work on behalf of getting ophthalmological research published as part of a larger mission to which she was happy to devote her time and energy. Kristin said, "She valued what my father was doing in terms of global humanitarian work and she felt her contribution to that larger effort of his — her mission — was to be his helpmate and that her part was behind the scenes."[33] Ruth Lee did not require praise or credit; she was selflessly and anonymously willing to contribute. Over time, she left the ranks of the doctors' wives and in an important sense became one of the doctors' professional cadre. This was particularly obvious at professional meetings. Other wives would socialize with one another; Ruth Lee would get out her typewriter and work. She preferred the conversation and company of the doctors to that of their wives, and some of the wives noticed and resented this. There may also have been a bit of sexual jealousy or threat in the air, not because she flirted with doctors, but because she was talented and able to talk about ophthalmology, and was poised, elegant, and beautiful.

On the home front, there was a different sort of jealousy. Phil was jealous of things that took his wife away from him. Tragically, that sometimes included his children. When they were very young, he was quite affectionate. But when they got older, they felt he resented them. Child-rearing conventions of the era were much less hands-on than they are today. The medical model was to teach children to be independent and not seek coddling. Phil encouraged this and, in Kristin's view, was "jealous of my mother's involvement with any other human being."[34] Ruth Lee was a very affectionate, involved mother who loved to read aloud to her children. Even when they were quite small, she would read sophisticated adult texts to them, from Shakespeare to the Greek myths recounted by Edith Hamilton. In her own childhood, Ruth Lee's father brought the dictionary to the table many times during meals to discuss the nuances of word definitions. A generation later, her children adored their mother's attention and the intellectual enrichment she provided. "She had a beautiful reading voice with wonderful inflection," Kristin said. "It was a rich and full voice, and she'd make everything just come alive ... as she read to me."[35] Early on, Fritjof began to understand his mother and her needs apart from those of her husband. "I think part of the reason she read to me so much was because it gave her a chance to think and talk about subjects she was interested in that my father simply didn't have time to talk about."[36]

Ruth Lee often read books to Fritjof that were well beyond his years in reading level and complexity. He was a very bright child and willing to discuss almost anything with his mother, so he learned a great deal from her. One of the most important books she read was Constancia de la Mora's autobiographical book, *In Place of Splendor*, which appeared in 1939. De la Mora helped rescue children in orphanages whose caregivers had fled during the Spanish Civil War. She was a mother, like Ruth Lee, and worked tirelessly to resist the Fascists' taking over Spain. "This was a passionate book defending the loyalist government. I don't think [de la Mora] was a communist, but she certainly was a fellow traveler of the communists," said Fritjof.[37] Ruth Lee identified strongly with de la Mora, especially with her being a woman writer and activist.

Both Fritjof and Kristin felt that their mother loved them unconditionally and had contributed a great deal to their educations and growing up. Their father competed with them for Ruth Lee's attention, was critical of them, and was at times openly denigrating. In their early years, he was like many men of his era—extremely dedicated to his career. He didn't pay nearly as much attention to world events as Ruth Lee did. "I'm sure he would glance at the paper in 1935, '36, '37, '38, the war in Ethiopia, the war in Spain," said Fritjof. "My father knew these things were going on ... but his focus was one hundred percent on ophthalmology and anything left over was focused on my mother." Perhaps more surprising—and definitely unusual for a marriage between a physician husband and a wife who had stopped just shy of her undergraduate degree—is that "the time my mother spent with him was all about ophthalmology."[38]

In the late 1930s, Ruth Lee appears to have had a rich dual life—her political and personal activities and her work with Phil and others on behalf of ophthalmology. Fritjof mentioned two other books that were extremely important to his mother and that helped form her political philosophy. The first was James Peter Warbasse's *Cooperative Democracy Through Voluntary Association of the People as Consumers*. Warbasse's vision of the future was based on "voluntary association in which the people organize democratically to supply their needs through mutual action, in which the motive of production and distribution is service, not profit...." The goal was "the creation of a new social structure that shall be capable of supplanting ... profit-making industry ... by the cooperative organization of society."[39] Ruth Lee told Fritjof she wished she had the time necessary to help build a cooperative society, with common ownership and shared decision making. "It's a system that works only if the people put in time and effort," she said.[40]

Ruth Lee saw the flaws in capitalism, and perhaps held it partially responsible for her father's financially related despair and suicide. She also saw flaws in socialism and communism. It was ironic, given how politically conservative Phil became, that his two sisters were both communists. According to Fritjof, both Mary and Ruth were "very active members of the Communist Party."[41] Their mother, Sylvie Thompson Thygeson, was also very sympathetic to communism and traveled to the Soviet Union with Mary in the 1920s to learn about the Bolshevik experiment. Once during the New Jersey years, Mary accepted an invitation to join Ruth Lee and family for Thanksgiving dinner and canceled at the last minute because she was invited to have Thanksgiving dinner with Earl Browder, head of the U.S. Communist Party.[42] This annoyed Ruth Lee, who thought it bad manners to throw over one invitation for another.

Phil rejected nearly all of his mother's political views and organizational affiliations, including her memberships in Planned Parenthood, the American Civil Liberties Union, and the National Association for the Advancement of Colored People.[43] He believed women were as intellectually capable as men and was supportive of skillful female scientists and physicians, but he was more conservative than his mother. On her side, Sylvie was very proud of her son's achievements in ophthalmology, but she lamented his political conservatism and acknowledged that her daughters were the more progressive of her children, for they became social activists like her.

However, the most important book of all for Ruth Lee during this period was Clarence Streit's *Union Now*. Streit was the *New York Times* correspondent to the League of Nations in the 1930s and was very disheartened to see that international effort falter and collapse. His connection to Europe was strong, as he had been a Rhodes scholar and had married a French woman in 1921. He had an insider's view of the rise of totalitarianism in Europe. His experiences convinced him that uniting a core group of democratic nations to form the nucleus of a world government — world federalism — was the best strategy for breaking the cycle of international war. His vision was to start small, with a handful of democracies, and expand the federation until the whole world was united by a common government. He saw this as a federal union of freely associated peoples. The model was to be the United States Constitution.

Union Now: A Proposal for a Federal Union of the Democracies of the North Atlantic first appeared in 1938. It argued that the goal of "securing individual freedom, democracy, peace and prosperity" could be solved through expanding the model of the wealthy northern democracies. Streit quoted Alexis de Tocqueville, Alexander Hamilton, and Thomas Paine. He wished for union in citizenship, defense, money, trade, and communications, and for each country to have autonomy. "The union would guarantee the right of each democracy in it to govern independently all its home affairs and practice democracy at home ... whether by republic or kingdom, presidential, cabinet or other form of government, capitalist, social or other economic system."[44] The requirement for joining would be to accept the Union's Bill of Rights. "The Great Republic ... would be achieved by Union when every individual of our species would be a citizen of it.... Then Man's vast future would begin."[45]

Essentially, Streit argued, individuals had sacrificed their freedom to that of nations, and this was a mistake.[46] He stated bluntly, "We can not be for liberty and against Union.... Tremendous world power brings with it tremendous responsibility for the world."[47] This is how Ruth Lee felt as well. The proposed founding democracies were the United States, the United Kingdom, Canada, Australia, New Zealand, Ireland, the Union of South Africa, France, Belgium, the Netherlands, Switzerland, Denmark, Norway, Sweden, and Finland. Streit claimed that none of the countries had waged war on another in over one hundred years. "Together these fifteen own almost half the earth, rule all its oceans, [and] govern nearly half of mankind," he wrote.[48] Through colonial holdings, they controlled more than half of the most essential resources and raw material—oil, metals, cotton, wool, coal, wood, rubber, international shipping, the automobile industry.[49]

Ruth Lee was a world federalist by day and a doctor's wife and medical editor by night. "She lived kind of a double life," Fritjof said.[50] During these years, Phil became more and more involved in science. He had some interest in the social sciences and in certain forms of ideology, but his interests were in many ways opposed to those of his wife. Phil was interested in the conservative individualist ideology of Herbert Spencer, whose collected works he owned to his dying day. Spencer was considered an evolutionist who was opposed to burdensome social welfare policies. It has been argued that he believed in "individualism, laissez faire economics, the abolishment of 'poor laws,' and the general restriction of most governmental intervention."[51] He believed that social philanthropy created dependence that would lead to more human misery rather than less. Phil shared these views and had a sort of a "sauve qui peut"—or "every man for himself"—mentality. You were to pull yourself up by your own bootstraps and make the best of your abilities.

In regard to science, Spencer held a view that Phil embodied beautifully. "In science, the important thing is to modify and change one's ideas as science advances," Spencer reputedly said.[52] He was considered a Darwinist and, unknown to most people, he is the one who coined the phrase "survival of the fittest."[53] Phil strongly subscribed to the notion that human characteristics, including personalities and behavior, are heritable. He obtained some of his ideas from Spencer, who in turn got some from the Chevalier de Lamarck, who believed that evolutionary changes could be passed in a single generation via "the transmission to offspring of all changes undergone by the parent generation,"[54] right down to changes in musculature or a specially acquired artistic or employment-related skill. If there was something wrong with the parent, woe unto the child!

Phil thought of his parents as genetically different from each other in more than the usual sorts of ways. "I have always been interested in heredity," he wrote, "and I see so many aspects of heredity in the current generation. My mother's heredity is dominant.... I wish the Thygeson heredity had been dominant and not recessive." On the Thygeson side, there were two judges and many successful business owners. "On the Thompson side, I can't remember a single success."[55] Phil wrote. He believed his children took after his mother rather than his father. He particularly regretted that he had been the vector of the "bad seed" of Sylvie Thompson Thygeson, whom he disliked. He didn't call himself the bad seed — it was a generation-skipping bad seed — but once went so far as to write that, for genetic reasons, he thought he should not have had children. He also came to believe that he was not a good father. Interestingly, in his autobiography, Spencer "would speak glowingly about his father's influence, and give only scarce mention to his mother."[56] In his personal life, Spencer was a rather extreme individualist. Phil, too, would want to have things his way and to have those around him bend to his vision and desires.

Spencer and Lamarck have been much reviled for publishing texts that have been used in the service of eugenics-based theories of social engineering and genocide. In so-called positive eugenics, the most "fit" members of society are encouraged to reproduce actively, and the least "fit" are discouraged from it. Even Ruth Lee subscribed to positive eugenics in a sense, as she was known to say that bright, educated people should have the most children and to openly lament that this was not the trend during her lifetime. Giving the poor money made the social situation worse, in Spencer's view. Negative eugenics, to which neither Phil nor Ruth Lee appears to have subscribed, was intended actively to prevent the "unfit" from having children.[57] Darwin initially coined the phrase "struggle for existence," which Spencer, with Darwin's blessing, turned into "survival of the fittest." As Eric Roark has pointed out, the two are not synonymous. "[A] 'struggle for existence' might be a battle to be waged in cooperative endeavor.... Alternatively, a 'survival of the fittest' sounds much more like an individualistic hierarchical battle."[58] In the end, the view had a certain cruelty to it. Spencer wrote of people, "If they are sufficiently complete to live, they do live, and it is well they should live. If they are not sufficiently complete to live, they die, and it is best they should die."[59] Of the "idle poor," he argued that it was not a question of not having access to employment, but rather of refusing to work. "They are simply good-for-nothings...."[60] In less admirable moments, Phil was known to apply this concept to whole continents.[61]

Some of Spencer's ideas were very popular in the first decades of the twentieth century and one can even see how their logic informs Clarence Streit's choice of the nations he hoped would form the core of the world federalist union. David Weinstein argues that in Spencer's view, exercising one's moral faculties improved them, improvement that would be passed on to future generations.[62] Thus, some societies became arguably more morally fit over time, while others, barring intervention and positive role models, might degenerate. Unfortunately, in the American version of the eugenics argument, articulated by Madison Grant in his 1916 book, *The Passing of the Great Race*, the gene pool of descendants of northwestern Europeans was considered strong and worthy, while the southern and eastern Europeans were considered a threat to the gene pool and a source of overpopulation.[63] It is surely worth noting that the "good" gene pool corresponds to the same countries of origin that Streit chose as the nucleus of the new world federalist union.

To be fair to all involved, we should remember how broadly accepted eugenic thinking was in the interwar period. Grant's argument and book "found favor with a broad spectrum of political leaders, who sent fan mail to Grant, from the former American president Theodore Roosevelt to the political aspirant Adolph Hitler...." Marks wrote,

> More interesting, however, is that the leading science journals in the world reviewed it. In other words, they considered it to be science. The journal *Science* had a geneticist named Frederick Adams Woods review it, and he — like the politicians — found very little to criticize. The reason was simple: much of what Grant was saying was not far away from mainstream genetic knowledge.[64]

The American Eugenics Society also embraced the message. "Eugenics was scientific, it was technological, it was modern," wrote Marks. "Every American textbook of genetics of the 1920s advocated it."[65] After 1929, all of this changed. The stock market crash proved that "wealth was not necessarily a good predictor of genotype."[66] It became widely apparent that "the eugenics literature was invested with the authority of science without being itself rooted in the science of genetics."[67]

Phil was more of a genetic determinist than a eugenicist. Late in life, he did favor, however, forcibly preventing pregnancy in teenagers. "There is almost nothing worse than a teenage pregnancy," he wrote. "It means a life of poverty and ignorance for the child. In this age of science, we should be able to provide a suitable contraceptive."[68] What did he propose? "We should have a one-shot contraceptive. Teenagers of today will never learn about continence or the dangers of HIV infection. Teenagers are, by nature and lack of education, unable to understand the hygienics of promiscuity."[69] Phil himself was a chaste teenager, which he attributed to having wholesome interests — his studies, ham radio, and scouting. He held the view that the world had gone downhill during his lifetime and that sometimes wise elders needed to intervene on behalf of foolish young people.

Phil was shockingly Lamarckian in his view of his own family. He believed that everything flawed about it could be traced to his maternal line. Of them, he wrote, "They were all radicals — far left of center publicly — and they tended to be religious nuts, either atheists or agnostics. My mother, for example, was a violent atheist, whereas my favorite aunt — her sister — was all tied up with a religious cult in Los Angeles, called the 'Big I Am.' My uncle Elmer was a socialist who ran for mayor of New York, and was a theosophist, a San Diego-based cult." Phil could rant about family failings — uncle Spencer was a "real eccentric who could not keep a job," aunt Gladys and aunt Gatie "were real nuts and always left of center politically," and one of them "had a real nut for a son." Anyone who had trouble with marriage, employment, or politics was also a "nut." "And my mother was the weirdest of all the Thompson family.... She looked forward to a Russian-type revolution here in the United States.... She was nuts about politicians and nuts about Freud, Jung, and the newer psychology.... And she could fly into terrible rages over almost nothing. And these rages seem to be a characteristic of the family."[70] This last observation was a good bit of personal insight if he had thought to apply it to himself, which perhaps he did. Fritjof's view that Phil couldn't empathize well with others resonates in this context. Perhaps Phil had such a hard time imagining political and other views different from his own that his own relatives came to look like a bunch of "nuts" to him.

"But the joker is," he wrote, "that my mother's heredity, her mind set, her philosophy carried over into my children. They are both radical, very much like my mother, with the same mind set and philosophy of life. My father's genes and philosophy have been lost, alas."[71] Phil's political complaint against his daughter Kristin was that she disagreed with former presidents Ronald Reagan and George Bush, Sr. Phil dearly wished the Thygeson genes — by which he meant his interpretation of the Thygesons' values, views, and behavior — had dominated instead. "Heredity plays tricks," he concluded. "Good qualities are sometimes lost and the bad genetics survive. And that is what happened in my family. I can see my mother's genes at work in almost all of my children and grandchildren."[72] Ruth Lee was quite different in this regard. Though she was hard on family members who behaved badly or made errors of moral judgment, she tried to see the best in everyone. She was deeply committed to her grandchildren and even took notes on who was doing what and what she wanted to say in the many letters she wrote to celebrate each grandchild's path in life. These letters, many of them lost, are her personal opus, for she never kept a journal or wrote essays about her own life.

At the age of ninety-three, Phil wrote a poignant essay entitled, "I Wasn't Programmed to be a Father." It began, "I had such a wonderful father," and talked about how hard Phil worked to emulate him. Like Nels Marcus, Phil saw himself as someone admiring of and committed to hard work. Then he poignantly confessed, "I have had no luck with my children." They were planned, wanted babies, but he felt that Ruth Lee "made one bad mistake. She considered that the children were her responsibility while my responsibility was to provide support for the family. I was not allowed to have any role in the discipline of my children and they took advantage of that."[73] Kristin's opinion is that this division of roles was created because Phil's disciplining of Fritjof was, in Ruth Lee's view, too harsh. Ruth Lee requested that she be the disciplinarian because the alternative scared her.[74] It is hard to know the actual context in which the decision was made, but it was clearly an area where Ruth Lee's will prevailed. Phil also felt that because of this division of roles, his children did not come to him with their problems. "I believe that as a result I did not bond in any way with my children. In a way I was considered to be a hazard to my children. They always turned to their mother."[75]

Phil did not have a natural ease with children. Even in an emergency, he was likely to erupt in rage. Kristin remembered being a young child in Tenafly — certainly not more than six years old — when Fritjof accidentally started a fire with a chemistry set with which he was doing experiments. Kristin ran screaming for help, "Fritjof's on fire, Fritjof's on fire!" Phil chastised her for the way she sounded the alarm. Fritjof was reprimanded as well. As adults, Kristin and Fritjof traded impressions of their childhoods. Fritjof expressed their shared view that "the biggest problem we had with our parents is that unintentionally they set very high standards for us. They were set at the wrong time." Fritjof perceived Phil as "very, very judgmental."[76] Kristin said, "I think he really didn't like kids. He didn't like kids after they had grown up to be more independent.... He liked the American Indian children because they didn't cry. He hated children crying." In fact, if she cried, he would make her go away, out of his range of hearing. He also often used the popular refrain, "Children are to be seen and not heard." As a result, Kristin said, "I was pretty silent around him."[77] Phil's first priority was Ruth Lee. When Kristin was very young, she would run to greet him when he came home from work. But, the story goes, he would say, "No, I kiss Mommy first."[78]

Sometimes Phil was friendly and generous with his kids. At times he encouraged them to follow in his footsteps and become doctors. "[M]y father's messages about who he wanted me to grow up to be were mixed. One was to be a good housewife. Another one was get trained to be a secretary, another one was to be a great woman ophthalmologist."[79] Fritjof was long-limbed, gangly, and, by all accounts, not well coordinated. He was the antithesis of athletic and even found it hard to do certain kinds of chores, Kristin said. "My father was really down on Fritjof for this.... There were times when he would just be screaming at Fritjof and it was a horrible thing to witness. There were other times when my father would be screaming at me and it would just destroy me."[80] When the kids were younger, he spanked them, but soon harsh words replaced the spanking.

Ruth Lee suffered from the situation, too, according to Kristin. "My mother ... reached the point where she couldn't take any more, so she would just be out in the kitchen. She could hear every word, but she wouldn't come out of the kitchen or intervene or be present."[81] As she grew older, Kristin confronted her mother over the family dynamic. "I'd say, 'Mother, how can you stay with him?' or 'How can you stand it?' And my mother would say, 'Well, dear, the only time I could have done anything about your father was during our first year of marriage. And now it's too late. I can't do anything about how he is.'"[82]

At the same time, Kristin — like many people — was moved by the obvious love affair between her parents. She had a "small picture in a silver frame of these two people when they were very young and together and married."

> My father ... had his Stetson hat and his high mountain boots on, and my mother was in her clothing for a mountain outing. They were absolutely a beautiful pair of young people.... So many times I wondered how my mother could stay with him, but when I saw this photograph, I saw this enormous attraction between them that brought them together in the first place and continued despite ups and downs and the upheavals of raising children and the war and many things that come into any married couple's life. They had this early obvious magic between them, and they were so beautiful.[83]

In an attempt to understand why his children did not conform to his ideas about how they should be, Phil posed the question, "Was the problem genetic or environmental?" He answered himself: "I believe the problem was mostly genetic. The children did not resemble me or my wife genetically. They did not like to work and they did not do well in school, unlike their parents."[84] The truth was that Kristin won an academic prize and was written up in the local newspaper in middle school; she was a straight A student in her master's degree program in rehabilitation counseling later in life, and she excelled in her work with people with disabilities. Fritjof, too, had high honors at different moments in his educational journey. Phil communicated his negative perception of his children to them over and over, causing harm to their relationships with him and to their self-esteem. He was not very skilled at seeing the shades of gray and the complexity of people — they were all or nothing.

The family's critical view of Phil as a father is echoed by some of Phil's colleagues, who observed that he set very high standards and was demanding of his children. It also became obvious to some that he did not hold his adult children in high esteem. In contrast, the family's perception of Phil as a difficult husband was not so obvious to outsiders. Ruth Lee and Phil appeared deeply in love, highly compatible, and congenial in their dealings with each other. "It was such love, it was unbelievable!" said Richard O'Connor, who knew them for decades. "It was at all levels. You'd be sitting at a conference and see him reach out and grab her hand and hold it. They were absolutely the ideal love pair, and were not ashamed of being lovey-dovey in appearance."[85] It was a great — and complex — love affair.

Ruth Lee was willing to compromise in order to keep the peace and to support her husband emotionally and professionally. She was unselfish by nature and believed in being flexible, perhaps in part because flexibility was not Phil's strong suit. At different moments after her children were school age, she expressed a desire to go back to college and finish her degree. She had various academic interests over time — ranging from history to chemistry to Latin American Studies to an elementary school teaching credential. As Marcus told the story, "She never finished Stanford and it was a bitter thing for her. Fritjof can tell the story in more accurate detail — they had a big fight over this and Phil made it clear that he was not going to have her going back to school. He needed her to tend to the home front and take care of him."[86] It was not the first or the last time the issue would arise.

During the years in Iowa City and the New York City area, Phil's professional identity and happiness came mainly from his research work and from being highly respected in his field. He identified himself as a "research man" whose strongest traits were "curiosity and energy." He had to have enough energy to do copious amounts of reading and library work. Most important, he had to be interested in the unknown and to create new knowledge. "It is fun," he acknowledged, "to discover something that no other person has ever seen or recognized."[87] He saw the medical researcher's life, at least during his era, as being stable and valuable, but not lucrative. He also believed that "research men" tended to be "erudite, delightful, [and] intelligent...."[88] The researcher needed to work hard and to travel. To cope with the inevitable politics of academe, Phil believed that "charisma helps. And even a charming wife helps. And a wife who understands and appreciates your career helps in a very big way." Looking back later in life, Phil wrote, "I had the ultimate in a wife. She was beautiful and charismatic, and she ... was able to edit all my papers."[89]

A number of family members felt that Phil thwarted Ruth Lee's attempts to pursue additional formal education. At least once, his strategy was to find more and more editing work for her to do, so she did not have time to go to school. Another strategy was to become openly upset. Asked whether he thought the marriage would have lasted if Ruth Lee had insisted on returning to college, Marcus said, "I think either they would have gotten divorced or life would be so miserable that.... She once said to me, 'You got what you wanted, so what have you got?' And I think that was a rule she lived by. She was at a power disadvantage with him because that's not how Phil operated. Phil operated by getting what he wanted. That was his M.O. What he wanted, by all means he was going to get it."[90] Other relatives thought that Ruth Lee actually made her choice not to go back to school and that it was not Phil's doing. Fritjof's former wife Ralda said, "I think that Phil has gotten a bad rap in the family for being the demon who wouldn't let Ruth Lee do this, that, and the other thing." But at one point, Ralda said, Ruth Lee confided in her, "I'm not going back. I don't know why.... I have no one to be angry at but myself."[91] Ruth Lee told her granddaughter Mara about her not returning to college, "This is my fault. I should have put my foot down."[92] Other family members disagree, saying that Ruth Lee said these things because she believed in taking responsibility for herself and because she would not complain about her husband, not because Phil supported her dream.

On the other hand, Ruth Lee knew she had a magnificent life full of adventure and opportunity thanks to her and Phil's collaboration and careers. Though Ruth Lee had a desire to pursue an independent path, it was clear that she obtained a lot of prestige and enjoyment from her collaboration with Phil. Also, by the time she was in her fifties, going back to college probably held less appeal. She was a tireless champion of her sister-in-law Mary, Phil's younger sister, who decided to pursue advanced degrees in anthropology after she turned fifty. Stanford rejected Mary's application to its graduate program on the grounds that she was too old and female. Mary thought about giving up at that point, but Ruth Lee insisted that she apply to UC Berkeley. Mary got her Ph.D. in anthropology and went on to become a highly respected expert in the Navajo and the Bonin Islands south of Japan.

Ruth Lee was able to make her peace with her life situation and take responsibility for her decision to acquiesce. Marcus observed, "I never detected any bitterness. I really didn't. I think he ended up giving her such an interesting, rewarding professional life despite the fact that she didn't have a [bachelor's degree].... I think she still remained embarrassed about the fact that she didn't have a college degree. She was after all one of the best educated people I ever knew, right?"[93] Ruth Lee lived with grace and a maturity that her husband often lacked on the home front. Of the mere thought of Ruth Lee leaving him, Phil said that if she "had divorced me, I would have jumped off the Golden Gate Bridge."[94]

On the work front, Phil was highly successful in New York. He was John M. Wheeler's second in command at the Eye Institute of the Columbia-Presbyterian Medical Center. Wheeler's passion was surgery, so he gave Phil a lot

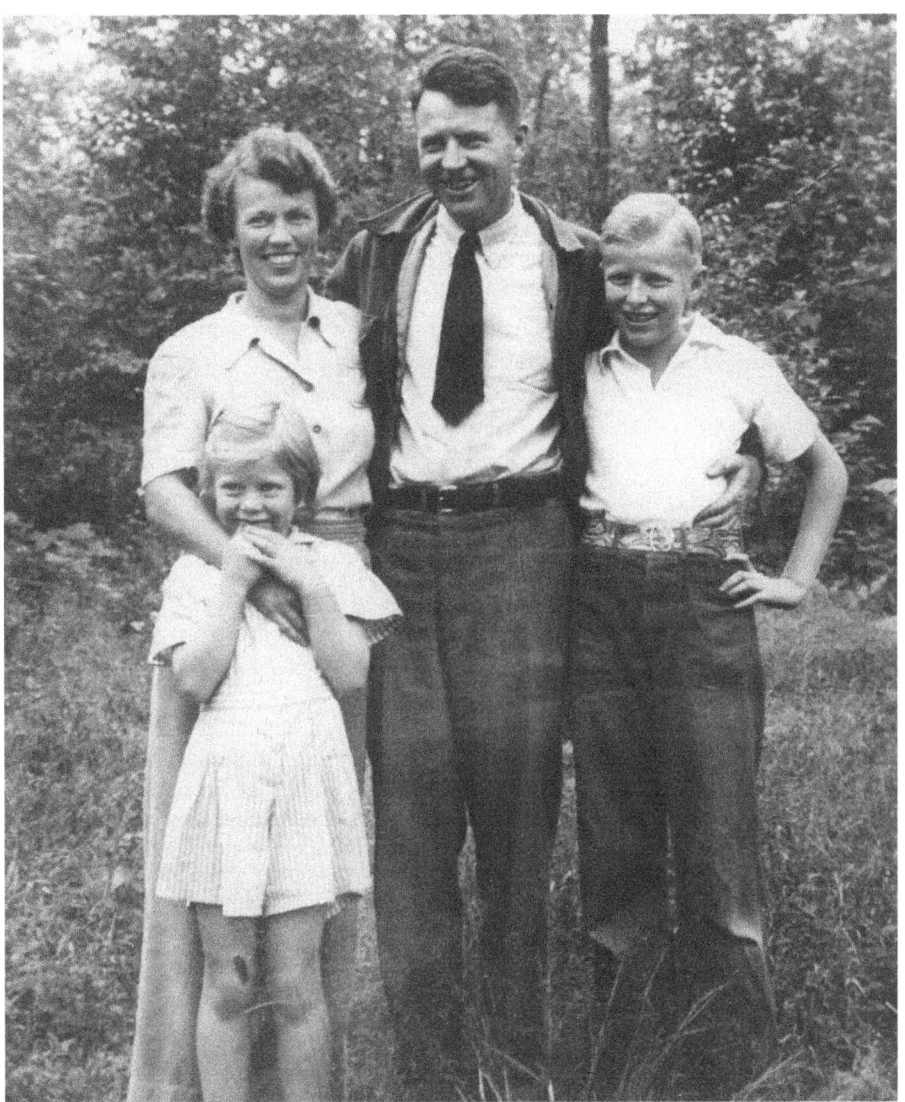

A happy moment for the Thygeson family during their New York–New Jersey years before World War II.

of administrative work to do. Because Wheeler's prowess with plastic surgery was so widely known and admired, visitors came from many parts of the world to see him operate in one of the elegant surgical galleries. This meant more visitors to entertain, more nonlaboratory time for Phil. He realized that he did not like this aspect of the work and that he greatly preferred "microbe hunting." Iowa City was where he had had the most uninterrupted laboratory time, and the fact that it was off the beaten track suddenly seemed very appealing. New York, in contrast, was the way station between Europe and the entire United States. Phil began to feel the loss of what he had given up for prestige.

By 1939, Phil held the titles of chairman of the Department of Ophthalmology and codirector, with John Dunnington, of the Harkness Eye Institute, Presbyterian Hospital. This happened in part because John Wheeler died unexpectedly. Phil's ascent to even more powerful positions did not bring him happiness. His new status "was a disaster for my laboratory work because of so many visitors."[95] Even the logistics of his work were problematic. The eye institute, the laboratories, and the clinic were located in different buildings, and Phil spent a considerable amount of time dashing from place to place. When a visitor arrived, interrupting Phil in his laboratory, "it would take me five or ten minutes to get over to the eye institute and then waste all the time on the visitor."[96] Asked whether this caused his research to "come to a standstill," he said, "Well, it was badly damaged."[97] Even his codirector, Dunnington, was very little help, as he had kept his office elsewhere in Manhattan and was conveniently off-site when most of the visitors arrived. Phil also had to handle personnel matters and office conflicts. "[I]t was really very annoying," Phil said. "I couldn't have lasted."[98] Phil later looked back on this transition with a sense of his own limitations.

> I have seen many examples of the Peter principle, where a good research man gets kicked upstairs to an administrative job that he is not qualified to handle. The Peter Principle happened to me. I had a good research job at Columbia, but when Dr. Wheeler died, I was kicked upstairs to be chairman of the eye department and codirector of the Eye Institute, jobs for which I was not qualified.[99]

Phil had additional duties as one of three members of the Board of Trustees of the Knapp Foundation. He had trouble getting along with Willard C. Rappleye, dean at Columbia, with whom he was forced to work. When Wheeler died, the $80,000 Wheeler gave every year from his private practice to support ocular research dried up. Dean Rappleye "either couldn't or wouldn't raise money,"[100] Phil said, so there was no money even to pay honoraria to those who were asked to teach the basic science course. Phil was supposed to cajole them into it. In addition, he did not like all of the egos with which he was forced to work. He believed that Dr. Roman Castroviejo was taking up laboratory space only for show. Phil claimed Castroviejo would show off his lab to visitors but not do any work in it, so he set out to wrangle it away from him. He succeeded, and turned the lab over to a very grateful researcher, Ludvig von Sallmann. All of this politicking added up to too great a burden. He began to look for a way out.

15. World War II in the Army Air Corps

World War II provided the perfect escape route. Phil was very patriotic and supported the Allied effort in the war. Ruth Lee did as well, though she had a deeper sorrow about the fact that a world war had come again a mere twenty-five years after the one that affected her childhood. In an effort to do something important to support their overseas allies, Ruth Lee and Phil offered during the London Blitz of 1941 to take in children being evacuated from London. They agreed to take the two children of a London ophthalmologist named Scott Brown. It never came to pass. "The girl got sick," Fritjof recalled, "and they missed the boat, which was later sunk. I think it was as a result of the boat being sunk that the parents decided it was safer for them to stay home." Indeed, the risk of German submarine attack was high. The offer to take in the children happened even before Phil enlisted in the Army Air Corps. If the plan had worked, according to Fritjof, Phil would have stayed at Columbia because he would have been unable to support five dependents on an army salary.[1]

Phil really wanted to be involved in the war, though at age 39 he was considered old for military service. He hoped to be shipped to North Africa, where there was a lot of trachoma, but he did not get his wish. "I was on the essential list [for Columbia University]," he said, "so I could have stayed out, but I wanted to get in so I volunteered. I got in in September of 1942."

Was all of this moving good for Phil's career? In an essay entitled "Stability," he actually posed the question, as he had a friend and colleague who absolutely refused to leave Iowa City. "In contrast, I was a mover. I started in Colorado, moved to Iowa, then to New York, then to the Army Air Force...." The siren song of some new possibility was what kept him moving, though he acknowledged, "It was hard for me to move." And yet, the family did keep moving, leading Kristin to attend eight grammar schools in as many years and feel shy and out of step with her peers. "I loved Colorado, the university, my mentors Finnoff and Jackson, and I loved the Colorado weather and gorgeous mountains," Phil recalled. "But on my move to Iowa, I got much better laboratory working conditions, a stimulus from O'Brien and others. And when I moved to New York, it was for better pay and more responsibility. And the move to join the Army was a big decision."[2] In the army, his salary declined dramatically and he had to bone up on general patient care and general ophthalmology. However, he loved it.

"The Army Air Force did me a lot of good. It gave me a much broader outlook on medicine…. As officer of the day, every eight days I had to practice general medicine, and that was good for me."[3] The Thygeson family also had the beach, the ocean, a tennis court, volleyball, and the companionship of other army doctors' families. The whole family loved their time in Florida. Was all of this moving good for Ruth Lee? Phil, on reflection, thought not. "It worked well for me to move around a bit," he wrote. "It was a bit hard on my wife, but she had a very sheltered early life. I believe that it was good for her to see more of the United States and the various aspects of academia."[4]

Asked why he chose the Army Air Corps, Phil talked about the "very attractive recruiter … who was making a kind of fetish of recruiting young university faculty" so the Army Air Corps could have the very best staff. "Wasn't there another reason?" Ruth Lee teased. "I don't remember another reason," he responded. "[T]he reason he wanted a commission," Ruth Lee said, "[is that] he wanted to fight those Nazis."[5] The recruiter did a little sleight of hand in promising that the Army Air Corps would have hospitals needing physicians in North Africa. This was Phil's dream, to be of the greatest possible service. It was not Ruth Lee's dream, as she did not want him near a battle zone. The U.S. Army, however, wanted to run all of the overseas hospitals and prevented the Air Corps from establishing its own. Thus, Phil was stuck stateside for the duration of the war. He said that the Air Corps had more physicians recruited from academe and that those doctors tended "to be a little bit snooty about looking down on the Army."[6] Also, unlike the situation in the Navy and Army, Air Corps doctors were encouraged to practice their specialties and pursue their research interests. Phil's rate of publishing journal articles and contributing to ophthalmological books did not suffer during the war years.

"I never felt better [than in Florida]," Phil said. "I was fighting Hitler."[7] In fact, though Phil never fought in the conventional sense, he had to learn how to be an army officer. That process began with three months of intensive training at Morrison Field, near West Palm Beach. The graduates were jokingly referred to as "ninety-day wonders" because they had been reincarnated as military men after, in Phil's case, nearly four decades of civilian life. "[W]e were green; we didn't know anything about the army. We had to drill, and we had to do parachute jumping and use a rifle and a revolver." The curriculum covered everything from tropical diseases to decorum.[8] Ruth Lee was given a book called *The Officer's Wife*, which she said scared her to death.[9] What was scary about her proposed role is unclear, but obviously it did not feel like a natural fit. According to Fritjof's reading of that book and others, her assigned role was to take care of other military wives by welcoming new arrivals, helping them settle in, and generally trying to keep them happy.[10] Ironically, she did that work beautifully, but not in the way the manual writers envisioned.

After his ninety days of basic training, Phil was assigned to be chief ophthalmologist and second in command of the entire hospital at Drew Field, located near Tampa. He was assigned the rank of major. The Thygesons rented a bungalow-style house near the beach at Clearwater Beach, next to other military families. It was paradise — swimming, sailing, bicycle riding, parties, friendly neighbors, and a shared spirit of collaborating against a common enemy in what they believed was a war the United States had to fight. On Clearwater Beach, Ruth Lee quickly found her niche among the wives and established a weekly book group that she led. It took place during the part of the day when husbands were at work and children at school. Whether Phil ever knew much about it is unclear. Fritjof and Kristin were old enough to be quite aware of what was going on in their parents' world. For instance, Fritjof remembered that his father preceded them to Clearwater Beach and he, Kristin, and his mother arrived together by train. On the train, a young lieutenant took a fancy to their mother. "[M]y mother was a very beautiful woman, but a unique kind of beauty.... This young lieutenant, I mean, two small kids, he knew he couldn't — [that] anything romantic or sexual was totally impossible. So he kind of hung around and then he said to my mother, 'The person you remind me of so much is Katharine Hepburn.' Of course, my mother just loved that."[11]

Ruth Lee's reading group took place on Wednesday mornings. The wives, according to Fritjof, almost never read anything. They were white southern women who lived on their side of the color line. Neighborhoods were segregated and Kristin saw almost no African Americans during their years in Florida. Ruth Lee instinctively felt it would be best if she read aloud to the group. She was a fabulous reader and loved to enthrall her audience. She also used her remarkable charm and personality to get away with taking risks with the other wives. The first book she chose for the reading group was Carey McWilliams's *Brothers under the Skin*, an important, popular book about the state of racial affairs nationwide and a direct appeal for greater social justice and racial equality. Bold and brave, Ruth Lee read to the conservative white southern women, never having lived in the South herself. As the wife of a ranking officer, she had some extra influence with the other wives. McWilliams has been described as a "self-styled American radical" who advocated for immigrants, migrant farm workers, and victims of racism and hatred, including African Americans, Jews, and Japanese-American World War II internees. He opposed big agriculture, Joseph McCarthy, and fascism.[12] He is credited with saving the venerable publication *The Nation* from McCarthy's henchmen and once described himself as "a radical democrat who might better be called a socialist."[13]

One of McWilliams's arguments in *Brothers Under the Skin* was that racial identity in the United States is a cultural construct in certain ways. McWilliams pointed out that in some cultures, a small amount of visible "black" heritage identified a person in that culture as "black," whereas even a small amount of visible "white" heritage did the same in a different country. He was ahead of his time in pointing out that racial identity is often based on cultural factors that transcend genetics and science.

What happened in Ruth Lee's reading group? According to Fritjof, "She read this [book] and they discussed it and they loved it. They couldn't have loved the political message, but they took it, they listened. And my mother's charm and friendliness, just so warm and friendly and loving, really, and then book after book after book."[14] Though a high school student at the time, Fritjof preferred to stay home and listen in on the reading group, so he would manufacture illnesses.

The group went on as long as they were in Florida—three years. Fritjof opined that as many as 200 or 300 women cycled through the group. Ruth Lee had become a teacher of sorts, encouraging women to open their minds to new ideas about social justice in the United States. Years later, a woman stopped Fritjof in Grand Central Station in New York City and said, "You probably don't remember me, I'm so-and-so, but I was in your mother's reading group. She changed my life." Fritjof agreed. "I think she changed lives. I think she had an extraordinary effect." On Tuesday nights before the group, she would prepare by going through the book and marking paragraphs that especially invited discussion.[15]

Ruth Lee was also a volunteer with the Red Cross. She would visit impoverished, stressed civilian families and offer support and instruction in basic health and self-care. The Red Cross gave her a gasoline ration card so she could make house calls. Kristin remembered her mother getting dressed up in "a very smart seersucker suit," her Red Cross uniform. "It was fitted and looked like a million [dollars] on her," Kristin said. "I remember my mother coming home one day and being utterly appalled and horrified at one poor white family." Ruth Lee said, as Kristin recalled the moment, "'They're dirty'.... My mother was dismayed to find this among a white family, whereas she didn't run into this with the Negro families. It was so illuminating to her that here was one more instance of misplaced prejudice...."[16] Ruth Lee's role was to find out what a family needed in terms of supplies and clothing — not cash — that the Red Cross could provide.

Kristin was not allowed to go on any of the visits, but her mother gave her an education in racial issues. She showed her daughter the segregated housing on the air base, indicating how black enlisted men were not allowed to live next to white ones. The two sets of barracks were separated by a road. "My mother went to great lengths to explain to me how this was wrong, how everybody's the same, everybody's equal. She just thought it was morally wrong."[17]

Ruth Lee also educated her children about racial discrimination in the arts. The great singer Marian Anderson was not allowed to sing in Constitution Hall in 1939 because the Daughters of the American Revolution (DAR), which controlled the hall, would not let a black woman sing there. Instead, at the invitation of Eleanor Roosevelt, Marian Anderson sang on the steps of the Lincoln Memorial to an enormous crowd, many of them there to protest the DAR's overt act of discrimination. That performance is remembered as a pivotal moment in the early Civil Rights movements. Later, after much apology and soul-searching, the DAR had a major role in the dedication of the commemorative postal stamp featuring Marian Anderson.[18]

Ruth Lee, who loved opera and many American musical traditions, was a great admirer of Marian Anderson. When she learned that Marian Anderson was coming to the town of Clearwater, she asked the people who were hosting the concert to introduce her. As Ruth Lee told the story, when the concert hostess introduced them, the hostess did what was customary in that part of the South at the time, which was to accord the white woman full respect and the black woman only partial respect. The introduction went like this: "Mrs. Thygeson, this is Marian." To this, Ruth Lee responded by breaking the code of dropping the last name of black people, and said, "It is an honor to meet you, Miss Anderson." She also held out her hand, another violation of racial protocol, to shake Marian Anderson's hand.[19]

Phil may not have liked his children's politics, but they were pure Ruth Lee in many ways. Ruth Lee was never a socialist or a communist, but she was progressive and egalitarian for her time. She taught her children how to treat other people in the world, and her main lesson was that every human being deserved care and respect. When Kristin was in the third or fourth grade in Clearwater Beach, she came home from school singing a racist jump roping ditty she learned on the playground. If "Negro" was the acceptable "n" word of the era, the song featured the unacceptable one. Kristin did not know what it meant and when her mother overheard her singing it, she stopped her, pointed out the word and said, "This is a terrible, terrible word. It should never be used by anyone."[20] Clearwater Beach was completely segregated and Kristin said that she never saw even one African-American child in the family's years of living there. She got to know only one African American during the war, Lottie, the woman who cleaned the Thygeson house once a week while Phil was away at work. Ruth Lee and Kristin and Lottie were friendly, but even that took place within the context of the employer-employee relationship. Lottie would often go home with a bag of groceries Ruth Lee gave her for her family, or with Fritjof and Kristin's outgrown clothing for her nephews and nieces.

Ruth Lee had another service-related activity during their war years. She was a plane spotter, trained in recognizing the make and insignia of airborne small planes. Fritjof related that he and his mother and perhaps Phil and Kristin as well "took a little course in identification of different planes. There was a tower within walking distance of where we lived. We would sign up for periods of time; usually it was a team of two people, so it was fun."[21] Kristin, who often kept her mother company during Ruth Lee's shifts, felt that her mother enjoyed the work and was glad to contribute in this way to the war effort. According to Kristin, Ruth Lee "had a telephone, binoculars, and a bank of windows, and every time a plane flew overhead she was to identify it if she could. Most of the time she would telephone in a familiar U.S. plane, a P-38 or something like this, or a fighter or a B-17.... [T]here were German planes flying out in the Gulf; it was known that they were flying in the Gulf of Mexico."[22] However, the Thygesons never spotted one.

During the Clearwater Beach years, Ruth Lee was deeply attracted to a man who was not her husband. She later confided that she had "been pretty smitten by this young medical professional." Kristin, whom she later told, was "surprised because at the time that we were in Clearwater, nothing filtered down to me that would have given me the slightest clue of this.... It was fairly serious the way she spoke of it. She was even sort of contemplating separating from my father because there was a mental component to this friendship with this man that she didn't have at all with my father."[23] Kristin believed her mother experienced a certain loneliness or isolation with her father. "She could get into my father's world and he required that she do so because he would talk endlessly about what was on his mind and about his experiences, but he never asked her a question or appeared to be curious [about her thoughts], and so my mother was not known to my father in terms of her values."[24] Other family members confirm this asymmetry in Ruth Lee and Phil's understanding of each other in certain areas.

However tempted she was by this man, however, Ruth Lee was basically conservative and very loyal to her family. Years later, she wrote in a letter, "As some perspicacious observer noted: you can terminate a marriage but a divorce goes on forever. And children of almost any age get wacky ideas about *reasons* for it, no matter how you try to put it over. And then the marriage you put in its place can be *soooo* disappointing. I've about decided that nobody has any sense about mating!" She went on to confide, "*Of course* I have been intensely attracted to other men — more than one. But measuring up the list of my husband's virtues has so much more than offset the differences and 'failings' (?)...."[25] She added, "I think we need to have very strict laws about getting married.... It's so easy to get divorced."[26] Essentially, she believed that divorce was a form of personal failure, but she was also a pragmatist and thought if couples tried all remedies and could not work things out, divorce was an option.

Ruth Lee and Phil loved each other dearly but there were ways in which Phil did not know his wife. Ruth Lee later confided in her daughter, "If he really knew me, he wouldn't like me."[27] To another relative, she said the same thing, but more gently: "If Phil really knew me, I don't know whether he'd like me."[28] Phil assumed he and Ruth Lee thought alike, and he assumed his values were her values, which was only partially true. He was happy in his belief in their similitude and Ruth Lee allowed him the happiness of this particular ignorance. It was, in a way, her gift to him.

Phil, knowing nothing about the threat to his marriage, was happily engaged with his medical work while Ruth Lee pursued her volunteerism and their children were at school. There was plenty to do at Drew Field because of the sheer number of airmen involved. "Aviation at that time was very risky, and we had all kinds of accidents, [including] aircraft falling out in Tampa Bay," Phil said.[29] There were also thousands of Army Air Corps members in training who needed eye examinations. The radar corps was channeled through Drew Field on its way to assignments overseas. The signal corps involved "disability" cases that disqualified enlisted men from combat duty. Given all of the different groups of servicemen, there were as many as 50,000 men at Drew Field at a given time. The radar men would develop eye strain from gazing into radar scopes for eight hours a day. The pilots had their own set of problems. Many were from the South, where they were exposed to a lot of sunshine. Some developed pterygium, a small growth on the eye that sometimes required surgery. Phil also reported pilots with "muscle imbalance," which affected depth perception and could make a pilot unsure of exactly where he was during an aircraft landing.[30]

Phil was a stickler when it came to enforcing military rules. Among his patients were Pan American Airlines pilots who were drafted into the Army

Air Corps to ferry large planes across the Atlantic. Phil examined one of these pilots in the dark, using the old-fashioned method of checking for ocular pressure by manually palpating with his fingertips. "His eye was hard as a rock," Phil reported. He discovered that the pilot was wearing hard contact lenses, which were brand-new technology and expressly forbidden in the Air Corps. Without the contact lenses, the pilot failed the vision test miserably. And though this particular pilot had already been ferrying military planes across the Atlantic for two years quite successfully, Phil did not make an exception for him. "He was perfectly safe, but I had to let him go just because of regulations. There were a lot of things like that."[31]

Phil also proved that trachoma had not been eradicated and was in fact alive and well in the Air Corps. In the course of doing eye examinations, he discovered about twenty previously unidentified cases and published a paper about them in *Military Surgeon*. He also described Drew Field's hospital as having "an epidemic of meningococcic meningitis," for which penicillin was a godsend once it became available. Early work on penicillin was done in England, but soon Pfizer and other American pharmaceutical companies were busily aiding the war effort by "building great big vats to grow the mold."[32] At the time, there was no resistance to penicillin or the sulfa drugs, so they were a great boon. "Penicillin was a tremendous victory. It saved a lot of lives in the war. It saved a lot of eyes that would have been lost from sympathetic ophthalmia, which was a terrible curse in World War I."[33] In the case of war wounds, one eye would be wounded or affected by disease in the uveal tract—the inside of the eye—and the other eye would, in time, "sympathetically" come down with the same sort of auto-immune granulomatous uveitis. Then both eyes would be at risk of going blind.

There were also eye injuries unique to the war. For instance, American gunners sometimes suffered from solar retinitis, sun-related burns on the retina. The Japanese pilots skillfully positioned themselves between their enemy and the sun so that the American pilots and gunners would be forced to squint directly into the sun for extended periods. Protective goggles were eventually developed, but in the meantime, there was no remedy for a burned retina. Nonpilots showed up at the hospital with a similar injury not caused by exposure to sun. It was a macular lesion known as "central serous retinopathy," which some thought was due to stress, but which Phil concluded was never fully understood.[34]

There was no shortage of interesting cases and opportunities for research papers. It helped that Drew Field had very high priority with the government. Whatever the doctors requested, they got, whether it was medication or equipment. "All I had to do was call the adjutant in Washington, D.C., and he would fly down the instruments from Washington, so it was very satisfactory," Phil said. "Anything we wanted we could get."[35] There were excellent lab facilities. Phil published a paper on blepharitis in 1946 that was a direct result of patient contact at Drew Field. The paper defined three distinct types of blepharitis and outlined their treatment. It won second prize in a contest for which first prize was $500, which Phil and Ruth Lee badly needed. Second prize, most disappointingly, was a lifetime subscription to *Military Surgeon*, where the article was published.

The group of ophthalmologists at Drew Field was called a "pool" because doctors frequently rotated in briefly, sometimes for training, before being reassigned elsewhere. There were as many as fifteen ophthalmologists working at a given moment during peak periods. Phil and his colleague, Alexander Rodman Irvine, who had been recruited from the University of Southern California, were permanent staff. Rod and Phil became great friends as well as next door neighbors on the beach at Clearwater. They carpooled together to Drew Field from home, along with several other doctors. The car pool was a lively affair. Doctors took turns driving, which meant that once a week Ruth Lee had to give up the aging family car because it was Phil's turn to drive. The doctors loved to talk shop during these thirty-mile drives, and Phil found the conversation highly stimulating. There were two "chiefs of medicine" who were part of this group. "The car pool was very valuable because we could discuss the cases of the day. It wasn't the usual boy talk. It was all medicine.... It was a rather remarkable unit because it was young university people, without exception."[36] Drew Field also featured a wonderful library, a weekly seminar, and a journal club. In a way, it was a bit like Iowa — the pleasures of academic and clinical medicine with a minimum of bureaucratic hassles.

Phil and Rod Irvine collaborated in interesting ways at Drew Field. They discovered that each had been trained directly by one of the two great national experts in physiological optics. Irvine had been trained at Harvard by Walter B. Lancaster in the "Lancaster method" and Phil had been trained by Edward Jackson in Colorado in the "Jackson method." The goal of each was to be able to test accurately and quickly for astigmatism. The Lancaster device had a dial on it with which one mapped out the axis and degree of astigmatism. Jackson had the famous cross-cylinder. Phil and his friend got into competitions about how fast they could refract a patient using the two devices. Phil always won — he was about twice as fast on the Jackson cross-cylinder. Soon, Irvine had crossed over, as all other ophthalmologists eventually did as well.[37] Phil and Irvine also teamed as a sort of joint preceptor for a young doctor in the signal corps named Joe Hallett. Hallett wanted in the worst way to be an ophthalmologist, but he hadn't been through the appropriate residency. Phil and Irvine devoted two years to giving him "all the training we

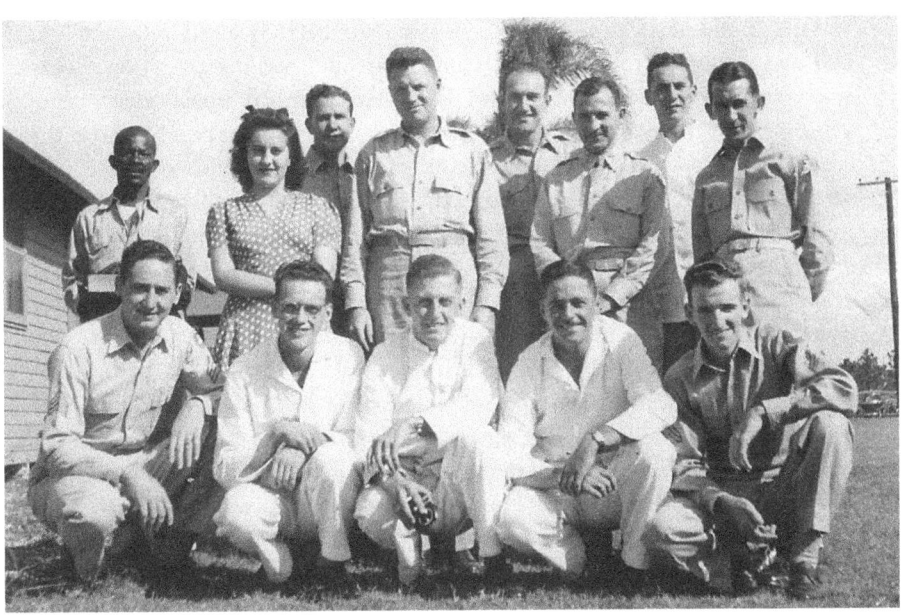

Phillips Thygeson, rear center, with other member of his medical group at Drew Field, Florida.

could" and telling him what to read at night to catch up in the field. In 1946, when Hallett took the American board examination in ophthalmology, he scored second best in the entire group of candidates in spite of never having done a residency.[38]

The Army Air Corps generally assigned physicians to bases near where they lived. This meant that most physicians stationed at Drew Field were Southerners accustomed to de facto segregation. When Phil observed that a Northern African-American physician had been assigned to Drew Field, he anticipated that other doctors might give him a hard time. He made a special effort to get him involved in ophthalmology, where the two of them would be able to work together and Phil would be in a position to intervene if anyone treated the doctor disrespectfully or unfairly.[39] This was the era in which Phil famously said that in a hundred years, there would be no more "race problem." "We will all be mulattoes," he told Fritjof.[40] Neither he nor Ruth Lee approved of mixed marriages, but he did foresee a future where there would be much more blending of racial groups and fewer related social issues. At the time, Ruth Lee had just read Eugene O'Neill's *All God's Chillun Got Wings*, which explored in painful detail the subject of miscegenation. Ruth Lee came to believe that mixed marriages harmed children, a view she held to some degree all of her life.

Back on Clearwater Beach, there was a wonderfully engaging social life. Phil was never one to love parties, but Clearwater was the exception. Every Saturday night there was a party, and Phil broke another personal rule by being willing to imbibe alcohol during these parties. "We had the best house on the beach, so everybody came to our house," he said. "We could go to bed, and then they would come in and wake us up." "Tell us it was Saturday night," Ruth Lee continued, not missing a beat. "Sometimes we would turn out all the lights and scuttle into bed early, but on the whole we enjoyed it immensely." The parties, by her description, were "purely social, but they were awfully funny because Saturday night we were out of school. The way we had never been in our lives and never would be again."[41] It is not clear what Ruth Lee meant by "out of school," though it was nearly the only time in their professional lives when they were not literally connected to a university employer and the sense of being "at school." It was also clearly the most carefree they had ever been together — the children were older, Phil and Ruth Lee's jobs and roles were limited and clear, the war was on, and for the moment there was no question of career ladder climbing or what major decision to make next.

When Phil was promoted from major to lieutenant colonel, his friends and colleagues threw him "the party to end all parties." They had gotten him to promise in advance to embrace their celebration party, so there was no escape for Phil. The family would remember it well. According to Ruth Lee, who laughed while recounting this story, it was the "one and only time in his entire life — I can testify to that since I've really been in on most of it — he was pie-eyed. He was gloriously drunk."[42] Fritjof concurred that theirs was the best party house. Not only did it have a tile floor that made a wonderful surface for dancing, but it had two large connected rooms, a living room and a dining room. On the night of the fateful party, Fritjof and Kristin were sent to bed. Fritjof recalled, "We woke up about two in the morning to the sound of marching men. We looked out the window and there was my father drilling these officers up and down the street in front of the house. 'March to the left! Column right, left!' Just having the time of his life giving orders and marching these men."[43] The awful thing for Phil was that his promotion had come through on a Thursday, and it was on a Thursday night that he became so gloriously drunk. The next day he had to work at Drew Field. He dragged himself to work, survived the day, and returned home, ashen, a little after five o'clock. Fritjof remembered that, too. "He was death warmed over.... He walked right past me, didn't see me, ... didn't say anything, staggered up the stairs, fell into bed, and we didn't see him until five o'clock the next afternoon. He had the worst hangover anybody ever had."[44]

The greatest family adventure during their years in Clearwater was shared by all four members of the family. It was the resurrection of their own sailboat, named *Before* and then, upon its first launch, renamed *After*. Fritjof discovered the boat, a mud-swamped wreck, half-buried along the shore. According to Kristin, it was a gaff-rigged cat boat with a round hull, no keel, and a center board.[45] It was a "racing cat" of sorts, because you could regulate your speed by pulling up the center board. When the center board was fully up, the boat could move easily in only a few inches of water. It needed a new deck and had at least one broken rib in its hull. The four-sided white sail was mildewed but salvageable, though all of the rigging had to be replaced. Ruth Lee told the story of finding the shipwrecked, sunken boat. "Fritjof came home and said, 'I found a boat; I found a boat! Can I have it?' We said, 'You can have it if you can find the owner and ask him if you can have it.'" Fritjof managed this beautifully and the owner offered to sell them the boat for twenty-five dollars. Kristin was only eight at the time, but pitched in with the others for an entire winter of boat refurbishment.[46]

Like most magnificent Thygeson projects, this one began as an act of construction. Where was the pleasure in a boat or, for that matter, a house they did not help build with their own hands? Phil bought a book on sailboats and everyone pitched in for long weekend days of getting the boat seaworthy. Ruth Lee's job was to procure the parts. She became very familiar with marine supply stores and various sizes of cleats and types of rigging. They bought copious amounts of sand paper, spar varnish, canvas to cover the new deck, combing to rim the deck, and special nails that would not corrode or rust in salt water. The biggest excitement was *After*'s maiden voyage. "My father had never sailed but he was a believer that if you had a book, a how-to book on any subject, he could do it," Kristin recalled. "As he'd say, 'It might be rustic but I can do it.'"[47] The book in hand was H. A. Calahan's 1932 classic, *Learning to Sail*. According to Jim Cadranell, a sailing enthusiast who reviewed the book, it is simple, clear, and filled with appealing wry humor. He quoted Calahan, "If, at times, the book adopts a preaching tone, it must be borne in mind that preaching (or profanity) is of the essence of all teaching of seamanship."[48] There's much practical how-to advice in the book as well as lists of warnings and advice for the landlubber, entitled "Seventeen Ways to Get into Trouble" and "Seventeen or More Ways to Get Out of Trouble." Phil took to heart Calahan's advice on how to be an effective skipper in his tiny boat. "The over-confident skipper is nearly always in trouble," Calahan warned, and "the under-confident, almost as frequently."[49]

With his family on board the 15-foot boat, Phil launched *After* from a dock in the estuary on the lee side of Clearwater Bay. The estuary was quite narrow, so it was necessary to tack back and forth across it in order to get to more open water. Kristin remembered the drama of that first launching and sailing expedition. "My father had the book literally in one hand and ... the far shore ... was coming closer and closer. I yelled, 'You're going to hit! You're going to hit!'" Her cries did not faze Phil because he was a confident skipper and he knew exactly when he wanted to give the command, "Ready about? Hard to lee!" so that when he moved the tiller, his crew would pull in on the sheet and the boat would go about in the wind.[50] It had to be done right so the sail did not get caught in the luffing, or flapping, stage. Phil would take fellow officers out sailing, and Fritjof discovered that the boat was a great way to impress girls.

Kristin loved to go into the extra-large cockpit and "just listen to the water on the other side of the hull go 'whoosh.' It was magical to me...."[51] She especially loved to sail with her parents in Clearwater Bay. "Very often there were dolphins in the bay and they would play with our boat. They would come along in a little school, three, four, five, six dolphins, and hop up on one side of the boat, ... dive under the boat, come up on the other side of the boat, turn around and then go under our boat again.... They'd look you in the eye ... you looked right back.... And so I felt pure wonder ... that this species would be interested in us.... Even as a child I thought it was amazing."[52]

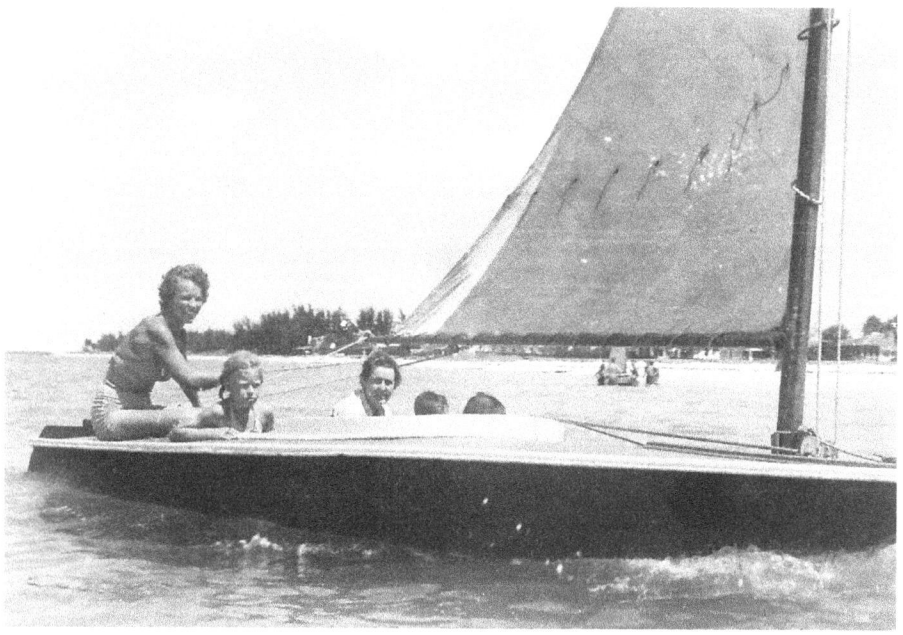

Ruth Lee sailing the restored sailboat *After* with Kristin and family friends in Clearwater Bay, Florida.

Now that the children were older, Phil and Ruth Lee had a different sort of relationship with them. Fritjof and his mother were very compatible intellectually and loved to read and talk about books together. This stirred up some jealousy in Phil. Marcus opined that Phil felt competitive with his own son. "There may have been a triangle going on there, because I think my father appealed to certain aspects of my grandmother's personality that my grandfather did not appeal to. In a way, I think she was living through him and his aspirations and ambitions."[53]

Phil still chafed under the edict that banned him from disciplining the children. He felt that Ruth Lee had spoiled both children. He managed to be a disciplinarian at times. "Whenever either one of us crossed the line, he would come in like a ton of bricks," Fritjof said. Their mother would "let us know there were certain things we should not do because it would upset him, and if it upset him we would all suffer."[54] There were a few memorable conflicts. In one, Fritjof wanted to participate in a Sea Scout group overnight. Phil said no. Fritjof rebelled, jumped on his bicycle, and headed off anyway. "And he comes after me and marches in there, grabs me, and pulls me out of there. Then tells me to get on the bicycle and drives behind me. It was a couple of miles, and he is right there with the lights shining on me."[55] Both of the children felt their father was capable of physical violence toward them. They feared he could become out of control.

Nonetheless, Fritjof continued to test the limits of his father's patience. He was a teenager, after all. He was friends with a girl named Ann who got a babysitting job "in a broken down hotel" not far from the Thygesons' bungalow on the beach. "I walked her there, planning to go home.... It was obviously a real dive with drunk sailors, and I thought ... she should not be there alone. There was no telephone there." Fritjof believed that if he went home and shared his concern, his parents would say, "That's not your business. Call her parents." And so, as Fritjof told the story, "I did not go home." That was early in the evening and the woman for whom Ann was babysitting did not return until midnight. All that time, Fritjof was A.W.O.L. and his father grew progressively more upset. Around ten o'clock that night, Phil started driving all over Clearwater Beach in search of Fritjof. When Fritjof finally appeared after midnight, Phil meted out a double punishment: he could not see Ann or go to the movies for two months. Fritjof thought he had done the gentlemanly thing, the noble thing, so he in turn was outraged. Ever the mediator, Ruth Lee stepped in. She suggested that Fritjof be allowed to choose one of the two punishments, which he did. He gave up the movies, but not his time with Ann. His choice impressed his father, as it turned out.[56] Phil and Fritjof enjoyed going to movies together, often favoring traditional westerns over other fare. Giving up John Wayne meant Fritjof really liked that girl.

During their years in Florida, the family kept close track of the war news. They saw government newsreels whenever they could and listened to the radio every day. "We listened to Edward R. Murrow from London," Fritjof said. "I'll never forget that. That was extraordinary."[57] Phil had a patient who was a top aide to General Douglas MacArthur and, as a result, Phil became a great supporter and follower of MacArthur's.

Phil and Ruth Lee had no reservations about the need to fight fascism and preserve democracy. Phil had supported the Republican cause in the Spanish Civil War even though socialists and communists were part of the Republican side of the conflict. However they could serve the American war effort, Ruth Lee and Phil served, which meant conserving resources and collecting bacon grease, newspaper, and other materials useful for the weapons factories. Although they did not always vote for the same candidate for president, both Ruth Lee and Phil considered themselves "New Dealers." They believed in Social Security and a certain level of government-provided social safety net for Americans. Phil had never liked the idea of socialized medicine until he found himself essentially practicing it in the Army Air Corps. He saw plenty about it to admire.

In spite of the sacrifices of the war years, Phil enjoyed life in the military. As he put it, "I liked everything about it; it was good experience, and I learned a lot of general medicine which served me later." He even enjoyed the financial stability of being essentially underpaid. His army salary was around $400 a month. "It wasn't enough even though my mother scrimped, saved and budgeted. We ate our meals very frugally and so on," Kristin said. Ruth Lee was a fabulous money manager and was expert at buying used clothes at thrift shops. Kristin received hand-me-downs from the older daughters of Ruth Lee's close friend, Libbie Green. Ruth Lee had managed to save about $5,000 before their Florida years. By the end of the war, they had spent it all and were "flat broke."[58] Phil, however, told a completely different story about the Drew Field years. "I really enjoyed it because I didn't have the financial worries that most of the people in practice had. We never had a big salary. We spent five thousand dollars over our income, but we made it up on sabbatical, because Columbia gave me a half salary, $5,000, for a sabbatical, and it just evened it out, so I ended the war even."[59]

During this period, they managed to replace the makeshift tar paper roof of their Colorado cabin with shingles. They had scraped together enough money to put on a shake roof, a cheap form of roofing that needs to be replaced every so often in harsh climates, and begged friends in Denver to get shakes put on the cabin. The friends mistakenly purchased shingles, an expensive error that worked out beautifully because the carefully oiled shingles have held up ever since.

There was a horrifying moment late in the war when Phil and a couple of fellow Drew Field ophthalmologists were presented with a bill for several thousand dollars for having prescribed glasses to Navy and Marine Corps personnel without proper authorization. They provided the care under orders from their commanding officer and supply sergeant, and were specifically told to give the Navy and Marine Corps servicemen the same level of care they gave to members of the Army Air Corps. The bill came with a demand letter that instructed Phil to pay a third of the sum due. The commanding officer and supply sergeant were expected to pay the remaining two-thirds out of their personal funds. This was a shock, especially to Ruth Lee. "We didn't have an extra dime. We were just living hand to mouth and taking care of these two children." Fortunately, the master sergeant said he would handle the problem. He did so with consummate skill, with Phil taking note of how these things were done. "He started a letter to St. Louis," Phil explained, "with reply by endorsement, and had these letters going back and forth. He got after the Navy in Washington, and after some months the Navy agreed to pay for this without charging us.... You couldn't hedge.... You had to answer. He knew just how to do it...." As with all of Phil's other moments of being mentored by great talents, he learned what he could. "He knew all the ropes. That's a lesson I never forgot, because I used it myself later on, handling the [U.S.] Indian [Health] Service bureaucracy. The Indian Service bureaucracy was pretty rough."[60]

When it became clear that the war was starting to draw to a close, Phil and Ruth Lee were faced with a decision: what to do next? Phil's position at Columbia was being held for him, but his years in Florida made him see just how unhappy he had been there. Nonetheless, he had planned to go back to Columbia until late in the war, when he and Ruth Lee realized they had other options. In March 1945, he made a trip back to Columbia to visit the eye institute and check in with his dean, Willard Rappleye. "Everything was very sad," he reported. "The school had deteriorated; many of the staff had left, and it was running very poorly. The weather was terrible. In Florida it was orange blossom time."[61] His conversation with the dean about his dream of a major basic science program at Columbia was more than a little dispiriting. The dean flatly was not interested. This rejection helped Phil give up any last thoughts of returning to his old position at Columbia. In addition, both he and Ruth Lee recognized that the eastern seaboard was hard on Ruth Lee's health. She had bronchial asthma and severe hay fever triggered by ragweed. In California, they had not encountered ragweed, so that was another strong argument in that state's favor.

Phil wasn't free to do whatever he wanted, however, because he had not been discharged from the military. When the war in Europe ended, Drew Field quickly became a much less active air field, with many fewer personnel. Phil's work there was ending. He was transferred into the regular army and moved to Valley Forge General Hospital in Pennsylvania. The hospital had a specialty in ocular plastic surgery, and Phil assisted in many surgeries and learned what he could. He did not particularly like doing surgery, but he understood that if he went into private practice, it would be important to be well-trained. To this end, he spent six weeks getting experience at the military hospital in Valley Forge. It was an enormous hospital — nearly 900 beds — and he got to see all sorts of interesting cases. His six weeks there were less than happy, for he was alone. Ruth Lee and the children, assuming that Phil's Valley Forge assignment would be short and the war would soon end, packed up and moved to California.

Even before the transfer to Valley Forge, Phil longed to go back to California, where he loved the climate, the fruit trees, and the casual friendliness of the people. Kristin remembered "this soul-searching period when my parents would walk the beach, just the two of them…. They would walk the beach and talk about what to do."[62] The decision was theirs alone, for that was their style of parenting. Kristin explained, "Fritjof and I were not consulted ever…. It would be unthinkable for them to consult us. We would just be told of the decision and we were going to do it."[63] Neither parent wanted to return to their old life in New Jersey. As Kristin told it, "My father really, really wanted to leave. I think my mother was very happy about it too, because she wanted to get back to her mother and her sister…. It was decided that my mother would go up to New Jersey and sell the house."[64]

At the end of the war, few people had money. Ruth Lee and Phil were able to get back the money they had put into buying the land and building the house in New Jersey, but no more. Another challenge was that there was no university job waiting for Phil out in California. He would have to go into private practice, a fate he had always worked to avoid. The first step, though, was to get back to the West. "We were just waiting for the Japanese to fold up," Phil said. "Valley Forge gradually slowed down. So I wrangled a transfer to Dibble, which is in Menlo Park…. I wanted to end up [there], so I manipulated it."[65]

16. California and an Experiment in Private Practice

The family moved in with Ruth Lee's sister Lib, Lib's husband Milton, and Ruth Lee and Lib's mother in Menlo Park-Atherton, a few miles from Stanford. Although the house was large by California standards of the day, there wasn't a lot of room in the inn. Ruth Lee and Lib's mother moved into the guest bedroom downstairs. Ruth Lee and Phil moved into the attic, which consisted of a large room, a small room, and a bathroom. Fritjof slept in the small room with the sloping eaves and his parents had the large room. Kristin slept behind a screen in Lib and Milton's room, a very generous arrangement designed to give Phil and Ruth Lee privacy. It did not provide Lib or Milton or young Kristin with any privacy, but she appreciated her little "cubby hole," as it was called. The newly enlarged multigenerational family cooked together in the downstairs kitchen, with Ruth Lee and Lib breaking into peals of laughter as they accidentally duplicated each other's work in their enthusiasm to collaborate. Because Ruth Lee and Phil were broke, Lib and Milton helped support the family.

At first, Phil and Ruth Lee planned to live close to the ocean in Carmel. On weekends, they would drive up and down the coast looking for property to rent or buy, though they had no money. Finally, Phil realized he did not like the climate of Carmel. It was too humid, too often overcast, too cold. They decided to settle in the sunny little town of Los Altos instead. They put down a deposit on a half-acre lot in Los Altos but everything changed when Dr. Proctor's widow, Elizabeth Proctor, came to visit. She "was used to acreage" and "was horrified at our half acre," Phil wrote. She told their realtor, Pat Carey, to "take the half acre back and to get us some acreage."[1] Carey found them a five-acre hilltop of beautiful apricot and peach orchard on the first row of hills behind the little town of Los Altos. It did not matter that they could not afford the land, which cost $17,500.[2]

Elizabeth Proctor beneficently provided the money necessary to secure the five acres, and Ruth Lee and Phil remained ever grateful to her for that.[3] Phil commuted three days a week to San Jose and three days a week to San Francisco. Given their new, more rural location, they needed a "commute car," which Elizabeth Proctor gave them as a present. Whether or not they paid her back for the land is not clear. In an undated letter written in the late 1950s or early 1960s, Elizabeth Proctor returned an uncashed check for a thousand dollars to Ruth Lee with the request that she spend it on care for Phil's aging mother, Sylvie.[4]

Ruth Lee fondly referred to the town of Los Altos as "the village" because its downtown was just a couple of streets with little shops lining them. Phil and Ruth Lee could not really afford another construction project, but they also could not inconvenience Lib and Milton forever. They took stock of the tiny house that sat on the hilltop they had just bought. The house was hardly worthy of the name. It was just two rooms; there was a nook that became Ruth Lee and Phil's study and there was a living room, which extended from the study but was two steps up. There wasn't even a kitchen; it was more like a makeshift kitchenette. As soon as it was even physically possible to live there, they moved in, though it meant washing dishes in a dishpan rather than in a sink with a drain. Ruth Lee took out three mortgages, "one for the driveway up the hill, one for a bedroom addition, and one for the kitchen."[5]

On the back of the house, they began to build two bedrooms, another tiny "cubby," this time for Fritjof, and a bathroom. The cubby was made very cheaply; its walls were covered with Celotex, a cheap, temporary material, and it was plumbed so it could become a second bathroom someday. That day never came. Living in the house was in essence a form of camping. "There was tar paper on the floor over the sub-flooring and there were just shells for rooms. There was no plywood or any kind of wood on the inside of the bedrooms," Kristin said. "Of course, we'd been well prepared because we had all this cabin experience, so it wasn't as hard on us as it would have been on some people.... It was a couple of years I would say before, gradually, the interior of the house was done."[6]

They walked on the tar paper floor so much that they had to replace it as they went along. When finished, it was a small, simple house. The kitchen had built-in steel-topped appliances — stove and oven — with an old ice box they had hauled all the way from the New Jersey house. There was a washing machine but no dryer, so they hung their clothes on a clothes line. Ruth Lee kept her mangle in the kitchen — a large, foot-pedal-operated machine for ironing sheets and Phil's shirts. She was very skillful with it and claimed never to want to sleep between cotton sheets that had not been ironed. They hung a framed handwritten note by Abraham Lincoln in the hall outside their bedroom. It was about a boy who wanted to work. President Lincoln asked the recipient of his note to give the boy work "if at all possible," given how rare he felt it was to find someone who truly wanted to work.

In 1949, the house finished, Phil and Ruth Lee built what came to be known as the "guest house," a separate building with a room and a bathroom (where Fritjof spent some of his teenaged years), a laundry room and workbench, and a carport. They bought redwood siding on sale and put in on the house themselves. In fact, they did much of the manual labor themselves, though Phil was very busy those days. They enjoyed the work and, when the house was done, they kept working. "Friends and neighbors brought trees, shrubs and plants for our garden.... We built two terraces, red brick with places for plants. Our library grew and we kept building shelves in the study, in the hall and in the bedrooms and guest house."[7]

Both Ruth Lee and Phil loved to garden, but Phil loved it the most. Ruth Lee would go to the nursery and buy plants; Phil was often the one to plant and water them. Because the property had been a vineyard before it had been a fruit orchard, there were still some old vines here and there. Phil and Ruth Lee planted rows of berry bushes and enjoyed fresh blackberries, raspberries, loganberries, and boysenberries with vanilla ice cream. Los Altos probably reminded Phil of Lake Minnetonka, except that the California winter was much milder. The tradition of planting and tending a vegetable garden continued. They had several rows of corn, chard, string beans, cucumbers, and tomatoes. Phil loved to water his garden by hand after a long day of work and on weekends. It was probably as close to meditation as he ever came. He once told Kristin that he would have chosen to specialize in plant science, rather than medical science, if he could live his life over again.

When they acquired the Los Altos property, the orchard was already well established and even considered an aging orchard. Still, the apricot trees lasted a long while before they died and some have survived to this day. There were also quite a few walnut and almond trees. Ruth Lee and Phil bought baby apple trees and planted a whole row of them along what became the driveway. They also planted a few plum trees and a wonderful assortment of peach trees. The orchard had to be sprayed for pests every year and rototilled so that the ground wouldn't become too compacted. According to Kristin, the orchard "fruit was sold to canneries and to dried apricot vendors. The net of it all was that my parents broke even because the sale of the fruit paid for the maintenance." Like many other family ventures, ranging from the Paiute cabin to the little sailboat *After*, the work gave the family a great deal of pleasure. "They loved that orchard and the beautiful green grass of oats that would grow up in the spring and the yellow mustard sprinkled through the orchard. In the spring after the rains would come, it was just beautiful." The oat grass grew three feet high and was a great place for kids to lie on their backs, dream, and gaze up at the sky, as Kristin loved to do.[8]

Work at Dibble General Hospital turned out to be quite fortuitous for Phil, as he met Crowell Beard there, his future private practice partner. Both Valley Forge and Dibble were large rehabilitation hospitals, including for blind soldiers. Their mission was similar, but they served the two different theaters of war. Beard was an expert ocular plastic surgeon and an army captain. He had been trained at the Mayo Clinic, where surgical training wasn't even an option, but he was born to be a surgeon and was largely self-taught. "Dr. Beard was a natural," Phil said. "He made his own curtains; he could sew.... He, of course, became the plastic surgeon of the [San Francisco Bay] area. He's by far the most important plastic man in this whole area."[9]

Phil and Beard had a very positive effect on each other. Phil went into private practice with Beard, and Beard went on to become part of the clinical faculty at the University of California at San Francisco (UCSF), largely thanks to Phil's influence. Phil and Beard opened a practice and, in time, were joined by another former army doctor, Daniel Vaughan, who became a lifelong friend of both and who ended up working with Phil as well at UCSF.[10] Phil would have preferred a full-time academic position, but there simply was no such thing at the time. After the war, "in California everything was volunteer; there were no full time appointments anywhere on the West Coast." There were not many on the East Coast either — he had had one of the few while at Columbia. "It was logical that I had to do a private practice," he said.[11]

It was now 1946, and Phil had been discharged from the Army Air Corps at the rank of colonel. Beard did not want to work in San Francisco and had lobbied to establish the practice in San Jose. This worked well with the Los Altos plan, so Phil had said yes. Opening a practice required a lot of cash, so it took quite a while for revenue from the small new practice to permit either doctor to take home a paycheck. They had to pay the office rent, acquire furniture and equipment, and pay salaries for the nurses and other office staff. Phil and Ruth Lee had so little money they borrowed from Lib and Milton to pay their expenses.[12] Even though the private practice was in debt for a solid year and Phil needed to work full-time, it was not long before he managed to slip away to San Francisco and do ocular laboratory research in the city two days a week. His true passion was calling to him.

17. The Francis I. Proctor Foundation for Research in Ophthalmology

The story of the Francis I. Proctor Foundation for Research in Ophthalmology, the greatest and longest chapter in Phil and Ruth Lee's lives, takes us back to the 1930s and Dr. and Mrs. Proctor. As mentioned earlier, the independently wealthy Dr. Proctor wanted to establish an important laboratory or research institute to study trachoma and other eye diseases affecting Native Americans. The Rockefeller Institute had been a major funder of teaching hospitals around the country, so in the early 1930s Proctor went to them for advice. According to Phil, he was told "it would be too expensive and that the only hope would be to tie it in with a university." But because Santa Fe, where the Proctors retired, did not have a university, Dr. Proctor gave up on the idea.

When Dr. Proctor died unexpectedly in 1936, he left directions in his will that approximately $300,000 of his estate was to be devoted to the study of trachoma and other infectious eye disease.[1] The money was held in trust at the Old Colony Trust in Boston, and the law of Massachusetts gave the estate only a certain number of years to spend it or have it become state property. Time was running out. Dr. Proctor's nephew Harrison Proctor raised the subject with Elizabeth Proctor, who contacted Phil during his war service years in Florida for a major consultation about what to do. Phil knew that the Army Air Corps flew B-17s back and forth from Drew Field to Denver for training flights. He managed to get a seat on board one of the planes and made his way to Santa Fe to meet with Elizabeth Proctor.

At first, the plan for the Francis I. Proctor legacy was to have a granting program to provide funds to ocular research projects of their choosing. However, so little eye research was being done during the war years that they received only two applications for grants. The plan never worked out.[2] Phil had a brilliant idea that would solve two problems at once—the problem of how to spend the Proctor money before it was too late and the problem of how to get back into academic medicine in California, where there were no full-time ocular research positions available. "I advanced the idea of a special laboratory in a western university under Dr. Proctor's name," Phil said. During the last years of World War II, with Harrison Proctor, Dr. Polk Richards, Dr. Arnold Knapp, and Dr. John Dunnington, Phil was the fifth person in a five-man research committee assembled to investigate possibilities. According to Phil, this committee did not last long, though he did not say why. Phil ended up doing most of the work investigating possible sites for the research institute by himself.[3] He arranged a short leave of absence from his medical duties at Drew Field and went to visit Stanford, the University of Southern California, the University of California, and the University of Oregon. Stanford seemed the best option in Phil's opinion.[4]

Unfortunately, the reception at Stanford was mixed. Hans Barkan and Dohrmann Pischel, the resident luminaries in ophthalmology, were quite enthusiastic, as was the dean, Loren Chandler. However, the plan could not proceed without the support of Stanford's president, Donald B. Tresidder. In preparation for what Phil and Mrs. Proctor thought would be Stanford's acceptance of the plan, Mrs. Proctor gave $25,000 to Stanford on the condition that a memorial laboratory be set up. Phil met with Dr. Tresidder to make arrangements. To his surprise, the president said he would be happy to take the Proctor money but that, in Phil's words, "He didn't want to favor any special department or unit because that would make the other units jealous." In other words, there would be no specialized, semi-autonomous eye research foundation at Stanford. Since that was not what Phil and Mrs. Proctor had in mind, they said no.

The process of finding a home for the future Proctor Foundation unfolded through the 1940s. The next step was to approach UCSF. With the help of Frederick C. Cordes, Phil met with Dean Francis Scott Smyth, a pediatrician who agreed with Phil that a specialized research laboratory would be a great asset to the university. Before long, Phil and a lawyer hired to represent Elizabeth Proctor's interests were collaborating on a plan for the future foundation. Phil consulted with Karl Meyer about what had made the George W. Hooper Foundation, a biomedical research entity at UCSF, so successful.

The lesson of the Hooper Foundation was that foundation directors come and go, but trustees remain, and thus a stable board of trustees is essential to a foundation's long-term health. Phil did not learn this the easy way. He deduced it because Meyer had eliminated his Board of Trustees. "Meyer

17. The Francis I. Proctor Foundation for Research in Ophthalmology

didn't like anybody to tell him what to do," Phil said, "so he managed to get rid of them. And then the university set up a faculty committee which was much worse for Dr. Meyer than the Hooper trustees. Meyer made a terrible mistake at the Hooper, and I recognized it at the time...." Meyer also "got rid of the Hooper family," which meant losing funding from that family—another big mistake.[5]

Phil did his best to keep the board of trustees for the Proctor Foundation quite small. He used the model of the Knapp Foundation in New York, which was just three people. In the case of the Francis I. Proctor Foundation, it was the dean (and later the chancellor), the chair of the eye department, and the director of the Proctor Foundation. This board configuration has endured for over half a century. It was soon known as the Board of Governors rather than the Board of Trustees so as not to be confused with the university trustees.[6]

Phil had a bit of Karl Meyer in him. He wanted to make sure the Proctor Foundation was separate from the ophthalmology department at USCF, and he was adamant about avoiding what he often referred to as a "takeover." He feared losing laboratory and clinical space, funding, and decision making to the larger entity. Phil wanted the foundation to be fully in charge of its own staffing and program goals and implementation.[7] He believed that its role model, the Lucien Howe Laboratory of Ophthalmology at Harvard, had met the bad fate of being taken over and "absorbed in the general purposes of the eye department."[8] Because the Howe Laboratory space had not been owned by the laboratory but was merely borrowed from the Massachusetts Eye and Ear Infirmary, in Phil's view it never had enough space, could not expand, and was in a sense doomed to tragic limitations.[9]

On September 15, 1947, Elizabeth C. Proctor and the Regents of the University of California signed an agreement establishing the Francis I. Proctor Foundation for Research in Ophthalmology. Phil tried to talk Mrs. Proctor into moving to the Bay Area so she could more closely follow the progress of her and her husband's biggest legacy, but she merely came for a visit and then returned to her beautiful home near Santa Fe. It was her last visit to San Francisco. "Because of crippling arthritis that struck her down soon after," Phil wrote, "she was never able to return, and thus never saw the laboratories in action or the growth that was to come. We kept in very close touch, however."[10] Phil communicated by phone and letters, reports were sent, and Phil and Ruth Lee visited Mrs. Proctor at least once a year whenever possible.[11] The humble beginning of the Proctor Foundation was a single room and a small, part-time staff. The mission was "basic and applied research on disease of the eye." Ophthalmologists served as the original core staff. "My understanding," said G. Richard O'Connor, "was that there were no true basic

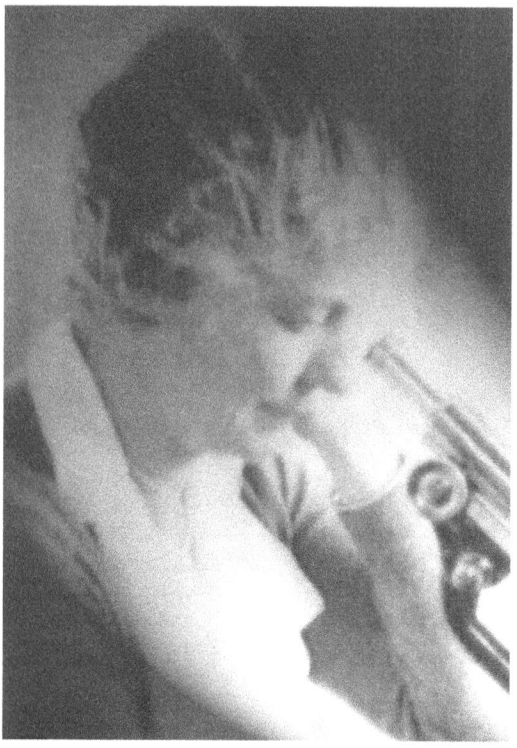

Elizabeth C. Proctor, Phillips Thygeson's benefactress, who helped establish the Francis I. Proctor Foundation for Research in Ophthalmology.

scientists in the beginning. There were no Ph.D.'s on staff. They were all ophthalmologists."[12]

After an initial period of working full-time in his private practice in San Jose, Phil chose to divide his time between private practice and part-time work at the Proctor Foundation. The plan was for him to work Monday, Wednesday, Friday, and half of Saturday in the practice, and spend Tuesday and Thursday at the University of California at San Francisco. He wanted to have two blissfully uninterrupted days to devote to laboratory work, but he also needed to earn a living.[13]

The private practice Phil established with Crowell Beard evolved in parallel with the early years of the Proctor Foundation. Phil and Beard had to build their practice from the ground up, but as the only board-certified ophthalmologists in the city of San Jose, they quickly had the market cornered. Phil had two fee schedules, one for patients who could afford the care they were receiving and one for patients of lesser means. He told a story to Marcus about a patient of his, an older woman who appeared to be in financially straitened circumstances. He charged her the lower fees. After he had been her ophthalmologist for quite a while, she had an emergency that required a house call. "He drove out to see her and her house was this fantastically luxurious mansion," Marcus said. "As he was leaving, he said, 'I've been charging you my low rate because I thought you were living with strained circumstances.' She looked at him and said, 'I fooled you, didn't I?'" After that, Phil charged her his higher rates.[14]

Phil never did like private practice, but he was dutiful. He knew his children would soon be heading to college. It took a year before he brought home a paycheck. It was for $100, the first grocery money to come out of his new endeavor. "I'll always remember that announcement when my father came home waving a hundred dollars in front of all of us," Kristin said. "Everybody whooped and hollered and rejoiced and celebrated that night."[15] From there, the practice built and built, permitting the family to live on a private practice income of a three-and-a-half-day work week. Of course, this also meant there was not a lot of extra cash. One day, however, Phil drove up at seven o'clock in the evening in a brand-new Studebaker. He had bought the car to surprise his family. Ruth Lee was naturally very frugal and a diligent money manager, so Kristin remembered her as being "kind of wide-eyed." "She had the philosophy that you save your pennies and pretty soon you have a dollar and then you have two dollars and you pay off the mortgage early."[16] When the private practice became too busy for the two of them to handle, they added Robert Cook and Daniel Vaughan, both of whom were ophthalmology residents at UCSF. Phil had to do some general ophthalmology, but he got many referrals in his favorite area, external disease. And though he disliked surgery, he had to spend a lot of time assisting Beard in the operating room.

During the brief period when he worked full-time in private practice, Phil managed to remain connected to ocular research. In the early days of the Proctor Foundation, Dr. Proctor's passion for supporting trachoma prevention and treatment among Native Americans was a major emphasis, especially for Phil. He continued to collaborate with the Indian Health Service, which at the time was administered by the Public Health Service. The Public Health Service was willing to provide ophthalmologists rather than general practitioners for the effort. The important laboratory work at Fort Apache continued. The doctor in private practice never had to give up his research.

18. Father and Son: From San Quentin to Steroids

Family life was changing around this time. It was a decade full of transitions for the Thygeson family as well. In fact, some of the transitions had begun in the late 1940s. Fritjof turned eighteen in 1947 and in his opinion "the most important conversation" he ever had with Phil occurred then. "He told me what his father's philosophy of life was. It isn't what you accomplish in the world that's important. It's what you do with whatever gifts you have been given. And the person who is somewhat limited in gifts, but fulfills them to the utmost, is more to be admired than the brilliant guy who just coasts on his intelligence."[1]

Fritjof was a young prodigy in learning from his mother and following her path into devotion to world federalism.[2] He got involved with the movement in Florida during the war, even though he was quite shy. After the war, he briefly attended Sequoia Union High School while the family lived with Lib and Milton in Atherton. One day in his high school home room class, he learned that the local Lions Club was sponsoring a public speaking contest. The topic was: "What is my responsibility as a young American to lasting world peace?" Suddenly, the shy Fritjof was moved to speak. He was allowed to read his speech and was one of three students chosen to compete in the local Lions Club competition.

The terror of public speaking — which at that point Fritjof shared with his mother — set in with a vengeance. Neither Fritjof nor his mother was convinced he would make it through the speech. In fact, on the day of the competition, Fritjof threatened to run away. In front of the audience, he froze. He could not remember a word of his speech. At last, the title came to him. Once he had uttered those words, he focused on a lone man at the back of the room and delivered his impassioned speech to him. The speech was a triumphant success.

18. Father and Son

In 1947, when he was finishing high school in Los Altos, Fritjof was invited by Harris Wofford, the head of Student Federalists and a future senator of Pennsylvania, to go on a national speaking tour. Fritjof managed to travel to New York to meet with him. "I was the coming leader of the organization and was elected chairman of the high school division," Fritjof said. "And then ... I graduated from high school in June of '47 and had been accepted to Stanford. I delayed one quarter and went on a national speaking tour the fall quarter of 1947. My father was absolutely opposed to that. He just thought that was terrible. He said, 'Who does some young punk think he is telling people how to go about changing the world?'" According to Fritjof, Phil "thought the world government idea was simply utopian." Fritjof suspected his parents argued over his participation and that his mother, who actually won the day, "paid a price for making it possible for me to go on the speaking tour. And of course, she was extremely proud of me. I don't think anything could have pleased her more than my doing that."[3]

Fritjof was an extremely successful speaker and advocate, and came home from the speaking tour to a proud mother and an unforgiving father. "To his dying day, my father said—the last conversation we had maybe two or three months before he died—he said it was the stupidest thing I ever did. He said it ruined my life. I just got off on the wrong track. That just led me off to socialism and being a marginal figure. You know, it was literally in one sense the greatest experience in my life."[4] Fritjof believes this episode represents one of the times when his mother's will clearly triumphed over his father's. She wanted him to go on the speaking tour and she saw that it happened.

In 1949, Fritjof met Ralda Lee and married her in December of that year. She was eighteen and he was nineteen. By nearly everyone's account, they were too young. Ruth Lee and Lib liked Ralda very much and though she might help Fritjof grow up. Ralda greatly admired Ruth Lee and Lib, who encouraged her to pursue a career but also to be a devoted wife and mother. The message was a bit confusing, but Ralda loved the sisters' sense of humor about their historical moment and their roles as women. "They were writing a book about housekeeping and running a home, being wife and mother. The title of the book was, *We Don't Like It Either*." In it, they pointed out that no one cared if your windows were clean, and that if you didn't have a paid job, as relatively few women did in those days, people thought nothing of interrupting you whenever it suited them.[5]

Fritjof and Ralda struggled financially, had two children, and Phil and Ruth Lee later ended up providing support for their grandchildren. The early years of the marriage included Fritjof's and Ralda's living in the Los Altos hilltop guesthouse—Fritjof's room. At one point, Phil becoming enraged at Fritjof's politics. "You're talking like a goddamned Red. Get out!" Phil yelled at Fritjof. The young couple moved out and lived briefly in a motel, but Ruth Lee helped broker a peace agreement and they moved back in. She appeared not ready to let them launch into emancipated adult life.

Ralda believed that Ruth Lee had a hard time letting her children grow up and become mature adults. "Fritjof's car would run out of gas — surprise, surprise — on the back roads, and Ruth Lee would come down and bring a can of gasoline.... Ruth Lee had a very hard time disciplining her children."[6] Ruth Lee sometimes held the same opinion and once went so far as to say that if Phil or Lib had brought up their children, things might have gone better for them.

Fritjof dropped out of Stanford in 1951 and joined the U.S. Navy. A high school classmate had been killed in Korea and Fritjof felt uncomfortable about his student draft exemption. He loved the sea, thought he could become a medic, and was fascinated by submarines. However, since submarines did not have a lot of medics, he had to choose. He chose submarine service. He outsmarted the psychological exam by figuring out what the desired answers were. He did beautifully on all of the aptitude tests except for mechanical skills. On shipboard, he charmed nearly everyone (except for some of the officers) and was quite popular as a member of the crew of the USS *Tilefish*.

Fritjof was a disaster as a sailor, however. All members of the submarine were supposed to be able to navigate and control the submarine's movements. In other words, every submariner was supposed to be a generalist. Fritjof, however, had never mastered the bow and stern planes that caused the sub to dive and surface. As a fairly new sailor, he was summoned from his perch in the conning tower to control a dive in the Pearl Harbor area. As the horns sounded and the commanding officer yelled orders at Fritjof, he took up his station at the stern planes. He adjusted them to cause a dive. The bow did not seem to dive, so he added a bit more angle. Still nothing — until he made another adjustment, at which point they were diving fast and hard. At that point, Fritjof and nearly all of the crew heard the captain bellow, "Get that man off those planes! He'll kill us all! He'll kill us all!"[7]

The USS *Tilefish* was transferred to San Diego from Hawaii in 1953. Ralda, Fritjof, and their two small children were able to live together again. The USS *Tilefish* was on daytime operations, so Fritjof enrolled in night classes at San Diego State College, graduating in the summer of 1956. He enrolled in the graduate political science program at UC Berkeley that fall, but found practicing politics far more compelling than studying them. With a friend who was a leader of the Berkeley student left, he cofounded "SLATE," an organization trying to break down the national two-party system in favor of a multiparty system.

By the late 1950s, Fritjof's family believed his zeal had gotten out of control. Ralda said, "I thought he'd really gone round the bend — when he ran for the U.S. Senate in the Peace and Freedom Party as a fisherman. He listed that as his vocation."[8] Fritjof had worked briefly as a fisherman, but at the time he was supposed to be in graduate school. In the election, he garnered 4,500 votes, carrying one tiny Northern California precinct where Norwegian was still spoken by some.[9] The Peace and Freedom Party was a socialist party, much to the delight of Fritjof's grandmother Sylvie.

Phil and Fritjof had other dramatic encounters. Fritjof, who opposed the death penalty, went to San Quentin in May of 1960 to participate in a vigil to save a death row inmate named Caryl Chessman, who had been nicknamed "the red light rapist." The charges were rape and robbery, not murder. Fritjof and his political compatriots were vehemently opposed to the death penalty as a state practice. They spent the night before Chessman's execution in a vigil with several hundred other death penalty protestors. The next morning, after it was clear that there would be no stay of execution, Fritjof and Frank Harper were arrested for civil disobedience, though Fritjof initially had not planned on taking that step. But when he saw his featherweight friend being carried away by police, he instinctively sat his much heavier body down where Frank had been sitting. This caused the police to drag him away and arrest him. "As Frank and I are being carried out of San Quentin, Marlon Brando and the Hollywood contingent arrives," Fritjof recalled. "The next day, my picture and Frank's picture are on the front page of the *San Francisco Chronicle*. My father's practice is in San Jose. My mother says it was the worst day of his life. Patient after patient comes in and says, 'Dr. Thygeson, are you any relation to that Thygeson who got arrested at San Quentin?'"[10] For his part, Fritjof enjoyed his brief experience in jail. He spent his time interviewing fellow prisoners and was soon bailed out by some sympathetic faculty at UC Berkeley. Two felony charges were dropped in exchange for his pleading guilty to a misdemeanor: unlawful assembly. The penalty was time already served.[11]

Though Phil disliked political notoriety, he did not mind being at the center of family or medical controversies. In fact, he seemed to attract and create them. The year Fritjof and Ralda married, Phil published several research papers on trachoma, but most of his publications were on other topics, such as epidemic and severe forms of keratoconjunctivitis, inclusion conjunctivitis, conjunctival disease, and basic science research in ophthalmology. The following year, he began to publish on herpes simplex, a disease about which he would stir up a good deal of controversy, particularly concerning ocular steroids as a treatment strategy. Phil's approach to treatment was based on his extensive experience before steroids were invented. As one of his protégés, Khalid Tabbara, said, "Before the use of steroids, patients were doing well and he was not seeing corneal blindness. All of a sudden when steroids became popular in 1952, he started seeing all these difficult problems with stromal keratitis."[12] Phil's friend Alson Braley had sent him cortisone acetate for treatment of eye disease. Braley reported that it proved effective in treating dendritic keratitis. Phil began his own experiment — he treated four of his San Jose private practice patients with the cortisone. Three of the patients did well; the fourth was a disaster. The patient developed "severe stromal keratitis, uveitis, and a rise in intraocular pressure."[13] Some months later, he was permanently blind in that eye, in spite of surgery to try to save his vision.

Phil was very disturbed by this blind eye. "This was the first time I referred a herpetic eye for keratoplasty, the first time in my experience that the outcome of an attack of herpetic keratitis was a blind eye, and the first time that blindness had followed steroid therapy."[14] Another patient, who had already been treated elsewhere with systemic steroid medication, was referred to Phil that same month. In spite of everything he tried to do to help her, she went blind in both eyes. "The disastrous effect of steroid therapy was so obvious I abandoned any further testing of this treatment in humans and turned to rabbit studies," Phil wrote.[15] A number of studies on rabbits done at the Proctor Foundation and elsewhere soon confirmed that steroids could be dangerous, especially in the case of herpetic eye disease. Phil and his colleagues published an important paper on the subject in the *American Journal of Ophthalmology*. "We were the first, I think, to recognize the bad effects of steroids in herpes. That paper went around the world, and I think did quite a bit of good. [It] didn't get to everybody the way it should have, but it got to a lot of people. It got me into hot water with the drug houses."[16]

Phil dubbed steroids "the heaven and hell drug."[17] His work was soon corroborated by others at the Proctor Foundation and by researchers around the world. Even so, Phil lamented, "this didn't get into the general ophthalmologic picture as it should have. The reason was that cortisone stopped all the symptoms of herpes, so patients were initially delighted — until they lost their eyes."[18] What helped Phil, of course, was his longevity. As a fellow ophthalmologist later pointed out, "He was one of the very few people who had experienced the disease process from 1926 all the way to the 1990s.... Other people witnessed it but didn't understand it like he did."[19] Phil was aware, for example, that during World War II, the Army Air Corps never had to resort to corneal transplant due to herpes simplex. The reason for that, according to Phil, was that steroids were not yet in use.[20]

Fritjof observed that his father was willing to risk the wrath of fellow ophthalmologists in his crusade to save patients' eyes from inappropriate use of steroids. "He made many, many real enemies. Not just people in the drug companies, but doctors who made that their primary method of treatment. One doctor grabbed him and threatened to hit him...."[21] The most upsetting aspect of the problem for Phil was that other doctors, including ophthalmologists, continued to use steroids in what he thought were very reckless ways. According to O'Connor, "many ophthalmologists, including prominent ones, thought that his idea about steroids was just totally irrelevant. If a person had inflammation, by God, give him steroids. A lot of doctors thought they were sued because of Thygeson's statements about steroids ... and were, therefore, very angry with him."[22] By 1956, two hundred cases of herpetic keratitis largely worsened by steroids were treated by the Proctor Foundation staff. The corneal ulcers that resulted were horribly painful. The Proctor doctors were led to conclude that herpetic keratitis had become the leading cause of corneal disease-related blindness in the United States. Most distressing of all was the fact that this had not been the case until steroids were widely used.

According to a story told at Proctor, Phil "went to the FDA and begged them not to allow steroid-antibiotic combinations to be approved. They didn't listen to him and they came out with ... horrible combinations."[23] Some ophthalmologists were not convinced by Phil's research, and others were fooled by the early effect of steroid use — eyes might temporarily look white and healthy again, before steroid-induced immune depression took over and caused a much worse outcome, at least in a percentage of patients. One partial solution was to lower the dosages of the steroids. However, it was hard to convince general practitioners to exercise caution.

> Pharmaceutical companies began a wide distribution of steroid and steroid-antibiotic samples to pediatricians and general practitioners for use in the "red eye syndrome." In northern California it became common practice for these physicians to treat undiagnosed "red eyes" with these drug-house samples. Only if complications developed was the patient referred to an ophthalmologist.[24]

Phil would talk about and teach the theory of the "compromised host." He differentiated between systemic immunodeficiency or compromise and local compromise. He also argued that herpetic keratitis was an opportunistic infection and that it did not occur unless the host — the patient — had compromised immunity. In a seminal essay he published later in life in an anthology aptly entitled *Controversy in Ophthalmology*, Phil used his careful record of cases throughout his career to argue that steroids could suppress the body's protective reaction to injury as well as suppress cellular immunity.[25]

That was the "hell" side of the "heaven and hell" drug. The "heaven" side was discovered at nearly the same time. During the war years, Phil had met Milo H. Fritz, an ophthalmologist working in Alaska. Fritz became a close friend of Phil's. They collaborated actively for years and then corresponded for many more. Fritz was a frontiersman of the first order — he would go anywhere and do anything. A bush pilot with a pontoon plane for landing on rural lakes, he was able to visit remote groups of Alaskan Inuits. He flew without instruments. He found that Inuit children had high levels of phlyctenulosis, an allergy to the tuberculosis bacillus that can damage the cornea, and high levels of pulmonary tuberculosis, which caused the phlyctenulosis in the first place. He loved Alaska, but his wife hated living there. The couple tried to live in the lower 48 states, but Fritz was so miserable they gave up. Phil and family visited them in Alaska; Kristin got to travel by ship to Alaska in 1949. Phil did field work with Fritz at Mt. Edgecomb School, a school for children with tuberculosis. Phil was convinced he had — or at least had been exposed to — tuberculosis in the course of his work in Colorado and Alaska.

Given Phil's experiences with Native American children at Fort Apache, Phil and Fritz had much to talk about. The only treatment for phlyctenulosis — a perfect treatment as it turned out — was steroids, though dietary changes to combat tuberculosis sometimes helped as well. According to Phil, phlyctenulosis was once "a principal cause of reduced vision in children all over the world."[26] It fit perfectly into Phil's life mission.

Fritz worked on the cause and treatment of phlyctenulosis under the auspices of the Alaska Department of Public Health. He invited Phil to collaborate, so when he was able to, Phil flew to Sitka and examined Inuit children at the Mt. Edgecomb School. In 1950 he and Fritz published a paper that showed the "heavenly" side of the drug. The paper, published in the *American Journal of Ophthalmology*, was called "Cortisone in the treatment of phlyctenular keratoconjunctivitis."[27] Phil had been thrilled to discover, with Fritz, that "overnight we could abort a phlyctenulosis attack by instilling a corticosteroid into the conjunctival sac. Only a few days of steroid treatment were necessary, thus avoiding the well-known complications of prolonged steroid therapy…. Steroid treatment never failed."[28] For this use, it was a miracle drug.[29]

In 1950, Phil published a paper that resulted in his having a disease named after him. The paper, "Superficial punctate keratitis,"[30] or SPK, differentiates between subtypes of spotty keratitis. Phil saw his first case of SPK in the 1930s. He asked Finnoff what it was and Finnoff recalled that his teacher Ernst Fuchs had said it was SPK. So Finnoff called it "Fuchs superficial punctate keratitis." That disease existed but it wasn't what Phil was looking at. Phil decided that SPK was an excellent way to describe what he was seeing and that it should have the honor of being called superficial punctate keratitis. The other related disease should have a new name, such as epithelial keratitis. A London ophthalmologist named Barrie Jones added Phil's name to the disease. Ever since, it has been known as Thygeson's superficial punctate keratitis.[31] In spite of his protestations to the contrary, Phil probably enjoyed having a disease named in his honor.

19. Mother and Daughter: World Federalist and Equestrienne

During these years in Los Altos when Phil was trying to find his way back to full-time academic medicine, Ruth Lee continued to be politically active. She also continued to keep her activities separate from Phil. She volunteered for Alan Cranston, a progressive politician involved in world federalism. The future U.S. senator lived in Los Altos, so Ruth Lee was able to work with him and his colleagues. The meetings Ruth Lee attended took place during the day when Phil was at work. "I don't know how much she told him about what she was doing," Kristin said. "My father didn't ask.... He probably got the drift that there was something going on but I think he didn't want to know because he was so opposed and my mother did not want a confrontation with him.[1] Whatever Ruth Lee did, she was sure to be home to greet Fritjof and Kristin when they came home from school. According to Kristin, Phil would drive up the steep Los Altos driveway at six o'clock every evening "expecting dinner immediately. The table had to be set."[2]

After the war, Ruth Lee was thrilled when the United Nations was created and was hopeful that it could further the mission of world federalism and international peace. For Phil, though, world government was too radical an idea. He feared that it would mean that the United States would have to give up some of its vast store of power and sovereignty. As Kristin put it, for Phil, "It was America first. America first, right or wrong."[3] Kristin saw his swing toward ultraconservatism—he had not been as conservative in his youth—as perhaps a belated additional reaction to his mother Sylvie's politics. Her politics were "very liberal, humanistic, all inclusive—women's liberation, women's right to birth control, equality of all the races."[4] Sylvie was also very sympathetic to communism and to the Soviet Union. While Ruth

Lee had sympathy for some aspects of Sylvie's politics, neither she nor Phil found anything to like about her communism.

Phil and Ruth Lee had been very sociable during their war years in Florida. When their building projects on the Los Altos hilltop were all finished, they kept right on socializing. "It seemed no time at all before we began to entertain in a big way," Phil wrote. "The Proctor Foundation in San Francisco had begun to attract visitors from all over the world and many of them were entertained by day or overnight in Los Altos. The guest house seemed always occupied and the patio was the site of many gatherings and even a few seminars." Among the visitors were Sir Stewart Duke-Elder of London, Milo Fritz of Alaska, and Dame Ida Mann of Australia.[5] Ruth Lee was a skillful hostess at all of the events.

Meanwhile, Kristin was growing up and developing her own passions. School had not worked out well for her because her family's many moves caused disruption to her education. Nonetheless, she was a good student. In seventh grade, she found herself at the Mothers of the Sacred Heart School. It was a convent school run by strict nuns. Kristin's greatest passion at this

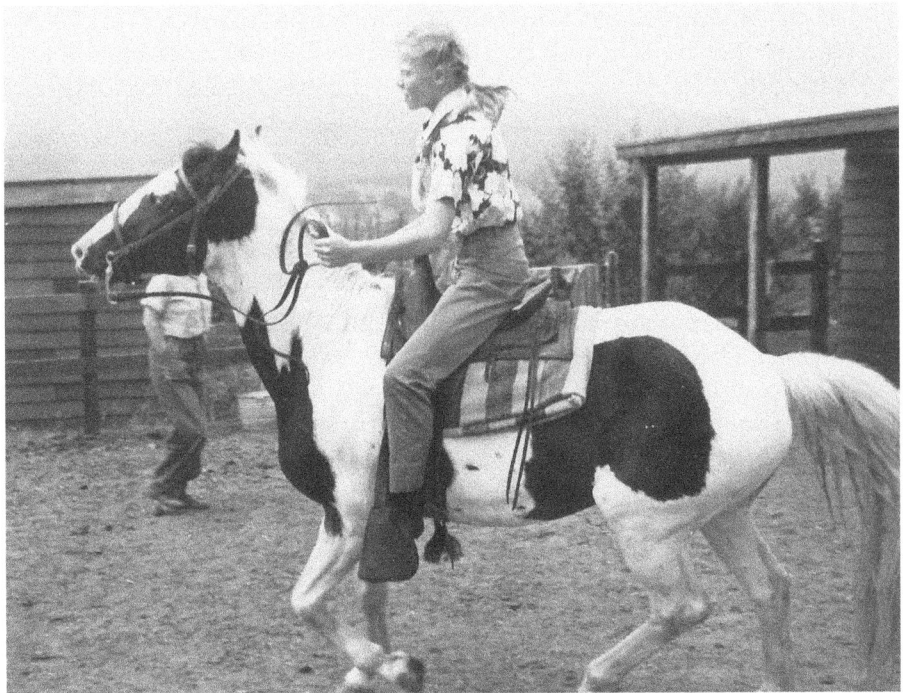

Kristin Thygeson riding her family's second horse, Pinty, in the paddock she and her father built in Los Altos.

time was to have a horse. She had saved $250 in silver dollars, which were worth exactly their face value. While they were still living at Lib and Milton's in Atherton, Kristin, then aged twelve, begged her parents to let her buy a horse with the money. A family friend, Sylvia Blackburn, helped with the enterprise. She owned horses and rode them in horse shows, so she found for Kristin a purebred American saddlebred mare, all black with a white star on her forehead. The mare, "Vivacious Lady," was nicknamed Vi. Sylvia taught Kristin to ride with an English saddle. "She really scorned Western riding as being an undisciplined, sloppy kind of riding," Kristen said. Vi seemed to scorn that sort of thing, too, and had a beautiful collected trot and other gaits that helped her and Kristin go on to earn many blue ribbons at horse shows.

At first, Sylvia boarded Kristin's horse at her barn, but when the Thygesons moved to Los Altos, which was perfect horseback-riding country, it seemed reasonable to move Vi over there. First, they needed to create a paddock and build a barn. Building the barn and paddock was perhaps the best experience Kristin and her father ever had together. "This was a wonderful and generous thing on my father's part," Kristin said. Phil was willing but only under the condition that Kristin work with him every step of the way. "He would never work on it unless I was out there pounding nails or holding the end of a board or grinding away with the hand posthole digger. It was all done by hand." Even though digging postholes in the incredibly hard clay was a grueling process, Kristin loved the work. "It was really the best part of any relationship I had with my father by far." It was Phil's expression of love, for the paddock and barn were purely for Kristin's benefit. Phil taught her a lot about how to build a structure. And he refused to buy precut lumber. He liked to cut his own boards and she had to help.[6]

The project took the better part of a year. When they had finished and there was a fenced paddock and a tack room, Vi came to live at the hilltop. Then Kristin wanted a foal. "The stud fee was fifty dollars for a beautiful Arabian stud, so the foal was half–Arabian, half-saddlebred." It wasn't clear for a while whether Vi was pregnant, but eventually she began to show. Before the family even expected it, she foaled. "What happened was my father heard Vi just out of her mind because the foal had slid under the fence and down the embankment next to the garage. Vi made such a ruckus that my father came out to see what was going on and found the foal. He picked up the foal … and scooted her under the fence and back to her mama, but Vi had never been a mother and she wouldn't let the foal nurse."[7] Even with the help of a veterinarian, Vi refused her foal. They tried tying her up with ropes, but she would kick the foal. Finally, the vet recommended that they bottle-feed. They used homogenized cow's milk, but after three days, the foal died. They were not sure why she died, but suspected that either she wasn't getting enough nourishment or got an acute case of colic from the cow's milk.

The loss was so devastating to Kristin that she could not go to school for a week. She stayed home and wept. She buried the foal herself under a fig tree on the hilltop. Her parents understood that she needed to go through the mourning process on her own.[8] She never bred Vi again, and loved her dearly all through her remaining school years. When she went away to college, she made the wrenching decision to give Vi to a family who wanted her. She knew her childhood had ended and she could not take her dear friend Vi with her.

20. The Glory Days of Academic Medicine

When it came time for Phil to work full-time at the new Francis I. Proctor Foundation in San Francisco, it reduced the family income. "My mother always said to any proposal of this sort, 'Of course we can live on less,'" Kristin recalled.[1] Ocular research work was *always* more important than money in the Thygeson family. Late in life, Phil shocked Marcus, who had gone into private practice in gastroenterology, by remarking, "I couldn't stand being in private practice. It was too much hard work." There was always a waiting room full of patients and not enough time to take care of everyone. Marcus, a Harvard-trained physician who was having his own struggles with private practice, remembered thinking, "Why didn't you tell me that ten years ago?"[2]

Phil also did not particularly covet the income that private practice physicians made. He believed that doctors were supposed to contribute to the welfare of human societies and the species at large without expecting a lot of money in return. O'Connor said, "I think he resented wealthy doctors. I think he thought they charged too much money, in many cases. This was particularly true of general surgeons. He would occasionally make some disparaging remarks about very wealthy doctors."[3] Phil and Ruth Lee never did accumulate much cash wealth, though they managed, with the help of Elizabeth Proctor, to acquire spectacular parcels of land.

Many of Phil's views on the creation of the Proctor Foundation were formed by his past experiences and observations. When he worked at Columbia University, there had been 3,000 square feet of laboratory space. That was not much, really, but it was a good start. Phil thus demanded at the outset 3,000 square feet of laboratory space for the Proctor. Fortunately, that space did not cost the Proctor endowment anything, as the family of Berthold Guggenhime, a grateful patient of Dr. Cordes, chairman of the Department of Ophthalmology, donated the money to purchase the space in the new Medical Sciences Building at UCSF.[4]

The Proctor Foundation's largest mandate was basic research, and this set it apart from other eye research foundations around the country. Its work included being a tertiary care facility for difficult cases, combining clinical and laboratory research where the combination was fruitful. The research emphases at the Foundation were three in number — microbiology, immunology and uveitis, and experimental pathology.[5] Dr. Proctor's great passion was infectious disease, so that was a common thread through much of the research.[6]

According to Phil, at the time of the Proctor Foundation's founding, "the etiology of trachoma was still in limbo."[7] For Phil especially, trachoma was an important research focus. Phil, Ruth Lee, and Dr. and Mrs. Proctor were devotes of preventive ophthalmology,[8] so the Proctor Foundation devoted time and resources early on to the prevention of trachoma in children.[9] The foundation's work later expanded from its original research mandate to include teaching medical students, residents in ophthalmology, and, especially, postgraduate research fellows from around the world.[10] Uveitis, "inflammation of the uvea" or middle structures of the eye, was the primary research interest of Phil's successor as Foundation director, G. Richard O'Connor, and remains a Proctor research interest today.

The first director of the Proctor Foundation, from 1947 to 1959, was Dr. Michael J. Hogan, described by Phil as Dr. Cordes's "right-hand man." Mrs. Proctor had initially insisted that Phil be the director, but he declined on the grounds that he would do better as a member of the board of governors and the staff, but not as lead administrator. Perhaps his memories of what happened to him in New York were still too fresh. However, Phil did not like the choice of Hogan because he believed he "was not really interested in external disease," the Proctor Foundation's specialty. Phil thought Hogan "kept the foundation going very well," but that his contributions — in uveitis and electron microscopy — were not what Mrs. Proctor had set up the foundation to pursue.[11] He also faulted Hogan for being a mediocre fundraiser, telling the story of how Hogan routinely kept his patients waiting thirty minutes to an hour before each appointment. A wealthy patient of his got tired of that, moved to Portland, Oregon, and gave her new ophthalmologist half a million dollars that, presumably, could have gone to the Proctor Foundation.[12]

Phil was not always tactful when recounting the mistakes of colleagues. He told others of the time Hogan took a cotton swab contaminated with infectious disease and absentmindedly introduced it into the patient's other, healthy eye. Ruth Lee was no more diplomatic. Dr. Hogan, she said, laughing, "didn't believe in the germ theory. None of this new-fangled stuff." Phil interjected, "He just paid no attention to...." Ruth Lee finished his sentence, "trivial things like that." The upshot was that there was an unacceptable number of post-cataract infections connected to Hogan's surgeries.[13] This was before the days of specialized infections committees in hospitals. Phil and his private practice colleagues in San Jose were scrupulous about avoiding doctor-induced infections. Phil proudly said that he had never caused a surgical infection. Hogan was considered such a good doctor and was so highly esteemed that he was forgiven for this particular lapse. Nevertheless, it bothered Phil that Hogan would not set up an infections-related committee at Proctor, and he tried to remedy that by teaching infection prevention there.[14]

Phil was so interested in preventive ophthalmology that he and his colleagues participated in writing and publishing a book entitled *Preventive Ophthalmology*. As O'Connor recalled, it was not a popular topic and it was not easy to attract a publisher. However, a publisher in New York agreed to publish it. In clinical settings, Phil was especially adamant about hand-washing. "He made a point of hand-washing, and he made a point of having the patient know he was washing his hands," said O'Connor. "That was an important thing to teach residents also, as far as preventing the contamination of a new patient's eyes with the products of an old patient." Phil wanted every society in the world to consider hand washing necessary and acceptable. The problem with his teaching style was that he "tended to be rather extreme in whatever he took on so that he tended to push certain things very much.... He was a proselytizer."[15] According to O'Connor, if postsurgical infections following eye surgery exceed one-tenth of 1 percent, it is appropriate to start asking if something is wrong with the sterile technique, the handling of the instruments, preparations put into the eye, or even ventilation of the surgery room. Phil understood that the cornea heals very quickly and that if there is a postsurgical infection, it is often introduced while the patient is in the hands of the medical professional.[16]

Phil was considered a wonderful teacher and diagnostician. "He was known far and wide for being a good bedside teacher, a good teacher at the site where the patient was being examined," O'Connor explained.

> Usually he would allow the student, a young doctor, to examine the patient first and say what he thought was going on with the patient.... Then he would correct or comment on, and lead the discussion in that way.... This was without laboratory. This was clinical examination, which was the fundamental aspect of the training program at the Proctor Foundation.... [I]n the case of external disease of the eye, it was always supported by laboratory findings. We always did cultures and scrapings on anything that was even remotely connected to infection or allergy.[17]

Phil loved routine microscopy — taking a scraping, making a slide, growing cultures and examining everything under a microscope. When fancier new technologies became available, such as the electron microscope, he was not very interested. He was an old-fashioned microscopist who had his microscope from the 1930s on his desk all of his life. He took a microscope with him when he traveled. He also loved his camera. As O'Connor explained, color photographs were a "big boon ... the idea that a given patient could be recorded very accurately by a photograph of the eye. Here's the way the lesion looked on December 12th. And here's the same patient three weeks later after steroid treatment. Look at what's happened."[18] The technology to take really good photographs of the eye became available in the early 1940s, but few doctors used it with as much enthusiasm as Phil and David Donaldson. Donaldson, of the Howe Laboratory in Boston, developed the "stereo camera for close-up pictures with a bright, simultaneously-triggered flash."[19]

Echoing Phil's sentiments, O'Connor lamented the twenty-first century loss of careful clinical examination followed by diligent laboratory work. "I think ... there tends to be a slacking off of that particular kind of examination, doing cultures and scrapings for diagnostic purposes. First of all, many ophthalmic facilities don't have their own laboratories any more." If they do scrapings, they have to send the material to commercial laboratories that may well not have technicians half as skilled as Masao Okumoto, long the chief laboratory technician at the Proctor Foundation. Instead, ophthalmologists may take an easier route, especially if they believe it's a common, curable infection. "Many people feel they can just treat those conditions with combinations of antibiotics and steroids and get away with it," O'Connor said. However, when this strategy failed to cure a patient, the next step could be a return to the way Phil practiced ophthalmology. O'Connor said, "[A]s a tertiary center at the University of California, we saw all the bad cases that had been failures in the outside practice, people who had been treated with steroid/antibiotic combinations and failed to get well or got worse."[20]

Phil believed it was impossible to treat anything effectively if you did not know what it was. He opposed guesswork and even opposed treatment unless absolutely necessary because he thought some drugs were worse than the natural history of the disease. O'Connor saw Phil as a sort of "therapeutic nihilist," because "he believed that very few conditions actually required active treatment. We often joked about that. He would see a patient and make a diagnosis, and I would say, 'Well, Phil, how did you treat that patient?' 'Kodachrome therapy,' he would say. 'We took a picture of the patient and he got better.' ... [Phil] used very simple remedies: zinc sulfate drops or something of that nature that was not likely to be harmful." Phil's ability to please patients while not offering much in the way of treatment gave rise to some envy among younger doctors. O'Connor said, "I always joked with him and I said, 'Phil, it's easy for you to do that because if you have gray hair, the patient tends to respect your opinion, and will not demand expensive medication.'"[21] Phil did not hand out placebo remedies and claim they were nonplacebo medications. He worked with patients psychologically, which is somewhat ironic given that he considered psychology and psychiatry to be fools' arts early in his career. He came to have a healthy respect for the power of the mind on a person's health. He even believed that glasses could sometimes be an effective placebo.[22]

Many patients, of course, wanted to leave an office visit with a prescription, as if that were the only way for the visit to be worth the time and money involved. Because Proctor was a tertiary care center, from time to time its ophthalmologists took care of patients who had received poor treatment from the doctors who referred them. Phil was aware of the rapid rise in medical malpractice suits late in his career, and he deplored them. He did not tell patients that their referring doctor had made a mess of their case, but he would privately tell the doctor what he thought had gone wrong. On rare occasion, he felt that malpractice suits were warranted, but that was only in the case of gross negligence. He understood that doctors were fallible; he never forgot the cases where he felt he had made a mistake.

To read Phil's oral history is to get a sense that establishing and maintaining a fairly autonomous, university-based eye research foundation was a struggle. Autonomous and university-based were, at least in his eyes, an oxymoronic combination. He claimed that Dr. Cordes never wanted to have the Proctor Foundation be "a separate unit." "He went along with my ideas because he really couldn't do anything else, but he didn't approve of it at all," Phil said. "He made one major effort to combine [the Proctor Foundation] with the [eye] department."[23] Phil's story of that takeover attempt has a bit of drama to it. At the elite, all-male Bohemian Club, Cordes went into a huddle with Dr. John B. de C.M. Saunders, a dean at UCSF who at one point served on the Proctor Foundation's Board of Directors, and purportedly "cooked up a deal where by administrative edict the Proctor Foundation would become a part of the department." Phil learned of this from Cordes's secretary and wrote a letter of complaint to the president of the university, Clark Kerr, who looked up the founding papers of the Proctor Foundation, saw that it could not be done, and reprimanded Saunders. The punchline of the story is that Saunders refused to speak to Phil for an entire year, and then became friends with him.[24]

That was not the end of the tension between the two of them, however. Saunders wanted to change the foundation's research emphasis to optics. According to Phil, Saunders "thought infectious disease had been taken care of by antibiotics and therefore had no future and that we should change to optics, which had a future."[25] By Phil's account, there were other takeover dramas, of greater and lesser degree of threat, and he fended off every one of them. The eye department and the Proctor Foundation ended up having a generally collegial relationship, with Proctor generously lending space to the department's pathology lab when there was a space shortage elsewhere. Phil's view was that over the years the Proctor Foundation did much more for the eye department than vice versa. The relationship was, he said, something of a "one-way street."[26]

The staff of the Proctor Foundation was not limited to ophthalmologists. It soon had Ph.D.s as well as M.D.s, which is as Phil wanted it to be. "The value of an institute," he said, "is that you have diversity in the staff and that you break down barriers between disciplines and so on. The trouble with a department is that you get really ingrown.... So we had consultants in dermatology, microbiology, physiology, and several others. Right from the first we wanted to take advantage of the university consultants."[27] The Proctor also got consulting help in electron microscopy and anatomy. These consultations led to research collaborations. Phil worked with staff of the Hooper Foundation at UCSF, including the staff of Karl Meyer's laboratory, and with Dr. Ernest Jawetz.[28] There was a generous exchange of information. Phil, for example, learned from Bernice U. Eddie, an assistant of Dr. Meyer, how to "cultivate the psittacosis agent."[29]

There were also good collaborations with the Department of Ophthalmology at UCSF. One of the best collaborations involved working with Lavelle Hanna of the Department of Microbiology. She worked on Chlamydia and adenoviruses. In those days, it was possible to inoculate human volunteers with potentially dangerous ocular diseases in order to study their natural history and treatment. Miss Hanna, who had an M.S. degree but who, in Phil's eyes, was equivalent to a star Ph.D., ran the culture lab and cultivated the disease specimens. Phil was unable to think in terms of pure collegiality between the Proctor Foundation and UCSF, so he described Miss Hanna as "a wonderful jewel" that "we stole from the pathology department." She did such a good job with the cultures that Phil was moved to say, "Without her we couldn't have handled it."[30]

During the early Proctor Foundation years, from 1946 to 1952, Phil served on the prestigious American Board of Ophthalmology. It had been established by the two luminaries in optical refraction, Phil's mentor Edward Jackson and Walter Lancaster. Their purpose was to regulate ophthalmology by making board certification available and to improve the quality of teaching in the field. Phil believed he was nominated to serve on the board by the American Ophthalmological Society. Board service consisted of three meetings a year, during which board members examined candidates for board certification.

When Phil took the board certification exam in 1930, it had happened all in one day. "It cost me twenty-five dollars, and in the evening I was told [by the chairman of the American board] at a cocktail party that I had passed."[31] By and large, he had an easy time taking the exam, though there were about ten subject areas to cover. Finnoff had told him he needed to take the exam, but he did not feel compelled to prepare in any significant way. However, he decided to read Ernst Fuchs's classic textbook twice through on the train on the way to the exam in Detroit.[32] He miscalculated the time zone, believing that Detroit was on Central Time when in fact it was not, and arrived when all of the other candidates were already well along in their written exam. The examiners let him start late, and he still finished ahead of most of the others.

"I remember going up for ophthalmoscopy, and they gave me one patient to examine. I examined her and gave her the correct diagnosis, and then the examiner said, 'Who trained you in ophthalmoscopy?' and I said, 'Finnoff.' He said, 'Goodbye,' that's all there was to it. Then I went up for refraction, and they gave me the cross cylinder to define, which I did correctly. And they said, 'Who trained you in refraction?' I said, 'Jackson,' and they said, 'Goodbye.'"[33] He also breezed through pathology, though he had a little bit of trouble with perimetry, the study of visual fields, which was not an area of strength for him. He got into an argument with the examiner in anatomy, Parker Heath, over "the attachment of the vitreous. It turned out I was right, and he was wrong." Phil laughed over this story, especially the part about Heath inviting him to play tennis after the exam.[34]

It was an honor to be asked to be an examiner. Phil was asked to examine orally in one of the subspecialty areas, but not in his own strongest field. "They figured you'd be too tough on the candidate," Phil explained. In the written exam, however, you could contribute questions from your area of specialty. Phil wrote microbiology and pathology questions. He was never allowed to examine orally in external disease, so he settled for "pathology or refraction or ophthalmoscopy...."[35]

Marcus tells a version of the evolution of the ophthalmology board exams. His mother Ralda Lee ran into an ophthalmologist who had either been examined by Phil or had heard through the grapevine about Phil's record as an examiner. Ralda and the ophthalmologist "got on the topic of Phil Thygeson, and this guy said, 'Phil Thygeson is the reason they changed the ophthalmology boards.' Basically, he was such an expert in external eye disease and had such high standards in terms of what people should know that he was flunking everybody. So they finally changed the ophthalmology board exam so that the experts did not test people in their own field."[36] This is an interesting counterpoint to Phil's version of the story. Ruth Lee indirectly corroborated Marcus's story, as she sometimes assisted Lea Stelzer, the secretary of the examining board. Ruth Lee would help check the candidates in, take their names and other information, and tell them how long they needed to wait. "They'd say, 'I've got Thygeson coming up. Is he terrible?' I'd say, 'I hear he's terrible.'" Ruth Lee laughed while telling this story. "The candidates were often terribly frightened," she noted.[37] One was so distraught he accidentally put a microscope lens through the prized slide of famous ophthalmologist Frederick Verhoeff. Phil was examining with Verhoeff in pathology, so he was an eyewitness to the event. Verhoeff was so upset he attacked the candidate and had to be pulled off of him. Verhoeff never examined for the Board of Ophthalmology again. In Phil's view, Verhoeff was a fool for using a prized slide in the context of an exam.[38]

Phil was criticized for being hard on some candidates. He did not say whether he failed a young female ophthalmologist from Canada for not being able to answer his question, but whatever he did, he got in trouble. He asked her about onchocerciasis, also known as river blindness, which is still common in Africa. He thought it was a good question about a cause of blindness outside the United States and Canada. The candidate thought that it was completely irrelevant to her and her future because the disease did not exist where she was going to practice. Evidently, she complained far and wide about Phillips Thygeson, MD, and the feedback circled back to him. He also got in trouble over another candidate, who made a terrible mistake during a clinical examination. The candidate, from the University of Pennsylvania, was asked to check for corneal sensation in a unilateral herpes case. He took a bit of cotton, swiped it over the corneal lesion in the infected eye, and then swiped the contaminated cotton in the healthy eye. That so upset Phil he flunked him on the spot. Phil was roundly reproached for being too harsh with a nervous candidate.[39]

Even though he never wrote a book on ophthalmology — to Ruth Lee's great chagrin — Phil was a frequent contributor of chapters to the books of other prominent ophthalmologists. His view was that writing a book took an awful lot of time and that any book would quickly become out of date. "Phil not only didn't write a book, but he kind of resented the efforts of others around him to write books and sometimes referred to these 'awful books' being written at Proctor," O'Connor said.[40]

Daniel Vaughan credited Phil with helping him publish what became a classic textbook of ophthalmology. In 1954, Jack Lang of Lang Medical Publications asked Phil to write a comprehensive book on ophthalmology. "Dr. Thygeson said he didn't have time, but [there was] this young, eager Dr. Vaughan who would be glad to do it. And that's how I happened to get involved," Vaughan said.[41] Some people thought of Vaughan as Phil and Ruth

Lee's surrogate son and as Phil's "heir apparent." *Ophthalmology*, currently in its sixteenth edition, has been published in many languages and has been touted as the world's most popular ophthalmology text. Phil finally got interested in it at around the eighth edition and contributed a chapter on the cornea, though he declined to sign his name to it. His comment to Vaughan about book writing was, "When you're over fifty, you're too old to write a [textbook]; if you're under fifty, you're too young."[42] The fact was that Phil did not want to do all of that work.

Although Phil was a diligent worker, he was known to balk at awkward times. O'Connor said,

> He didn't like doing anything because it was a duty. For example, on papers on which he collaborated he would agree to be coauthor and then when the deadline approached, he wouldn't have done his part of the paper, and I would get after him.... He would say, "I'll just finish it on the weekend." And then Monday would come ... and I would say, "Well, Phil, have you got your part ready?" "Well, I just had a mental block on doing that," he would say. "Mental block" would mean that he recognized that he had promised to do a piece of work and he didn't feel like doing it....[43]

In other words, Phil was as human as the next person.

21. World Health Organization and World Class Editing

The 1950s was a decade of great success for the Proctor Foundation, which attracted federal funding and launched successful research initiatives. The National Institutes of Health (NIH) grew a great deal after the war, and large grants were awarded to Proctor research projects.[1] This era of expansion in world public health and medical research offered Phil new opportunities as an international traveler.

In the 1950s and 1960s, Phil was a consultant to the World Health Organization (WHO) and served on the organization's Expert Panel on Trachoma. Trachoma was one of several infectious or preventable eye diseases in which the WHO invested time and energy. It was, and is, "the most common cause of infectious blindness in the world."[2] Phil had to travel to Geneva for general WHO trachoma meetings and was assigned to visit a number of countries struggling to control trachoma. The focus included some southern European countries, such as Italy, Yugoslavia, Spain, and Portugal. In addition, Phil said, "North Africa was pretty bad; Egypt was the worst."

The geography of trachoma was a product of poverty and warm climates, and especially of flies spreading the disease from person to person. "If you did nothing but just improved the economics, you could completely change the trachoma picture. You wouldn't have to treat the trachoma; it would just disappear on the basis of personal hygiene and fly control," Phil remarked. Of course, changing the economics of a developing region was beyond the scope of the WHO, so the focus was on prevention and treatment, especially on controlling "periodic epidemics of bacterial conjunctivitis which spread the trachoma."[3]

For the WHO, Phil was an expert consultant rather than a field doctor working with patients. "I did a lot of surveys, and I surveyed the laboratory work [in Tunisia, Algeria, and Egypt]. One year I made a survey of the whole Mediterranean area, and another year I surveyed South America."[4] The surveys were in no way definitive; Phil did what he could to get a sense of the scope of the problem in a few weeks on each trip. Elizabeth Proctor made it possible for Ruth Lee and Kristin to accompany Phil to Egypt when Kristin was seventeen, a trip she never forgot. More often, Phil and Ruth Lee were apart during these trips. When that happened, he wrote her postcard after letter after postcard, virtually every day.

Phil's letters and postcards to Ruth Lee are interesting because they were brimming with their collaborative work. On balance, they were more work assignment than anything else. They rarely expressed only the personal, though Phil told of his sightseeing adventures and his local hosts, who sometimes became his and Ruth Lee's friends. In a letter he posted from Lisbon in the summer of 1966, he wrote a couple of short descriptive paragraphs about arriving in Portugal and then changed the subject to a medical meeting that he and Ruth Lee were in charge of organizing. "More thoughts on the August program: 1. Should we look into transport from the hotel to medical center?? 2. American Airlines has a superb booklet on California which each of the foreign visitors should have. Can you write or call American Airlines to see if these would be available? ... 3. As to drinks — in Asilomar — we will need Brandy for a late snifter and sherry along with Bourbon and Scotch...." From there, he moved on to the abstracts and program, for which Ruth Lee was responsible. He even asked her to review a scientific paper he had not read to "see if it should be duplicated for transmission." Finally, he told her to go ahead and buy a station wagon on "bank terms." These work instructions were followed by, "Love you madly — Think of you every minute of the day and long to get back into your lovely arms where I belong."[5]

In an undated letter written soon after, while he was in Geneva en route to Algiers, Phil asked Ruth Lee to go to Asilomar to work out details of the conference. From Algiers, he dictated the list of sponsors that should be listed on the final program. And finally, he asked her to take his scribbles and turn them into decent business letters. "I'm enclosing a couple of letters for you to write — my Darling." He closed the letter with the words, "Love you madly — I really need you desperately. No life at all without you. Thank the good lord you still love me. I adore you."[6] The personal was completely interwoven with the professional. Neither of them ever wished it to be otherwise. Phil recognized that he deeply needed Ruth Lee, for affection and companionship and to do the thousand and one tasks he wanted to delegate to her and her greater competence. "I'm really a 'dependent' because I need you every minute of the day," he wrote.[7] Among other roles, Ruth Lee was his executive secretary, in charge of passing on his orders to colleagues. One person was to make sure the geraniums were in flower for a special occasion; another was to make sure the projectors worked in the meeting rooms. Sometimes he wrote to her twice daily. In one such evening letter, he called himself her "dependent" and added, "It is so wonderful to be married to an angel wife.... And how did you ever love me — It's a miracle."[8] When things went wrong, he sent a letter with a paragraph full of sentences that began "Sorry...." The paragraph ended, not insignificantly, with an oblique (but pre-feminist) compliment to Ruth Lee: "*What a staff I have!!*"[9]

The WHO did not run its own laboratory in Geneva, but instead provided grants to support laboratories in trachoma-endemic regions. Phil reported to Dr. Peter Maxwell-Lyons, who served in the virology department of the WHO. A British citizen, Maxwell-Lyons became a good friend of the Thygesons and went on to become the WHO liaison for the United Nations. The initial WHO trachoma committee was an illustrious group of eight or ten ophthalmologists, including Roger Nataf, with whom Phil had worked in Tunisia, and Giambattista Bietti, a famous Italian ophthalmologist. Phil prepared a lot of "working papers" before the meetings of the committee in Geneva. Ruth Lee was often at the meetings, if not actually in the meeting room, working with her typewriter up to the last minute. The WHO handled the travel arrangements for its expert committee members, and Phil had to insist that he be identified as a professor rather than as an American doctor. "[T]he American doctor was supposed to be wealthy, and the hotel rate would be raised about ten or twenty percent ... whereas the American professors were well known to be poverty-stricken."[10]

Later, Ruth Lee did not travel so much, either internationally or domestically. However, travel, especially exploring other cultures, held a place in her heart all her life. When she was no longer traveling, she counseled her granddaughter to make the most of her own first trip to Europe. To Mara Thygeson, she wrote,

> It is bound to change you and change your life a little, and I want you to savor every minute of it. You are stepping into HISTORY.... Your own world you have always with you, so please let this trip give you that other world — that rich world of the great past that is your heritage. Read and think and *feel* about all that while you are there. We go to the moon today, but we aren't building Notre Dames or Canterbury Cathedrals. Sense the *dreams* as well as the labor that built them.... Try to catch the poetry of it all, my darling.[11]

Phil had fewer opportunities to consider the romantic side of history. He was busy doing his lab work and writing. He occasionally got into and then out of stressful situations with his friends and colleagues. Nataf, with whom he was collaborating on a report on etiologic problems of trachoma

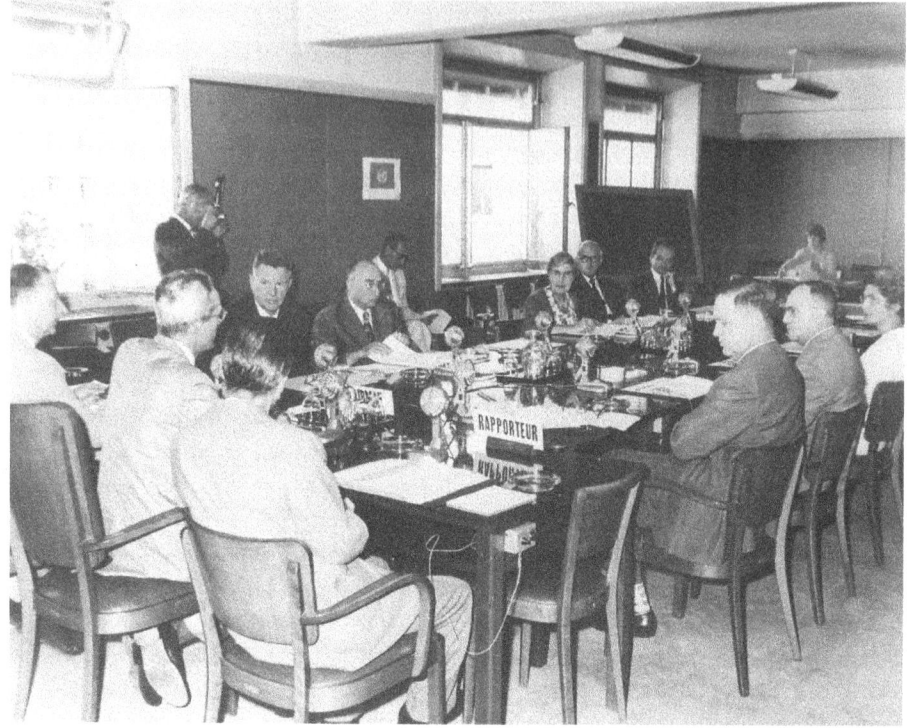

The 1952 meeting of the World Health Organization's Expert Committee on Trachoma in Geneva. Phillips Thygeson is first on the left of the left side of the table.

for the Ligue contre le Trachome, wrote in 1957 to say that he was surprised and upset that Phil had agreed "from the very first day" to write the first draft of their report and had apparently changed his mind. "You put me in a position of great embarrassment and my work plan for the year is upset.... I ask you, dear Phil, instantly revert to our original plan.... I insist that you write the Report.... Write to me right away to reassure me and confirm the dates."[12] This Phil did, thanking Nataf for his "good letter." Phil's letter was almost exclusively about trachoma, especially about the points of disagreement between himself and Nataf in their views on trachoma transmission and clinical manifestations, and on the report in question. As Nataf had, he closed with a gesture of friendship: "With warmest regards to you and your family, in which Ruth Lee joins me."[13]

As part of the WHO Expert Committee on Trachoma, Phil wrote the reports for the Second and Third Expert Committee meetings, in 1958 and 1963, respectively. He published the 1966 Report of the Fourth Scientific

Group on Trachoma.[14] Phil was also involved with a related WHO project, "Trachoma Reference Centres," and was its director from 1965 to 1970. Through this project, laboratories in the field could send specimens to more sophisticated labs for analysis and data cataloging. The Proctor Foundation became one such lab. According to Phil, it was the flagship lab. Others were located in London and Tunisia. The centers "had all the strains of Chlamydia that had been isolated and the pathologic specimens and the microbiology of the secondary infections, all the organisms that were found in the eye."[15] The work brought prestige to the Proctor Foundation and gave it an important international role in trachoma.

Phil liked being so international in his work and was very interested to see what happened in different countries. In Brazil, for instance, there was a tremendous amount of trachoma but there was also good cooperation from the Brazilian government. Together with the WHO, the Brazilian government managed to treat over a million cases of trachoma with sulfonamides with great success. In Australia, in contrast, there were treatment complications in the form of an allergic reaction, erytheme multiforme major. The problem was so upsetting, Phil said, that "the public health service of Australia cancelled the whole trachoma program."[16] Phil noticed a real difference between programs managed by the WHO and those managed by less skillful and experienced agencies. American Samoa, for example, had a "very poorly done" trachoma control program administered by the U.S. Department of the Interior.[17] Phil mentioned in various contexts that the Department of the Interior did not have the personnel or experience to manage medical programs well, unlike the Public Health Service and the WHO.

The WHO work was connected with other international trachoma-related efforts. Phil was an important member of a group of world experts who were the trachoma luminaries. The International Organization Against Trachoma, established in 1930, had Phil's early mentor in Tunis, Charles Nicolle, as its first president. It was connected with International Congress of Ophthalmology meetings and with the *Revue Internationale du Trachome*. Phil published in the journal in French in 1933, in English in 1955, and with Nataf in 1958. The International Organization against Trachoma had a prestigious gold medal it awarded from time to time. The Proctor Foundation was the first laboratory ever to receive the medal. Phil and his younger Proctor colleague, Chandler Dawson, were also awarded medals.[18]

Elizabeth Proctor had personal funds in addition to those earmarked in her husband's will for eye research. After the Proctor Foundation was well established, she generously gave large gifts that enabled the foundation — with the help of matching funds from the National Institutes of Health or the Regents of the University of California — to expand its physical space. In

1953, she gave a substantial sum to acquire space in the Medical Sciences Building. This gift was matched by the National Institutes of Health. Phil and O'Connor worked very hard to raise funds as well. By the 1980s, the foundation had expanded from 3,000 square feet of laboratory space to over 17,000 square feet. Three lots purchased on Kirkham Street in San Francisco, nestled right against a foliage-covered hill, became the core of the Proctor Foundation. The building, completed in 1954, was initially made possible by a $60,000 gift from Elizabeth Proctor matched by a gift from the Regents of the University of California. A significant sum was donated by Phil's grateful patient, Harry Hind, after whom the Harry Hind Research Library at 95 Kirkham Street was named.[19]

When time permitted, Phil was a prolific gardener at his and Ruth Lee's home in Los Altos. For their home garden they eventually hired Mr. Horiyuchi, a Japanese-born gardener, who spent many years tending their acreage and teaching them about plant care. The 95 Kirkham Street building is a reflection of Phil and Ruth Lee; it is flat-topped, surrounded by a beautiful oriental-style flowering garden, and is landscaped like the area around their house in Los Altos. Both 95 Kirkham Street and the Thygesons' Los Altos home featured flowering trees, camellia bushes, and wonderful outdoor patio spaces for sitting and having coffee. Phil loved to photograph both gardens. There is a deck on the second floor of the Proctor building where people can eat their lunch in the sun on days when the San Francisco fog has lifted. Mathea Allansmith, a former fellow trained at Proctor, loved the ambience. "We'd go upstairs and see the beautiful trees, the beautiful gardening, the planting, the cleanliness, the warmth of the wood in the building...."[20] Even now, the Kirkham Street building is a handsome oasis among more traditionally institutional UCSF buildings.

Forrest Davidson, of the well-known optical house Jenkel-Davidson, donated several thousand dollars to help set up an electron microscope on the bottom floor of the Proctor Foundation. A number of wonderful new technologies became available. What was exciting about the electron microscope, according to O'Connor, is that it made it possible to "actually see the infectious particles in some detail and see how they attack cell membranes." There was also fluorescence microscopy, "the labeling of antibodies with fluorescein so that you could look at sections of a tissue and see where antibodies had settled out by the fact that they fluoresced in ultraviolet light — a big boon." Finally, the scanning ultra-microscope "allowed us to see in three dimensions organisms like Toxoplasma attacking a cell," O'Connor said. "That was all very exciting."[21]

The lure of doing experimental inoculations with disease, in the tradition of Lavelle Hanna's work, drew some of the Proctor ophthalmologists to begin going to the Vacaville prison to get research subjects. The actual name of the facility was the State of California Department of Corrections Medical Facility at Vacaville. The proposed Proctor project had to pass a review with the Human Ethics Committee at UCSF.[22] A prison-related committee in Sacramento reviewed the proposed project for safety and scientific value and it was then passed to the director of Vacaville for review. The director was a psychiatrist sympathetic to their research aims. He approved their work and helped facilitate a call for volunteers. Phil gave oral presentations about proposed projects directly to the prisoners, explaining the risks and benefits. Volunteers were examined to make sure their eyes were healthy and suited to the study. They were paid $20 per infection.[23] Phil, Ernest Jawetz, and, in time, Chandler Dawson and perhaps some of the young fellows who were doing graduate training at Proctor went once or twice a week to Vacaville to examine patients. The doctors chose not to experiment with trachoma, considering it too dangerous, but they did inoculate inmates with inclusion conjunctivitis. "We were trying to work out everything with regard to the experimental infection, the incubation period, how the organisms behaved in the incubation period, how long the natural history lasted, what the clinical signs were, how long we could recultivate the Chlamydia."[24] They discovered something valuable, which is that if a case got well and they reintroduced the same pathogen, the disease would be milder the second time and might not appear at all the third time. In other words, there was some acquired immunity.

Phil thought that participating in these experiments did the prisoners good. He believed the ones he labeled "social misfits" appreciated being able to contribute to the benefit of others. Phil was convinced this program had a "therapeutic effect," as it "gave them something to think about."[25] The work was already well underway in 1964, when Chandler Dawson returned from England and joined the group. Dawson reported that the treatments given the prisoners were either oral sulfonamides or topical tetracycline. Dawson withdrew from the work when Jawetz "wanted to do one experiment that I thought was just too trivial." By then, he reported, Phil had already stopped working at Vacaville. "I think he felt uneasy about those experiments." Dawson definitely came to feel uncomfortable. "I got to feeling uneasy and started reading the Nuremberg War Crimes business, which is about human experimentation.... You know, we were very innocent about all that stuff in those days.... And then there is the whole ethics of people in prison."[26]

Dawson had noticed that Europeans were more conservative about this ethical issue than Americans were. Asked whether the prisoners' infections cleared up, he acknowledged that occasionally something surprising and disturbing would arise. "A couple of our patients got iritis—uveitis with it—

who knows what to do about that! It turns out there is a lymphocyte subtype ... that's associated with uveitis. Chlamydia is one of the triggers for that.... We had another guy who had a very peculiar corneal lesion and he had a monoclonal spike in one of his immunoglobulins, which suggested a pre-lymphoma condition of some kind. And again, we didn't know what was going on."[27] They made sure that all of the prisoners received antibiotics and steroids as needed, but because there was not extensive follow up after the experiments were run, they were not able to verify that no prisoner suffered harm.

It is not clear whether Phil had as many reservations as Dawson about human experimentation. In his oral history, he said of the experimentation that the prisoners "liked it, and the director of the hospital liked it, but then it was all thrown out by the writer Jessica Mitford. She was able to squash the whole program."[28] Mitford, an investigative journalist, argued publicly that it was abuse of prisoners to subject them to medical experiments as they were not really in a position to consent. This was not a new idea; the 1947 Nuremberg Code had set out the requirement that no coercion or constraint be involved in the consent process, a condition that was a contradiction in terms where prisoners were concerned.[29] Mitford's work received a lot of attention in 1973, when she published an article in *The Atlantic Monthly* that quoted a physician as saying, "Criminals in our penitentiaries are fine experimental material — and much cheaper than chimpanzees."[30] According to the Alliance for Human Research Protection, the Pharmaceutical Research and Manufacturers of America (PhRMA) acknowledged in 1976 that 85 percent of Phase I and II drug trials were being conducted on the nation's prisoners.[31] The FDA soon laid down the law that doctors receiving federal money for research could do only two kinds of research with prisoners. The two kinds were experiments that related *only* to conditions in prisons and experiments that had "the intent or reasonable probability of improving the health or well-being of the subject."[32]

The issue of human experimentation was also relevant to the work by Proctor researchers being done with Native Americans, especially children. Again, the ophthalmologists did their best to treat and cure. Phil thought it was a great loss to stop experimentation on humans. After all, chimpanzees and monkeys are different from human beings. "[V]olunteering for experiments did the prisoners good," he said. "It was all a mistake to stop the volunteering."[33] O'Connor made a cogent argument for why experiments on humans provide crucial information that can be obtained no other way:

> [I]f you really are to discover the cause of a human disease, you almost have to do some of those experiments, which seem dangerous and not fair to the experimental subject, but they ultimately accomplished the goal that you

needed to accomplish. It is true that apes, for example, have an immune system very similar to that of a man's, but it's not quite the same. So ultimately, those experiments with volunteers, particularly with blind volunteers, were necessary and justified.[34]

The advantage of blind volunteers, of course, was that they had no vision to lose and yet the natural history of an ocular disease could be followed by studying their eyes. If we remember the case of Clarence Brown, the experiment provided *the* long-awaited definitive proof of the cause of trachoma. O'Connor concluded, "I don't think that Phil Thygeson would have made the discoveries that he did make, if he hadn't had a freer hand with the use of human volunteers."[35]

Today, there is something unsettling about the idea of intentionally infecting a human eye, even a blind one, with a devastating disease that may or may not be fully treatable. As late as the 1960s, however, experiments with "volunteers and prisoners" were common. Whether prison inmates could ethically be said to be able to volunteer didn't seem to invite much debate decades ago. "If a prisoner would volunteer," Phil said in the 1980s, "we could either pay him or commute his sentence.... We can't do it now."[36] Medical students and residents also volunteered. Americans who volunteered to be infected with yellow fever in an effort to study the disease were considered national heroes at one time. During World War II, some conscientious objectors who wished to demonstrate their patriotism along with their commitment to pacifism volunteered for risky experimental infections with malaria, parasites, pneumonia, and extreme dietary, climatic, and altitude conditions.[37]

It is important to place this experimental practice in historical context and to recall that using human volunteers was strongly connected to World War II. Illinois prisoners were infected by the hundreds with experimental cases of malaria in an effort to find ways to treat the disease in American soldiers serving in the Pacific. A committee known as the Ivy Committee evaluated the experiments and pronounced them "ideal" in their conforming to American Medical Association (AMA) rules.[38] In fact, the Ivy Committee and the AMA rules influenced each other. In Europe, the Nuremberg Code discouraged certain kinds of medical experimentation; in the United States this was not the case. "It is difficult to overemphasize just how common the practice became in the United States in the postwar years," O'Connor said. After the Food and Drug Administration (FDA) revised its drug-testing guidelines in 1962, O'Connor continued, "prisoners became almost the exclusive subjects in non-federally funded Phase I pharmaceutical trials designed to test the toxicity of new drugs."[39]

This situation went on into the 1970s until Jessica Mitford and public opinion changed everything. When volunteers were no longer available in the

United States, and Phil and other Proctor researchers wanted to test adenovirus type 8 experimentally, they turned to two volunteers in other countries, one in Japan and one in Italy. In Japan, the volunteer was isolated in a special room, everything went as planned, and the volunteer was treated and cured. In Italy, however, the renowned ophthalmologist Giambattista Bietti was "very careless," Phil said, "and the virus spread all over the hospital. They had to close the hospital. He got a reprimand from the state health department for letting this thing go through the hospital."[40] The paper that resulted from the experiments did not include Bietti as author; the Japanese doctor, Yuhihiko Mitsui, was listed as third author, with Phil listed fourth.[41] Proctor doctors also did research using animals. The Proctor did not have animals of its own, but would use UCSF's supply of research animals. The researchers mostly used monkeys, mice, rabbits, and guinea pigs. Over time, there were three accidental infections among lab technicians and an animal handler — one with trachoma, one with adenovirus 8, and one with parakeet psittacosis.[42]

Throughout these years, Phil was very active as a researcher. In spite of declining the Proctor directorship initially, Phil found he cared a great deal about how the foundation was run and became convinced that no one could or would do the job exactly as he wanted it done. He was named the Proctor Foundation's second director, with a tenure lasting from 1959 to 1970. The new position meant giving up his private practice in San Jose and becoming a full-time Proctor employee. It also meant a loss of income because private practice paid better. A letter from UCSF chancellor J. B. de CM Saunders dated May 17, 1966, advised Phil that he had been advanced to "Professor, Step V, without salary in the Department of Ophthalmology," and that, as director of the Proctor Foundation, he would have a salary of $23,500 a year.[43] Phil was more than willing. He had always been a commuter, and now he had to drive nearly eighty miles a day to get to and from work. He and Ruth Lee favored red cars and for many years he commuted in an orange-red Chevy and a fire engine red Ford Falcon station wagon.

Phil had good reasons for having faith in his own abilities. He was, by all accounts, exceedingly talented, especially as a diagnostician and synthesizer of information. Like his father before him, he was a tireless reader. In Fritjof's view, Phil "had this encyclopedic knowledge, he had a fantastic memory, but most important, he was a voracious reader. What I remember more than anything else was that my father, when I was a child, ... every evening after dinner he would spend at least two or three hours reading journals. Every Saturday, every Sunday."[44] O'Connor said of Phil, "One of his talents was being able to remember things that he read and learned, and to dissect the wheat from the chaff so to speak, to discard that which was not really important ... and stick with a central line of what seemed correct. He had a prodigious memory." He was, in, short, "a very cogent observer," if not a remarkably original thinker.

Phil particularly admired "The Four Stumbling Blocks to Truth" penned by Roger Bacon in the thirteenth century. They are:

I. The influence of fragile or unworthy authority
II. Custom
III. The imperfection of undisciplined senses
IV. Concealment of ignorance by ostentation of seeming wisdom

O'Connor believed Phil's cockiness served him well. "[C]hallenging the observations of Noguchi — that took some doing."[45] Phil's willingness to say that anyone could be wrong helped him move his research along faster than if he had been more in awe of the great scientists who came before him. He was also willing to admit his own errors and make fun of himself, at least some of the time.

Phil had a charming, folksy quality, especially when he told stories. It probably helped him put people at ease. According to O'Connor, his stories "all had the quality of a Will Rogers character — a story that has some human interest, but not a lot of emotion put into it.... The story was told in an understated way, in kind of a Western idiom." Will Rogers was, in O'Connor's words, "part Indian in background ... and a hero of Western lore. Phil admired him tremendously."[46] Phil's former daughter-in-law Ralda Lee said he loved John Wayne and identified with the heroes and heroines in Western novels by Zane Grey and Louis L'Amour.[47] As often as not, Phil would laugh heartily at his own jokes. For sophisticated people from the East Coast, Phil had a way of coming across as "a kind of country bumpkin, which may be a reflection of Phil's upbringing in Minnesota. He wasn't worried about appearing polished or accomplished."[48] He certainly entertained his friends. In the 1980s, Vaughan said, "I'm always threatening to write down some of the things he says. He has sort of a macabre sense of humor."[49]

Phil got along beautifully with colleagues who never crossed him or challenged him. Given human nature and Phil's will to power, they were few in number. Phil had no conflicts whatsoever with his chief laboratory assistant, Masao Okumoto. Phil hired Okumoto very soon after he received his master's degree in microbiology from UC Berkeley. Okumoto ran the laboratory at Proctor and was by everyone's estimation extremely skillful. According to O'Connor, he was "every bit as good a cytologist and microbiologist as Phil by the end.... The two of them were like Ike and Mike in the laboratory."[50] Because Okumoto eschewed conflict, he did Phil's bidding for many years with nary a murmur of protest. Phil deeply appreciated Okumoto's talent and loyalty, calling him both "meticulous" and "extraordinary."[51] He pleased Phil by being a tireless worker, not stopping for coffee breaks and taking only one week of vacation time a year. He taught Proctor fellows and consulted with ophthalmologists needing sophisticated diagnostic assistance. He was such a wonderful ambassador for the Proctor that his nickname, according to Phil, was "Mr. Proctor Foundation."[52] Okumoto's name was on a number of papers coauthored by Phil, at first as a last author and later as an author whose name sometimes came before Phil's own.

A Thygeson family myth suggests that Phil gave away his thunder by letting younger, less experienced colleagues put their names first on published papers. It is said that Ruth Lee encouraged him to share credit with newer doctors working to make names for themselves in academic medicine. O'Connor agreed that Phil was generous in this regard, but opined that he was also always fair. "[I]f his work was the principal work, he made sure his name was the first name. That, of course, is all-important in writing.... [I]n that regard, it's a shame that Ruth Lee didn't have her name on some of these papers. One of the problems was that she didn't have a degree. So the editors of certain journals wouldn't have accepted her as a reasonable co-author...."[53] Like many others, O'Connor lamented that Ruth Lee was not formally credited with her significant contribution to many publications by Phil and other scientists at Proctor. "It's too bad in many ways," said O'Connor, "because Ruth Lee was extremely talented and articulate, and might have done a good deal of writing on her own if she had had that degree."[54]

As for how much ophthalmology Ruth Lee knew, not having been to medical school, O'Connor said that "by exposure all those years, she actually took on the knowledge of a medium-talented ophthalmologist...." She "knew all the vocabulary, which in ophthalmology is staggering.... She became absolutely indispensable as an editor."[55] She was also a coauthor who never got credit for one very sad and remediable reason: she did not have a college degree. If she had been able to put the letters signifying a bachelor's degree in science after her name, she would have been a multiply published coauthor of seminal ophthalmology papers.

Ruth Lee's editorial strengths included making sure that meaning was unambiguous and words were chosen with great care. She also admired brevity. To O'Connor, she often said, "Richard, too many words. Cut it down to the essentials." He was such an excellent writer that he and Ruth Lee were able to collaborate with great mutual respect and admiration. However, for lesser writers, her feedback could sometimes be overwhelming. "I think she was a pretty good diplomat," O'Connor said. "There were some who were incensed by what she said. That was a question of a conflict of egos, I think. A lot of people think that they are hot shots in writing, and they aren't in fact.... She was not at all namby-pamby. She insisted on what the correct usage here or there was. That offended some people."[56] Ruth Lee's role at Proctor extended beyond her editorial work. "Ruth Lee was tremendously important to the whole organization and worked very well and hard for the whole Proctor Foundation. She trained us, taught us how to write, and really was the glue that kept things together in many ways."[57]

During these years, Phil attended a considerable number of professional conferences. Ruth Lee often went along, with her manual typewriter in tow. "One of my persisting memories of Ruth Lee," O'Connor said, "is dragging that typewriter with her on trips — for example, to the American Ophthalmological Society ... still doing the very last version of Phil's paper (before he presented it) on her typewriter in their hotel room." She helped as many other ophthalmologists as her time allowed. Those in "other cities, for whom she did editing ... would write her notes and compliment her on her work and praise her for her devotion."[58] One of her authors said, "If you give her a rough draft of a paper, when it comes back it reads like a poem."[59] As with Algernon Reese, whose book on ocular tumors she edited, Ruth Lee's contribution was rarely acknowledged publicly. She was liberally praised and thanked privately, however.[60] A letter she kept in her files from Frederick C. Cordes, chairman of the Department of Ophthalmology at UCSF, read: "Thank you so much for editing the paper. I appreciate it no end and now will you please, as was our agreement, send me a bill for the work. It certainly has made all the difference in the world in the way the paper reads. Many, many thanks."[61] It appears that it was hard for her to bill her professional authors, so she often waited for them to raise the subject. Her devoted client Algernon Reese wrote a note to her with the salutation, "Dear 'Ghost.'" In it he mentioned how many compliments he had received on an article she had edited for him. "I am flying under false colors, dear ghost writer, but I love it. Thanks for the ride."[62] The lack of public acknowledgment was partly because there was no mechanism for acknowledging editing in individual papers published in medical journals, and partly because Ruth Lee did most of her editing work in an era when women were expected to serve selflessly, often on a volunteer basis.

For Proctor fellows, being edited by Ruth Lee was a rite of passage and, for most, a requirement of the fellowship. According to O'Connor, "if you wanted to publish this paper, you had to go through this process. That was the general rule. It was also the general rule that presentations to the public should be practiced in front of our own little Proctor group before they went out."[63] Though Ruth Lee spent many years volunteering her time to the Proctor Foundation, Elizabeth Proctor eventually decided it was not right for her to be a volunteer when everyone else was being paid. She wrote a letter, probably in the early 1970s, to the president of the university to argue that a salaried staff position be created and to articulate why Ruth Lee's position was not in violation of the university's policy against nepotism. Ruth Lee thus became a full-time paid editor until her retirement. After she officially retired, she kept on helping the Proctor fellows, a volunteer once more.[64] One of her more significant editorial contributions was the *Proctor Bulletin*, an elegantly designed newsletter that featured articles on the activities of the Proctor Foundation.

Ruth Lee also found time to assist international luminaries in the ophthalmology world. She saved a thank you letter from 1954 from the famous Bietti of the Clinica Oculistica dell'Universita di Parma. Bietti thanked her and then expressed his deep admiration for her ability to edit without changing his intended meaning, an issue that was critical for scientific publications. "May I ... congratulate you for the amazing way you exactly capture the meaning of my italo-english, transforming it to readable language? You have always found the proper expression without changing what I wanted to say. I was *never* misunderstood! Unbelievable!"[65]

22. International Fellows and Fellowship

Phil and Ruth Lee's work together spanned over six decades, beginning with his needing help getting through anatomy class. He would tell people that he had been a "B" student until he met Ruth Lee, after which he became an "A" student.[1] Perhaps because of his own history, he had a lot of compassion for students and their struggle to learn. As a product of first-rate preceptorships, he was a great believer in continuing education. Most important, he wanted to see top-notch research ophthalmologists in every region of the world. After all, discoveries were made where the problems were located. To be effective, an educational model had to be created, replicated, and carried on through generations. "[H]e was very much interested in spreading knowledge to all parts of the world, and he thought that the best way of doing that ... was bringing those men and women here to study for a year or two in a post-residency situation and have them go back and teach in the countries where they came from. It was very important, he thought, to have follow-up on what the eventual product was," said O'Connor. "Did they go back to teaching or did they just go back to some lucrative practice somewhere with a shingle on their wall saying they'd been to the Proctor Foundation for a year? ... He didn't like that idea."[2]

The Proctor Foundation Fellows program, established in the 1950s, is one of the Proctor Foundation's most important contributions to international ophthalmology. The program was designed to give bright, promising young ophthalmologists top-notch training in external eye disease and other Proctor specialties, such as uveitis, and have them pass their learning on to others in their home countries. Applicants to the Fellows program were carefully screened. "We always tried to get a commitment from the people we brought there to train, that they would go back and devote their lives to teaching others in the field," O'Connor said.[3] The strategy did not always work, but that was not due to lack of effort by Proctor staff. Phil and Ruth Lee were especially involved with the fellows and Ruth Lee did her best to offer them social support. She was aware of how lonely it was for young doctors to be far from home, perhaps for the first time, and often without family or friends.

The Proctor Fellows program was not an official part of the initial Proctor Foundation plan. However, very soon after the foundation was established, the first somewhat unofficial fellow appeared. He was Necdet Sezer of Turkey, and he went on to become the head of an eye institute in Istanbul.[4] He was very interested in trachoma, which is how he came to the Proctor in the late 1940s. In the early years, sometimes there were only a few fellows per year. Later, there were as many as eight at a time, and the one-year fellowship was extended to two years so fellows could complete their research projects. Funding was patched together from a variety of sources, both public and private. NIH money could go only to U.S. doctors, but other monies, such as the Cecilia Vaughan Memorial Fellowship, in honor of the daughter of Daniel Vaughan who died in a car accident at age seventeen, was earmarked for foreign fellows.[5] Early on, it cost only about $12,000 a year to support a fellow, though the cost became many times higher. Some of what was taught was tailored to what was possible in the home countries from which the fellows came. For instance, if a country did not have sophisticated laboratory facilities, it was not particularly useful to train ophthalmologists to be dependent upon them. On the other hand, every ophthalmologist would benefit from learning how to prevent eye disease.[6]

The first official fellow came to the Proctor in 1957. He was Prasanta Kumar Basu, born in 1922 in what is now Bangladesh. He was trained in India, and went to Canada in 1955 for "advanced corneal work." After his research work at Proctor, he returned to Canada and worked at the University of Toronto.[7] In 1958, Sigurd Ry Andersen, who was very talented in pathology, came from Denmark to spend five months at Proctor. According to the official account of the fellows, published as *Phillips Thygeson and the Proctor Fellows* on the twenty-fifth anniversary of the Proctor Foundation, Dr. Andersen "was so impressed by Dr. Thygeson and his staff that he decided to set up a Danish laboratory on ocular virology at the State Serum Institute in Copenhagen."[8] This was exactly the kind of outcome Phil hoped for. Andersen also sent to the Proctor Carl Mordhorst, a promising young Danish ophthalmologist who became, along with his wife, a lifelong friend of Phil and Ruth Lee. The third official fellow stayed and stayed. Chandler R. Dawson arrived in 1959, got involved with research on trachoma and other diseases, went to the Southwest repeatedly to do field work, and eventually became director of the Proctor Foundation after G. Richard O'Connor retired.

It took a while for the Proctor Fellows program to become internationally diverse. By 1971, fifteen years into the program, fellows had been selected from Canada, the United States, Denmark, Puerto Rico, Japan, Yugoslavia, Switzerland, Indonesia, Australia, Japan, Germany, Taiwan, and Italy. Men outnumbered women, but it is interesting to note that the first woman fellow came early in the program's history, in 1960, at a time when there were fewer than ten female ophthalmologists in the entire country.[9] Mathea R. Allansmith did six months of an ophthalmology residency at Stanford Hospital before doing a pediatric residency at UCSF and Stanford. She focused on pediatric allergies during her early years, but went into ophthalmology full-time in 1967 when she was an acting assistant professor at Stanford.[10]

Phil was able to come up with $3,000 in support for Allansmith's fellowship in exchange for her working on "some aspect of the combination of childhood and ocular problems and allergies." Phil suggested she work on vernal conjunctivitis, which she did, becoming one of the experts in the disease. By her own estimate, over time she wrote about a hundred papers on vernal conjunctivitis and giant papillary conjunctivitis (GPC), a sort of "false vernal conjunctivitis from contact lens wearing." She came to work at the Proctor in the summer of 1959, a moment she remembered clearly. "The reason I am so clear about the time is that Phil Thygeson never seemed to notice that I was nine months pregnant," Allansmith said. "And I always appreciated that he never, throughout all the years I knew him, cast sexism in my direction." Allansmith had the baby, her first, and went back to work soon thereafter. She had gleaned from sources other than Phil that it was unwise to take time off after the birth of a baby. "I really got that message loud and clear that maternity leave—you don't want to do that! When you come back, your turf is gone! So I stayed right on line the whole time."[11]

Allansmith loved getting clinical experience at the hands of Phil Thygeson.

> [T]he fellows would be upstairs in the Proctor Foundation, and Thygeson would be downstairs seeing patients. When he found someone who would be interesting—he knew each of our interests—he would have a person call us. And we would swoop from upstairs to downstairs as fast as we could go, and he would allow us to look at the patient. Then we would dart out of the room. We would discuss the patient that day or another day—he had to keep his practice moving....[12]

Other fellows were generous with their time, showing her how to use the slit lamp to visualize cross-sections of ocular tissue and so on. By the time Allansmith became a full-fledged ophthalmologist, she was forty years old and had six children. In support of her teaching during the years 1965–1973, Phil and Masao Okumoto provided special support in the form of lending her precious slides. "I would do [the] excellent quiz and microscope showing" that

Phil and Okumoto had prepared for the Proctor fellows, Allansmith said. "I would do that for about three hours and hear the discussion, which I wrote down as fast as I could." The miracle, as Allansmith saw it, was that Phil would allow Okumoto "to scoop up the whole thing — all the slides, explanations, extra pictures, and teaching guides — and I would cart the whole thing down to Stanford and teach it to the residents there the following day.... This was very generous of Phil Thygeson because these were his precious slides of very important cases that he had — one of a kind."[13] Jeffrey D. Lanier, another former fellow, reported that fellows were allowed to copy slides to create their own teaching materials. "We copied those slides and made teaching folders.... We made several hundred teaching slides that we took with us to teach. It extended the education we got for generations to come."[14]

Fellows particularly appreciated Phil and Okumoto's mentoring in how to take a good cytological specimen from a patient. To get a good conjunctival scraping,

> [y]ou put a drop of anesthetic in and then you flip the lid so you see the underside. You use this little flat spatula. You gently scrape off — you don't want too much or too little. And how much was too much or too little — Mas [Okumoto] was good about that. Thygeson was the main teacher but his work was enormously expanded by Mas. And then smearing the scraping on a slide and going through how to stain it and read it.... Mas did that — he taught us how to do it. But he wouldn't do it for us.[15]

Like other Proctor fellows, Allansmith was moved by Phil's dedication to her education and ongoing career path. "I think his primary motivation was to pass it on. Pass on the message of good scientific learning.... He was unconditionally generous. It was a while before I realized how precious his generosity was." Her borrowing from Proctor for Stanford residents bore fruit. "The residents, who took the national examination while I was teaching, scored higher in external disease than in any other subject. So [Phil] did that. He was enormously generous."[16] She had learned some of the finer points of the Phil-Masao Okumoto teaching method, a method frequently referred to as "show and tell." "You show what it is, then the person guesses what it is, then you tell what it is. Then you discuss its meaning," Allansmith said.[17]

Another thing she appreciated was the collegiality of the teaching environment. She called it a "community method." "We would all sit around this great big huge table ... maybe 20–25 people," eat brown bag lunches, learn and discuss. "Phil Thygeson fostered a collegiality that was more than that of any other faculty member I dealt with as a teacher, colleague or student."[18] Lanier, who sat at that table as well, recalled how comfortable the atmosphere was. "There was never an embarrassing situation in the entire time I was there. There were plenty of times when I didn't know the answer...."[19]

Phil also taught about how to survive and flourish in academic medicine. Allansmith learned about the art of grant writing and how to be a self-supporting self-advocate. Phil was very open about where funding for the Proctor's daily operations came from, so fellows were able to learn about the financial side of ocular research — what one could expect from the NIH, from a university, from industry, and from grateful patients.

Allansmith described Phil as personally charismatic. "He was enormously charismatic to attract people to come and share what they had to share.... He did not seem to be caught up in trying to control our lives.... A loving parent is the best way I can describe the way he was toward us."[20] But he was not very personal. "As far as I could see," Allansmith said, "he did not deal in personalities or what was going on in people's lives. I don't think we had a personal conversation."[21]

Phil could be very personal in some contexts, however. He became quite involved in Elizabeth Proctor's care as she encountered the problems of old age. She lost the central vision in her right eye to macular disease and, in the early 1960s, was faced with losing the vision in her right eye due to cataract. At one point, she checked into a hospital because she could not see well enough to care for herself at home. Phil arranged for her cataract surgery, and made sure all went smoothly. She suffered from severe arthritic joint pain and gastric pain. Before her final decline, she wrote in 1957 to the chairman of the Board of Trustees of the Proctor Foundation and to the chairman of the Executive Council of the American Ophthalmological Society to say that she wanted Phil to continue as trustee until he resigned or died. After that, she wanted David G. Cogan, the director of the Howe Laboratory at Harvard University, to continue in Phil's place as Proctor Trustee.[22] The letters are without dates or specific names, a sign perhaps that Elizabeth Proctor wrote them at a time of declining health.

Ruth Lee has been described as an affectionate parent figure in the context of the Proctor fellows. She was more personal with the fellows than was Phil. "There was a social life attached to Proctor," Allansmith said. "[T]he family-ness of the Proctor Foundation was very strong and I did not find that elsewhere in my career. It extended to all Proctor fellows and students of Proctor fellows." Ruth Lee's expressiveness and affectionate nature made her the matriarch and nurturer of the Proctor staff and fellows. She brought flowers for the seminar room table every time she came to the Proctor. Phil picked fruit from their orchard and brought peaches and apricots in buckets to share with everyone. "I respected and admired and I owe a great deal to Phil Thygeson. But I loved Ruth Lee," Allansmith said. "She was such a good human being. And she just had such good moral, internal characteristics."[23]

When Allansmith showed Phil a paper that she and others at Proctor had worked on, "he taught me a lesson which I never forgot — very quietly and without criticism of me, he said that I had not put Mas [Okumoto's] name on the paper, whereas Mas had done some of the work. And he had — he'd done a big part of it. And so I learned from that respect for co-workers, regardless of what their title was."[24] The lesson Allansmith took away was that it was wrong to "create a class system in research — this is this class of person, this is this class of person." Allansmith appreciated the lesson and made a commitment to pass it on. "I had 44 fellows whom I trained, and the lessons that Phil Thygeson taught me, I passed on to them."[25]

Allansmith got the advice commonly given to Proctor fellows directly from Phil: when writing a paper, consult Ruth Lee. "What happened was, for a year I took lessons from her in how to write a paper, how the paper is constructed, how to push the paper along, and how to get the thing published.... I used to go to their house in Los Altos and spend the afternoon on a manuscript with her.... I learned an enormous amount from her that I was able to pass on."[26] When it was time to say goodbye, Phil was the one who kept in touch with Allansmith — and many other fellows — over the years. "One of the lessons I picked up from him was, 'Don't let the world happen to you. You happen to the world.'"[27]

23. Lake Tahoe and the Alta California Eye Research Foundation

In 1956, after the Los Altos hilltop was well established and the Proctor Foundation building had been renovated and expanded, the Thygesons were ready for another building project. They loved wilderness and Phil loved canoes, so the sparkling blue waters of Lake Tahoe beckoned. On weekends, they would drive up Highway 50 to the south shore of Lake Tahoe. In 1956, Kristin found and Phil and Ruth Lee bought a beautiful piece of lakefront property several miles north of Camp Richardson, not far from Fallen Leaf Lake. Mt. Tallac loomed majestically in the background. Their land was part of a group of parcels known as Cascade Properties because it was so close to Cascade Creek, which flowed out of Cascade Lake. As with the Paiute cabin in the Colorado Rockies, Phil and Ruth Lee defied prevailing wisdom about what sort of roof to have in snow country — a peaked roof was strongly recommended — and instead built yet another flat-roofed house. Fortunately, it was a strong roof that sagged but did not buckle under the weight of what was sometimes several feet of heavy Sierra Nevada snow.

The Sun-Moon House, as they called it, was beautiful and simple in its design. It was built in 1957 into a steep hillside. The side facing the lake was on stilts while the other side was practically dug into the hillside. The house had a wall of floor to ceiling windows overlooking the lake. The downstairs was a great room that served as living room and dining room, and was dominated by a large brick fireplace on the side that faced the bank of windows. The galley kitchen was so small it made cooking a challenge, but Ruth Lee was expert at preparing meals in tight spaces. Upstairs, there was a master bedroom with a small deck, a bathroom, and a loft with beds for three or four people. The loft had no wall dividing it from the great room below, so those sleeping there woke to sunlight sparkling on the surface of the lake. They also could not have a conversation above a whisper that would not be heard by people downstairs. This was the year of Kristin's marriage to Douglas Strong, who subsequently did a great deal of patio-building, painting, and maintenance at the Sun-Moon property.

Ruth Lee and Phil decorated the house with Native American artifacts they had collected over the years: hand-woven Navajo rugs on the floors and the walls, a full chief's headdress at the top of the stairs, an old long-barreled flint-lock rifle, and a handmade doll — a woman sitting at a loom weaving a blanket, a papoose on her back. Outside of the house, there was a large deck with tables for eating meals and a wooden walkway that wrapped around and extended almost to the front door. The deck was visited by wildlife — blue jays and camp robbers, raccoons, foxes, deer, and even bears. Ruth Lee loved birds and had field guides to try to identify what she saw.

The Sun-Moon house became her and Phil's special place of refuge. In the light of dawn, they would take one of their Old Town canoes and slide it off the small dock they built into the lake. The lake's surface was often still and smooth in the first light of day, before the summer breezes had picked up. Phil and Ruth Lee developed an ability to paddle absolutely in unison. To onlookers, the sight of them setting off in the early morning light was beautiful. They paddled perfectly. They appeared effortless as they dipped their paddles, completed each stroke, raised their paddles dripping from the water, and prepared for the next stroke. Phil always sat in the stern, Ruth Lee in the bow. He was masterful with the J stroke, a traditional way of steering a canoe by creating angles and degrees of drag that turn the canoe to the left or the right. Each morning, they would head either south or north. To the south were Baldwin Beach and Taylor Creek, which they could paddle up most of the summer season, observing birds and fish as they quietly made their way inland.

If they headed north and were feeling energetic, they would paddle all the way to Emerald Bay, the exquisite teardrop bay that is now a state park. Vikingsholm, a large castle-like home built in 1929 featuring traditional Scandinavian architecture, is an unusual feature along the shore far into the bay. The home and its small stone teahouse on the tiny island in the middle of the bay now belong to the state of California. Phil admired Vikingsholm because it was designed in the tradition of buildings erected as far back as 1000 A.D. in Scandinavian countries, such as the old wooden homes of Lillehammer, Norway.[1] Phil loved being reminded of his Norwegian ancestry while at Lake Tahoe. He and Ruth Lee wanted Emerald Bay to remain pristine. When there was a proposal to build a highway across the mouth of Emerald

Bay, allowing cars to make the trip around the lake more quickly but damaging the wilderness, they joined the public struggle to prevent the highway bridge. Along with many other committed wilderness conservationists, they helped win the battle.

Not long after completing the Sun-Moon House, Phil and Ruth Lee bought the strip of land up the hill and to the west. There they built a small A-frame cottage that came to be known simply as "The Cottage." They were very generous with their Tahoe properties, inviting family members, friends, and colleagues to vacation there with their families every summer. Many people cherished their annual week of vacation time at the Tahoe house. When the house and cottage passed out of the family's hands in the 1990s, many people mourned their passing.[2]

For many years, ophthalmological meetings were held at the Thygeson homes at Tahoe. They featured Proctor staff and fellows, as well as other ophthalmologists and scientists, and were not put on by the Proctor Foundation. Phil had been dismayed to learn that USCF had rules on its books that cramped his style. He attributed this to the fact that the University of California was over one hundred years old and had accumulated too many "outmoded" rules and regulations.[3] The solution to this was the establishment in 1968 of the Alta California Eye Research Foundation, which was made possible by a grant from Elizabeth C. Proctor. The intention was to provide the flexibility that the Proctor could not, given that the Proctor Foundation "was not allowed to hold seminars off campus and could not pay consultants from other branches of the University for special lectures or consultations."[4]

The first slate of officers of the Alta California Foundation consisted of G. Richard O'Connor as president, Phil as treasurer, and Ruth Lee as secretary. They determined to hold a seminar at Tahoe each September. The group would be small, the tenor informal, and there would always be time set aside for hiking, swimming, and canoeing. There were two named lectures, one to honor O'Connor's work in uveitis and the other to honor Okumoto's "world-class" work in microbiology.[5] Phil had a fairly inclusive view of who could participate. The house next door to the Sun-Moon House was owned by Robert Cello and his wife. Cello was a veterinarian interested in animal eye disease. He and Phil created a collaboration whereby Cello led the first September seminar. They shared an interest in zoonoses, agents that infect both animals and humans.

Each September, they chose the seminar topic for the following year. Topics ranged from ocular immunology to herpetic infection to the "compromised host." They would set up a screen for projection of slides in the cottage and have coffee and conversation on the deck during breaks between presentations. Proctor fellows were encouraged to give papers on their research projects, and Proctor staff and invited guests scientists also presented. When there was a particularly good set of papers, the Alta California Foundation would turn it into a monograph. Over the years, published monographs included *Herpetic Diseases of the Eye, Immunologic Diseases of the Mucous Membranes, Antimicrobial Agents in Ophthalmology, Animal Models of Ocular Disease,* and *Prevention of Eye Diseases.*

On the twenty-fifth anniversary of the Alta California Eye Research Foundation, it published a volume that included essays on women who had contributed to Proctor and passed away, an essay on named trees at the Los Altos hilltop, medical papers and, in keeping with the spirit of historical curiosity that was characteristic of Phil and Ruth Lee, an essay by O'Connor entitled, "Is Ithaca the Island of Homer's Odysseus?" and another, "Indian Medicine," about Phil's interest in Native-American culture and eye health.

Phil and Ruth Lee did their best to make the experiences of the meeting attendees happy and memorable. "We could canoe to Emerald Bay and Vikingsholm or to Taylor Creek, where we could see the beaver dams, the ducks, and Canadian geese and sometimes, in September, the run of the salmon," Phil said. "I always enjoyed the Rubicon Trail, which overlooked the deepest part of the lake, where the old [paddlewheel] Tahoe Queen used to ply within 50 feet of the shore." Other outings included a wonderful fish profile exhibit on Taylor Creek, where you would watch salmon head upstream to spawn, a Washoe Indian Museum with early buildings and artifacts, and a sunset dinner at the top of the Heavenly Valley ski lift.[6]

Even recreation mishaps became good memories. Two Proctor fellows, one American and one Chinese, had an adventure in a canoe together. The American fellow, Gary Holland, told the story of his and Wenhua's capsizing in the lake:

> She wanted to go out even though she had never been in a canoe and didn't know how to swim. So Dr. and Mrs. Thygeson got her fit with a life preserver and I offered to paddle her out. We probably got a little farther from shore than we should have. We went out far enough that the wake from a passing water skier caused the canoe to become a little unstable. Wenhua lost her balance and we tipped over. I could not get her to let go of the canoe from underneath so that I could right the canoe.... Finally I just decided I was going to swim ashore and drag the canoe while holding onto it. Dr. and Mrs. Thygeson were cheering us on from the dock. Everyone was laughing—including me and Wenhua in the water. As soon as we got out, they took really good care of her and personally saw she was okay. It just showed how warm they were and how much they cared about the fellows.[7]

24. Ripened Souls Tend Their Orchard

Letters Ruth Lee wrote to family members reveal important aspects of her values and beliefs. Though she did not follow the artist's path, she was able to share her vision of it with her granddaughter, a budding painter, dancer, and writer. Of Mara Thygeson's artistic pursuits, Ruth Lee wrote, "Keep it up, Love, and don't be afraid of the discipline of the basic techniques. To my mind, they are any artist's *launching pad*—whether musician, dancer, painter, potter, writer—gotta know *how*, and gotta have that pad firmly in place before you can take off. Wish we could see the things you are doing now. I bet they're lovely."[1] Years later, she offered feedback on a short story Mara wrote, telling her that she had wonderful storytelling ability, which many aspiring writers do not have, but that she needed to keep working on the craft of writing. To that end, she wrote out by hand a seven-page list of suggestions and corrections, ranging from "1. Watch vernacular words" to "29. ecstasy: mean one to spell — Memorize it!"[2]

Both Phil and Ruth Lee had what are considered traditional Christian moral values — no sexual activity before or outside of marriage, no illegal drug use, and utter obedience of the law. Though he put on a lot of weight in his later years, Phil believed in taking good care of the body — with exercise and temperance. He had reason to believe that he would have a long life. His mother Sylvie celebrated her hundredth birthday in 1968 with three of her great-grandchildren. Her three surviving children bought her a little house in Palo Alto when she was old enough to need help. They hired a caregiver to live with her. Phil still disliked his mother. When she was donating money on behalf of Fidel Castro's Cuba, he was donating money to Barry Goldwater. He would not even speak to his mother unless she was directly in front of him, in which case he would avert his eyes and mutter, "Hello, Mother."

Phil let Ruth Lee provide the care to Sylvie that he might have provided to her in old age. Ruth Lee and Lib had strong personal ethics about caring for ailing or financially needy family members. Sylvie was sometimes cantankerous and demanding, and had special dietary needs that led Ruth Lee to cook great pots of soup and rice custard for her every week. Her care required frequent visits. An undated letter from Elizabeth Proctor to Ruth Lee begins, "How did you ever *do* it! Taking care of Phil's mother when you had one leg in a cast, all the housekeeping chores to do too!"[3] Phil appreciated but did not help his wife. In a letter he wrote to her from Tunis, he said, "You are so good to do all that [medicine-related] work and to take care of mother, who is so difficult. Without you, she would really be finished!"[4]

Ruth Lee was deeply loyal to family members. She may also have felt a debt of gratitude for Sylvie's important financial support decades earlier. Thanks to their mother, all four of Sylvie's children graduated from Stanford, and three of the four obtained advanced degrees. From her, Phil got his genes for a long life. Sylvie's mother had died at the age of 101. She still rode the Los Angeles trolley at age 100. At 101, she broke her hip and decided to stop eating rather than endure the recovery. Sylvie had a similar experience in that she outlived all of her friends, lost her vision and hearing but not much of her lucidity, couldn't seem to die of old age, and finally chose to stop eating near her 107th birthday in order to die. The family respected her wishes.

In 1970, Phil, nearing retirement age, gave up patient care and passed the role of director of the Proctor Foundation to his assistant director, G. Richard O'Connor. It was the beginning of a harder period financially for the Proctor Foundation, as inflation skyrocketed and federal research dollars dwindled.[5] Phil continued to go to San Francisco with Ruth Lee on a regular basis, give seminar-type presentations to the fellows and residents, and work on correspondence and other matters in his small office. He was not easy on his successor. As O'Connor remembered, "He was at times quite interfering with my decisions and activities as Director. And so we had some arguments and unpleasantness about that. I recall particularly that he objected to my idea of alphabetizing the books in the library. They had always been in a completely helter-skelter arrangement in the library so that no one could find a book if he was looking for it. I thought this was intolerable, and many other people did too.... But Phil regarded that collection as his personal collection."[6]

O'Connor's view of Phil, which was shared by others, was that it was hard for him "to yield control. Part of that was egotism. Phil had the idea that he was the source of all good ideas. And the ideas that other people had were suspect...."[7] Phil essentially concurred with this assessment. In an essay he wrote at age 93, he confessed, "I am a man who likes to be the captain of my ship. I will seek advice but I don't always have to take it. I like to make my own decisions in life. After all, I was an executive for many of my years in academia and in the four years in the Army. I am used to telling people what to do and not being told."[8] In O'Connor's words, Phil was a "fierce autocrat" who "didn't suffer any kind of argument with what he had in mind" and who "definitely made the regulations." O'Connor added that Phil was "considered by many people, including those who respected him, including me, to be very feisty."[9] Phil would have been much better off not retiring so soon, as he had a great deal of creative and teaching energy left and an unflagging desire to control.

Phil demanded a high degree of stoicism and cooperation from others. He told O'Connor that he never accepted anesthesia at the dentist's office. When O'Connor explained that Novocain helped him avoid wincing while the dentist worked with a drill, Phil rebuked him with, "Don't wince!"[10] Ruth Lee called Phil the ultimate Boy Scout, for he never lost interest in the service ethic and stoical values of scouting. He also never lost interest in radio and frequently listened to talk radio in the middle of the night.

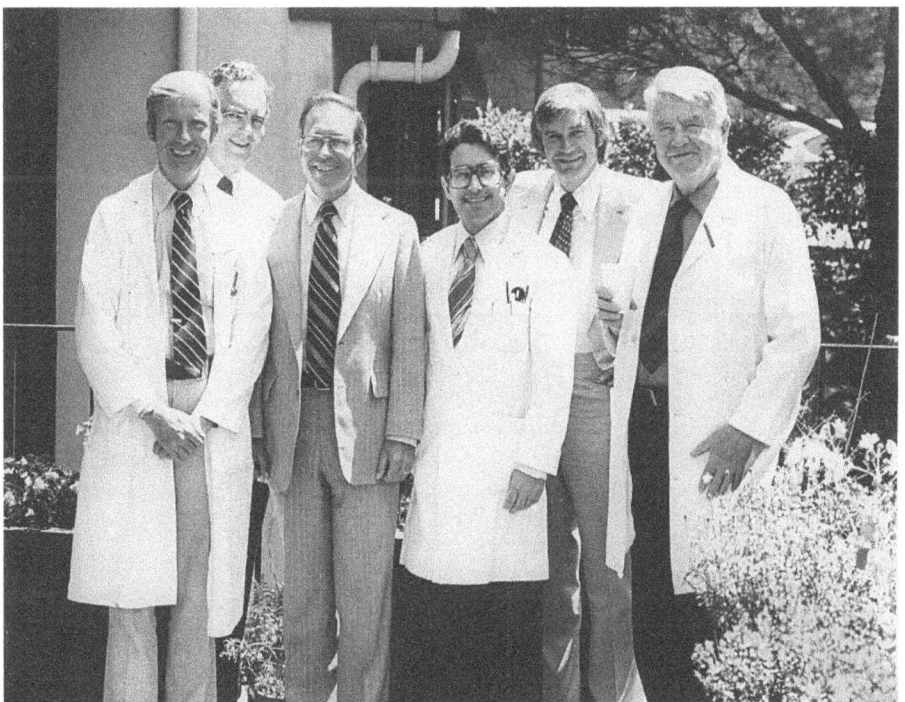

Ophthalmologists gathered at the Proctor Foundation, from left to right: G. Richard O'Connor, Daniel Vaughan, Richard Foerster, Khalid Tabbara, Jeffrey D. Lanier, Phillips Thygeson.

The scouting values to which Phil subscribed as a boy were clearly part of his leadership style. He expected obedience, loyalty, and collaboration, and expected those he saw as subordinates to act in accordance with his wishes. In other words, he was an old-fashioned boss and leader, though there were plenty of moments when he lacked the charisma great leaders exhibit. As former Proctor fellow Emmett Cunningham remarked, "We all have ... some narcissism.... Phil was further along the continuum than others. I don't mean that necessarily in a bad way. The narcissism allowed him to focus on what he thought was the right path."[11] Dawson recalled that Dr. Hogan, the first Proctor director, "always buckled under to anything that Dr. Thygeson wanted." He added,

> But I think anybody in their right mind would do it at the end of the day, because Phil could sit out anybody on the committee. You never saw a man who could be so stubborn. And at the end of the day, most people have to go home, and they have other things they have to do in this world, but Phil is going to go on to the end of time. He's been quite successful that way.[12]

The downside of this was that it caused divisiveness among the Proctor staff and fellows at times. "There is a pro–Thygeson group and an anti–Thygeson group," remarked former Proctor fellow Paul Riordan-Eva. Phil had "to a large extent polarized people around him."[13]

Even when he retired from his role as director of the Proctor Foundation, Phil wanted to be the boss. It did not appear to occur to him that it was someone else's turn to carry the torch and make his or her own decisions. When his successor G. Richard O'Connor retired, Phil continued to try to call the shots. In the tradition of his former boss and friend at the University of Iowa, Al Braley, he exercised

> the Braley approach to getting what you want. When he wanted Chan [Dawson] to be the next director of Proctor, he wrote to all the famous ophthalmologists he could think of and had each of them 'send an unsolicited letter of support' for Chan to the search committee. Chan got in when he had these ten or twenty glowing letters from these famous ophthalmologists from around the world. [Phil] called that the Braley approach and told that story every chance he had.[14]

Phil believed that he was always right and, further, that "there always is a right side in medical politics."[15] To this end, he remained on the Proctor Foundation Board of Governors until 1990, when he was nearing ninety years old himself.

On the other hand, Phil did not need a glamorous office or laboratory. When Khalid Tabbara, an ophthalmologist from Lebanon, came to visit the Proctor for the first time in 1972 and to meet the man after whom the disease Thygeson's superficial punctate keratitis was named, he was surprised to see Phil and Ruth Lee sharing a tiny office. "I was astonished and amazed that he was such a humble individual."[16] Tabbara chose to stay on as a Proctor fellow and later became one of its most famous alumni. Tabbara appreciated Phil's teaching style and historical approach. "He ... tried to make a complex clinical problem very easy to comprehend and solve. He gave us excellent differential diagnosis and management.... He talked about what happened to him in Egypt in the twenties and some of his experiences in the thirties and forties. We are talking about a man who lived a century and gave us all his expertise in a selfless manner."[17]

Even his more skeptical colleagues found Phil's diagnostic ability hard to match. Dawson said, "When he gives you a diagnosis, you really know he's right. He'll give you totally the wrong reasons for it, and you don't believe it.... I've argued with him again and again, but yet at the end of the day, he's right."[18] Phil loved to teach, and Ruth Lee greatly admired his easy ability with it. "To know a subject well," she once wrote, "and a subject you love at that, and to be qualified to impart it to others, and by so doing to encourage them to make the most of their talents ... what could be more soul-satisfying than that?"[19]

Phil also passed along his philosophy of not overtreating. Tabbara recalled Voltaire's dictum: "The art of medicine consists of amusing the patient while nature cures the disease." Tabbara collaborated with Phil on screening Native-American children for trachoma in Tuba City, Arizona. What he saw there reminded him of patients in Lebanon. With Phil's support, he began to publish on trachoma in the Middle East and eventually became a luminary in ophthalmology in Saudi Arabia. He also trained over a hundred ophthalmologists in research techniques in much the way Phil taught him.

In spite of graciously welcoming talented fellows from around the world to Proctor, Phil sometimes generalized about groups of people. "Effete" and "danged Easterner" were terms he would use to describe people he felt were physically weak and overly urban. Young men with long hair, some of whom might have been considered "hippies" in the late 1960s and 1970s, were "punks" to Phil. By this he meant they were unkempt, and possibly also hoodlums and miscreants. It bothered him when his grandsons grew their hair long. He disliked aspects of the Civil Rights movement — especially Black Power, race riots, and affirmative action. He also was prone to generalizing about racial groups, though he probably refrained from making comments around his colleagues at the Proctor Foundation. To his family, he would sometimes say, "No good ever came out of Africa," an ironic statement given the history of innovative ophthalmological treatments, including treatments for trachoma, used in ancient Egypt. As they grew older, Phil's values were

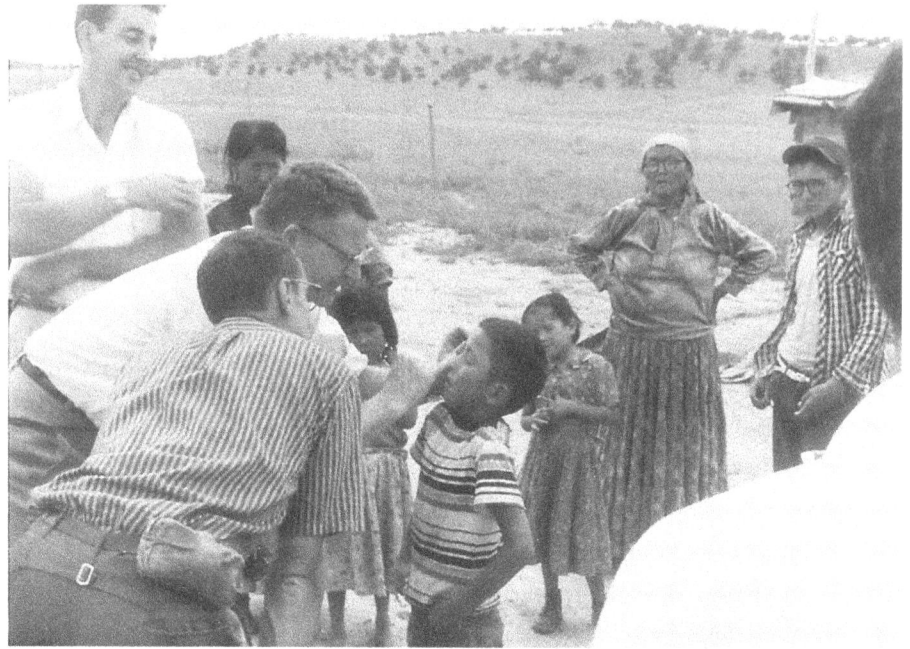

Phillips Thygeson examines a Navajo boy's eye for trachoma.

increasingly out of step with those of younger generations. Phil talked about his "good old days" and lamented that the youth of America had become degenerate. At the same time, he gained insight into himself in his old age and was able sometimes to apologize to family members about things he said or did.

Even Phil's conservatism mellowed in older age. His apparent atheism softened. He wrote, "As my vision fades from cataract and old age, I realize what a wonderful thing vision is and how it has made my life very wonderful.... I thank the Good Lord for my vision...."[20] After long years of being a staunch Republican, Phil voted for Clinton for president because of Clinton's commitment to protecting the environment. In general, though, he was very conservative most of his life. A letter from the U.S. Department of State began, "Dear Dr. Thygeson, President Nixon has asked me to reply to your letter. Thoughtful messages like yours are always a source of strength to the President. You may be sure that you have his deep appreciation for your understanding and support of his policy in Indochina."[21] Phil also wrote to President Carter about U.S. policy in South Korea and Taiwan. Hodding Carter III, the assistant secretary for public affairs, replied personally. To his U.S. senator, Alan Cranston, Phil wrote to ask him to protect Lake Tahoe from

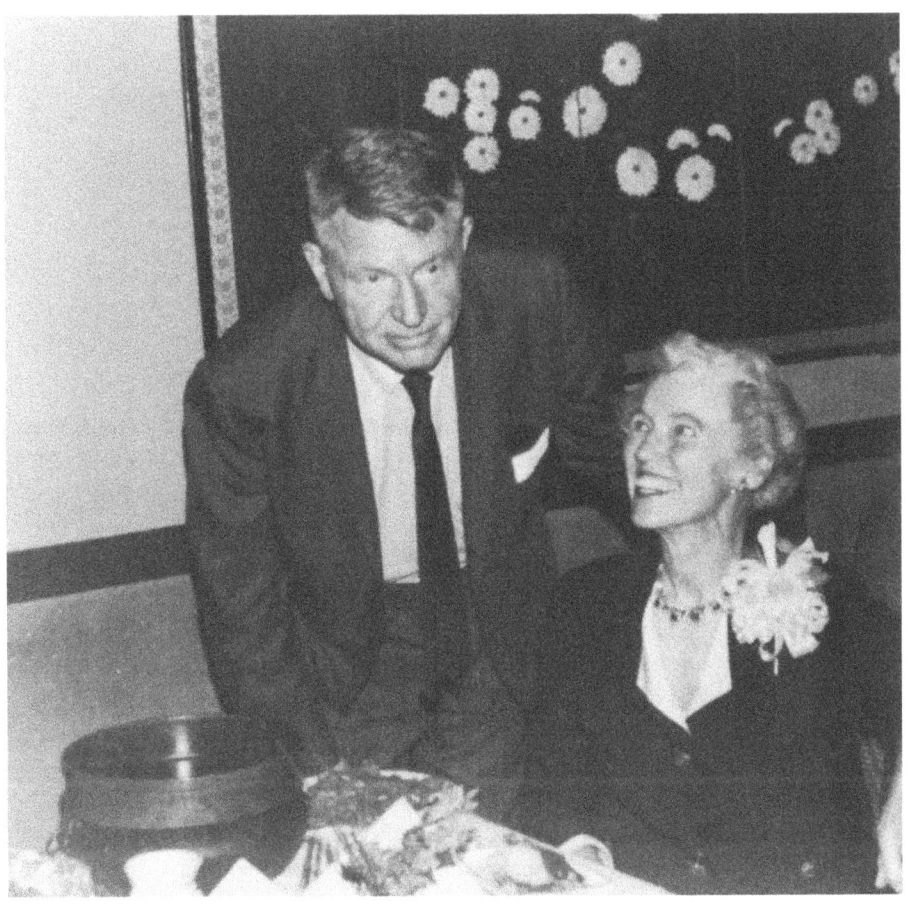

Phillips and Ruth Lee Thygeson at a party, 1972.

development and pollution. Cranston wrote back, reassuring him that they shared the same goals and values when it came to Tahoe. In contrast to Phil, Ruth Lee tried to stay connected to the experiences of the young people in the family. She was traditional in ways common to her generation, but she was also a liberal thinker. Her granddaughter, Mara, once fantasized about the life Ruth Lee could have led. "I think she would have been another Marie Curie. She was brilliant. She would have been a pioneer. If she had had a kind of husband who was more liberated, I think she also would have had five children *and* a brilliant career."[22]

25. The End of the Journey

Ruth Lee and Phil enjoyed slowing down a bit in their later years. They still made the trek to the Proctor Foundation once a week so Phil could teach a lunch-time seminar on ocular microbiology to the fellows and Ruth Lee could confer with her authors. Finally, though, they stopped going altogether. At first, it was hard for Ruth Lee to have Phil home all the time, but they fell into a pleasant rhythm. They would rise before dawn, have a bath together, light a fire in the fireplace, and share a breakfast of coffee and hot cereal. They both loved opera, especially the arias of Puccini, and often Phil played opera and classical music on the stereo for hours at a time. Asked how she could stand to get up every morning before dawn, Ruth Lee answered, "Believe me, my basic nature is very, very lazy. I would sleep in until eight o'clock if I could, but I get up because [Phil] wants me to."[1]

They were frugal even in old age. Ruth Lee's kitchen was full of collections of recycled paper bags, baggies, and rubber bands. Food was never wasted and Ruth Lee made casseroles with leftovers. After their retirement, Phil and Ruth Lee's income was approximately $40,000 a year, a combination of Social Security and their retirement from the University of California. Ruth Lee never bought herself expensive clothes or jewelry. She saved her small inheritance from her mother. It grew from the $7,500 she inherited to $300,000 at the end of her life due to being invested in Hewlett-Packard stock that split several times. She saw it as her and Phil's old age "insurance" money, and her plan, as shown in an early will, was to share it equally among her daughter and Fritjof's two children. In fact, most of it was spent on Phil's old age care.

Phil read the *San Francisco Chronicle* faithfully and clipped articles to mail to various friends and relatives or save in one of the many boxes where he kept papers he wanted to save. Over time, his inability to throw out newspaper clippings, old magazines, and much of anything in print became a significant problem. Boxes and boxes of yellowing paper began to fill the old horse barn and then the little carport where they parked their red Ford Falcon station wagon and orange-red Ford Maverick. Eventually, even the space behind the living room couch where Phil spent hours reading every day was filled with boxes of clippings. Ruth Lee gave up trying to persuade him to throw out the paper and the house gradually filled up with his decaying personal archive. As the situation worsened, Ruth Lee gave the guest room the nickname "the chamber of horrors" because it, too, had filled with boxes. She was able to reframe the problem as a good-humored joke.

Phil also loved to photograph people and nature. He subscribed to dozens of journals, loved to buy books, and shot hundreds of rolls of film. He was an avid correspondent with friends, family, and former fellows, and would often include photographs and newspaper articles with his letters. He especially loved to keep in touch by means of postcards, a practice he picked up from Charles Nicolle in Tunis.

For many years, Phil continued his decades-long correspondence with his dear friend Milo Fritz, the bush pilot-physician in Alaska. Like the Thygesons, Fritz had land he cared a great deal about and wanted to preserve from development after his and his wife's death. His idea of how to preserve the land was much like Phil's hope that the Los Altos hilltop could be kept intact. Fritz tried to sell his land to the state of Alaska.

> The only requirement being that Betsy and I be allowed to stay here until we passed in our dinner pails and then that the State would use it for a means of studying oceanography, riparian life, volcanology, forestry, agriculture, with no motor vehicles allowed except those of the family that would be caretakers of the place.[2]

This was similar to the dream Phil articulated repeatedly in writing about the Los Altos hilltop. Of his and Ruth Lee's dream, he wrote that they jointly wished after their deaths "to support the Alta Foundation in its educational effort and to save the hilltop forever from subdivision and the bulldozer." They hoped their beautiful five acres could "be saved forever as a place of beauty and a place of enjoyment...."[3] It was much more easily said than done, however, because of the economics of preserving a large parcel of very valuable land without having the capital to do so. Both couples were environmentalists and preservationists, but both shared the problem of a sea of paper invading their homes. Fritz wrote, "I don't know whether you folks have ever had to do it but Betsy and I are now in the throes of filing, collating and throwing away tons of outmoded papers, journals, correspondence and other flotsam and jetsam that we have accumulated...."[4]

Ruth Lee was an extremely devoted grandmother to her five grandchildren. Her eldest grandchild, Mara, remembers how Ruth Lee was the one who helped her get ready for her transition to college. "She's the one who went out and bought everything I needed.... I still have the sewing kit basket that she put together for me.... She took me on several trips [to the Sierra Nevada] to find housing. She was involved in all of the phases of my life."[5] When Mara married and had her first baby, her grandmother offered her support. "She also gave me brilliant advice.... She told me, 'Here are the mistakes I made. I didn't let Phil get involved because I didn't think he could diaper the baby right. You keep your mouth shut.... If you criticize, he won't want to help.'"[6] Both Phil and Ruth Lee — but especially Ruth Lee — trained their grandchildren in an ethic of service, first to family and then to community. Mara helped take care of her great-grandmother, Sylvie, and any grandchild wanting paid work could earn money working at the hilltop or at Lib's.

At lunchtime during their retirement years, Ruth Lee and Phil would have soup or sandwiches and watch television. Their favorite programs were "Perry Mason" and "Bonanza." They would discuss the characters as if they were family members. Phil spent hours out in the garden watering the vegetable garden, flowers, and trees. As the orchard had no irrigation system, the fruit trees were left to fend for themselves. Except in periods of extreme drought, they did fine. When a medfly infestation threatened the California fruit crop and state authorities demanded that all trees be stripped of their fruit, Phil tried to comply. Short of hiring a squad of day laborers with ladders, it was impossible to harvest all of the fruit, but Phil, ever law abiding, tried all the same.

In the late 1980s, Phil was approached by Sally Smith Hughes, Ph.D., a historian of science who did oral histories for the Regional Oral History Office at the University of California at Berkeley. She asked whether he would be willing to be interviewed. At first, she said, he was not warm and welcoming. In fact, he told her he didn't want to talk about himself.[7] He had her attend one of his last teaching seminars at Proctor. She was very impressed. "Microscopes were set up and the young fellows were clustered around," she recalled. She watched him teach and eventually joined in the discussion. Later, she realized that she had passed muster, as he invited her to Los Altos. She interviewed him over a period of months and interviewed a number of his colleagues.[8] Ruth Lee participated in a couple of Hughes's interviews with Phil. The Thygesons enjoyed the process and became friends with Hughes, who was soon receiving clippings and cards from Phil. "I'd get whole packets, usually from medical journals, of things that he felt I would be interested in — usually of a scientific nature, but not always."[9]

Hughes was impressed by how Phil and Ruth Lee collaborated. "It was an extraordinarily close relationship. In fact, I know of few others, if any, that were as close. They spent almost every working moment together."[10] In an essay penned in his waning years, Phil wrote, "In the 69 years of our marriage, we had no major conflicts or disagreements. We had no secrets from each other."[11] While neither perception was exactly true, his beliefs gave him peace and comfort.

Phil and Ruth Lee made other new friends late in life. Phil was introduced to Ralph Heintz, an inventor who had built radios for the Richard Byrd expeditions to the Antarctic in the 1920s and 1930s. They remained friends until Ralph died. Phil and Ruth Lee continued the friendship with Ralph's widow, Sophie. In his retirement years, Phil would chat with her on the phone, tapping out Morse Code messages on the old brass telegraph key that sat on his desk. She would tap back. The Heintzes donated significant sums to the Proctor Foundation.

Ruth Lee and Phil continued to go to Lake Tahoe as long as they could, which meant as long as Ruth Lee could negotiate the winding hillside path down to the house and Phil could drive them up Highway 50. They had long since stopped going to their Colorado cabin, but they still cared about its fate. At one point, they proposed selling it, but Kristin could not bear the thought of losing her most stable childhood home and asked that they let her maintain and care for the cabin. It was nearly lost again when Forest Service administrators issued an edict in 1979 to move it within ten years or let them burn it down in preparation for a new Wilderness Area designation.[12] "If we did nothing, [they] would set fire to it and bulldoze it and send us a bill for their trouble," Kristin said.[13]

In the summer of 1987, she undertook to move it to a purchased tract of fourteen acres of private land, a choice that turned out to be riskier and more perilous than she imagined. On the back of a flatbed truck, the cabin was moved from its original location at 10,200 feet[14] down a thousand vertical feet to the highway that runs past Ward. The road had to be closed in the pre-dawn for the move down the steep road to the Peak-to-Peak highway. The cabin was hauled a few miles and deposited at the top of a steep, homemade road on a promontory with a beautiful vista of the Indian Peaks. The dirt road up to the property was cut through virgin forest. Dozens of trees had to be removed and the road was steeper than public roads are ever allowed to be. There was a great deal of concern that the heavy cables holding the cabin onto the truck bed could snap during the slow crawl up that hill. Kristin had visions of a runaway cabin careering downhill and killing some of the crew who were helping with the move. Fortunately, all went well. Ruth Lee's sister Lib gave money to put in a huge picture window facing the peaks to the west, as the fireplace was not easily moved and had been knocked down. A magnificent view serves in its place.

Phil and Ruth Lee nearly always took adversity in stride, even in old age. Fritjof went through multiple divorces and was estranged from his parents for two decades. Kristin, too, got divorced and nearly died of internal hemorrhage in 1979. Her parents took her from the Colorado hospital, where she had been in intensive care, home to Los Altos for a long period of recuperation. There were various dramas with the grandchildren, and Ruth Lee did her best to support everyone through all of it. During these years, when Mara asked her which she felt was harder, raising toddlers or teenagers, she shook her head and said, "My dear, it never ends."[15] And for her, it didn't. She took her responsibility to each member of her family very seriously, and her family drew enormous benefit from her loving attention. She made each grandchild feel like the center of the universe. She had a way of paying deep attention to what a child said and conveying unconditional love.

The 1989 Loma Prieta earthquake shook the Los Altos house with great violence. While nothing broke at Lib's house in Atherton a few miles away, most of the dishes and crockery fell off the open shelving in the Thygesons' kitchen and smashed on the floor. The precious gifts they had received from colleagues around the world smashed as well, along with the old hand-carved cuckoo clock and many of their books. The floor of their house was literally covered with broken glass, books, and favorite possessions. Their wonderful friend and accountant, Mary Leihy, hurried over to help, as did their neighbor, Margot Lawrence. Leihy reported that Phil and Ruth Lee were calm, but calm in a way that suggested a degree of shock. They surveyed the ruins, but did not try to pick things up. Margot bloodied her hands scooping broken glasses and dishes into trash bags. It was the beginning of a friendship between the two neighbor couples that lasted for the rest of the Thygesons' lives. Eventually, Margot's husband Gerry would be crawling around in the dirt under the Thygesons' house doing electrical work, helping them with their finances, and giving Phil a large television when he became confined to bed.[16]

In another episode involving their closest neighbors, Margot called one day in a panic to say that a man had just burst into her home through an unlocked door. She screamed and he ran away. She believed he was headed up the hill to the Thygeson house. Phil "very calmly said, 'Well, he's already been here. We gave him something to drink.'" The man was shirtless and had lain down on the floor of Phil and Ruth Lee's house to hide from the sheriff. "Here I was so worried about this guy running up there," Margot said, "and he had lain on their floor so he wouldn't be seen. So I thought that was kind of cute — they were totally calm about the whole thing."[17]

The vulnerability of his and Ruth Lee's old age brought Phil to a new place, in part because they began to need outside care. Ruth Lee suffered from hypertension and after a time did not take beta blockers because of her worsening asthma. Though she tried to control the hypertension with daily relaxation meditation and dietary changes, she still ended up sliding into a hypertensive dementia in her mid-eighties. By 1990, she needed help. Phil did his best to become a caregiver for the first time in his life. At first, he was very unhappy about this reversal of roles, but in time he became a devoted caregiver. Grandson Peder Strong moved in to the guesthouse and helped maintain the property, and especially the garden and orchard. He remembers Ruth Lee as loving to do several kinds of work at once, and especially to work with her hands. His favorite memory of his grandparents was watching them from the shore of Lake Tahoe as they paddled rhythmically in the direction of the marshy nesting grounds of the Great Blue Heron. Her canoeing days had come to an end.

When Ruth Lee's personal care needs became too much for Phil, Earlene Chapman became Ruth Lee's home-based nursing assistant. Chapman deeply admired Ruth Lee, though the two did not meet until Ruth Lee's ability to speak had largely slipped away. "She was the most beautiful, charming lady I'd ever met in my whole life. She was the epitome of love — that smile just burst out so beautifully," Chapman said. "People felt it, and that's why they liked and loved her so much.... She made everybody feel good by just being in her presence." Ruth Lee had the effect of a warm sun brightening a darkened room.

Through the course of nursing Ruth Lee, Chapman got to know Phil pretty well. He confided to Chapman that Ruth Lee had been instrumental in helping him feel connected to the beauty and joy of life. "What happened to me is I lived through her," he said.[18] Chapman did not feel that Phil had been as generous with Ruth Lee as Ruth Lee had been with Phil. When she asked whether Ruth Lee had friends of her own, Phil made it clear that he had discouraged independence in Ruth Lee. In regard to whether she ever visited her personal friends, he said, "Oh no, we can go together. I don't want her to go any place by herself." Chapman responded, "Don't you think that's a little mean, because I think she'd like to have some women friends to go and have tea with or something." Given this prompting to share Ruth Lee more with others while there was still time, he said, "Well, I don't know if I can do that...."[19]

Traveling to visit other family members was more problematic. As Ruth Lee wrote in a letter to her granddaughter, "[Grandfather] is terribly dependent on me these days, and as much as I'd love to spend a few days with you all, and unfair as it seems, I just can't do it. So no use including that lovely idea in your plans."[20] Phil walked around their orchard during those years quietly saying "Mommy, mommy, mommy," his way of expressing his longing for Ruth Lee's presence. Ruth Lee responded with kindness and humor. "Isn't he a nut?" she told family members, laughing.[21]

When Ruth Lee wanted to see the musical *Evita*, about Eva Perón, Phil objected on political grounds. In his view, Juan Perón was a dictator and any artistic portrait of the lives of Juan and Eva Perón should be shunned. In one of her rare moments of defiance, Ruth Lee went anyway, but Phil was said to sulk for weeks to punish her for it. He was also hard on his devoted longtime friends and former private practice partners, Daniel Vaughan and Crowell Beard. He was especially hard on Vaughan when he made a financial decision, in his role as president of the Alta California Eye Research Foundation, that was his right to make but with which Phil vehemently disagreed. Sadly, the ensuing rift was never fully mended. Beard, on the other hand, forgave Phil for his orneriness and visited him often when they were both ancient of days.

When Ruth Lee no longer felt comfortable driving, her and Lib's devoted housekeeper and assistant, Jan Harwood, drove her back and forth to Lib's home. Everyone who worked for the Thygesons became honorary family members; care and loyalty were shared by all. Harwood drove Phil to the grocery store when he could no longer drive. She enjoyed her time with the Thygesons and their siblings. "They were just lovely, loving, funny, great people. It completely enriched my life. People say, 'You cleaned houses. How was that?' I said, 'Exhilarating!'"[22]

Phil had a hard time sharing Ruth Lee with her sister Lib, who was in many ways her best friend in life. Lib lived in Atherton, a twenty-minute drive from Los Altos, and for many years Ruth Lee visited her one morning a week. Phil could stand that for a couple of hours and then he would call Ruth Lee, urging her to come home. Lib was fond of her brother-in-law and gave him the nickname "Philly Buster." She often joked with him about his shortcomings and he would laugh. Ruth Lee deeply needed her intimacy with her sister. It was the one relationship where she could be exactly who she was and be entirely candid.

With the help of Chapman, Jan Harwood, and Jan's husband Sam, each week an "old folks luncheon" was served out by the goldfish pond on the brick patio at the hilltop. Phil's sister Mary, Lib and, occasionally, Mary's niece Barbara, completed the party. They read aloud from a newspaper about the "olden days" called *Old Times* and joked about the trials and tribulations of old age.[23] At one point, when Jan Harwood took Phil to see a doctor about pain in his leg, he reported his diagnosis to her as "ASF." She thought that was some sort of syndrome, but when she asked him, he said, "I have All Systems Failing." And then he laughed at his joke.[24]

Ruth Lee went into a long, slow decline. At first, she couldn't go to

Tahoe any more because it was too hard to navigate the steep hillsides and the stairs. She understood much of what people said, but had trouble putting her own sentences together. Since she was a master of language, this was painful for her and those who loved her. Her file of special quotations held the following, a quotation from the apostle Paul that she wrote out for herself: "I have fought a good fight — I have finished my course — I have kept the faith!" Ruth Lee's ethic in life was to give as much of herself as she possibly could, for the benefit of as many as possible. Hers was a tireless and completely committed effort. She considered herself fortunate. "You know," she told her granddaughter, "I've had a wonderful life. I've been to Egypt. I've been all over the world."[25]

In time, Ruth Lee had trouble walking and, especially, eating. She struggled to swallow, even when she progressed to a liquid diet. Kristin and Phil disagreed over Ruth Lee's care when she was ill and Kristin sued her father for legal custody of her mother, claiming he was providing inadequate care. She did not prevail, but it was a painful passage for everyone concerned.

Ruth Lee kept her radiant smile until the end, but gradually lost her awareness of who was who, except for Phil. Their grandson Peder, who lived on the hilltop during her last years, became "that nice young man." When Ruth Lee lost her language altogether, Chapman intuitively knew what she wanted and was able to treat her with great kindness. She saw that Ruth Lee needed her modesty and privacy respected, and she took care of her in a way that respected her dignity. Ruth Lee grew thinner and thinner and made it clear she would prefer not to struggle to take in nutrition. In keeping with the family ethos, artificial methods of nutrition and hospitalization were not even considered. While the hilltop was in full spring flower in 1994, she died peacefully in bed at the age of 89.

After her death, the following quotation was found in personal papers. She entitled it "The Ethics of the Flock."

> A flock of wild geese had settled to rest on a pond. One of the flock had been captured by a gardener who had clipped its wings before releasing it. When the geese started to resume their flight, this one tried frantically, but vainly, to lift itself into the air. The others, observing his struggles, flew about in obvious efforts to encourage him; but it was no use. Thereupon, the entire flock settled back on the pond and waited, even though the urge to go on was strong within them. For several days they waited until the damaged feathers had grown sufficiently to permit the goose to fly. Meanwhile, the unethical gardener, having been converted by the ethical geese, gladly watched them as they finally rose together and all resumed their long flight.
> — Albert Schweitzer, *Reverence for Life*

Phil was acutely lonely after losing Ruth Lee. As his general health slowly deteriorated, he had a gift of old age — his chronic migraines finally disappeared. He attributed this to the natural hardening of his blood vessels. Chapman was his regular companion. In all, she spent a decade helping Phil and Ruth Lee navigate the challenging waters of old age and end of life. She also helped nurse Lib and Phil's sister Mary until Mary's death. Toward the end of her life, Mary moved in with Phil at the hilltop, where both could receive care. She died peacefully in Kristin's childhood bedroom in 1997. Chapman was considered the family's angel. Phil was a sociable person and loved to talk during daytime hours. According to Chapman, "He started to open up and talk about people where he had done things kind of wrong. He was not happy about what he had done to a lot of people."

Phil's last years were a period of reconciliation with himself and some members of his family. When Fritjof tried again to reconcile with his father after nearly twenty years of estrangement — he knew his mother was nearing the end of her life — Phil refused to let him see her before she died. She and Fritjof had had a close bond, but both mother and son lost out on knowing each other for many years. Fritjof had not had reason to believe his father truly loved him. A gift of Phil's old age was that after Ruth Lee's death, Phil mellowed considerably and he and his son became close friends.

In 1996, Fritjof and his wife Cheryl arrived from New York and moved into the Los Altos guesthouse to help care for Phil. At first he resisted, and then he was grateful. Phil expressed his love for Fritjof before he died. In the tradition of Ruth Lee, Fritjof began to read aloud to his father, including in the middle of the night when Phil had trouble sleeping. One of their favorite books was the biography of William Osler, considered by many to be the greatest physician in Western medicine of his time, the mid-nineteenth to early twentieth centuries. Phil's relationship with Kristin, however, remained painful for both father and daughter. There was no true reconciliation. Fritjof had the advantage of living with Phil, and so their healing had years of daily contact on its side.

Like Earlene Chapman, Fritjof's wife Cheryl Stoll Thygeson was considered African American in the United States. She was actually from a Caribbean island and had lived in England, but the important thing for Phil was that both of these women caregivers were members of a racial group he had sometimes disparaged to his family. He came to respect, love, and depend on both of them. He also became very fond of two Latina nursing assistants who cared for him part-time. As Chapman said, "He learned to accept other people."[26] He became more curious about other people and would ask them about their lives. He confided in Chapman, "I'm learning about Mexicans and Americans."[27] Fritjof viewed his father as having been relatively unprejudiced about race until the 1960s, when he was deeply upset by the more radical aspects of the Civil Rights movement. Late in life, he again became more accepting of all people.

This evolution to giving up racism was very important in the life of the Thygeson family because Phil had caused great distress by rejecting his granddaughter Mara's interracial marriage and children. Mara and her husband had four handsome, talented sons who were half African American. They were not welcome at the Los Altos hilltop for years because of Phil's strong objection during his later decades to "miscegenation."

Whether or not Ruth Lee shared his views on this question — there's a difference of opinion about how she really felt — she did her best to support Mara's family, though she would not go to battle with her husband to try to change his mind. She showered her granddaughter's family with love and, to Phil's unhappiness, insisted on going to visit them at their home in Oregon to hold their firstborn great-grandchild. She wrote to her granddaughter, "All my love, my darling. You are the Light of my Life, and I'm with you all the time...."[28] The exclusion of this one family sent shock waves through the clan, as this was the only grandchild's family to be unwelcome at the hilltop. Very late in life, Phil changed his mind and invited these great-grandsons and their parents to visit, which they did. During this period, and through long, sometimes heated conversations with Chapman, Phil mellowed and became more loving.

To their careers, Phil and Ruth Lee gave a great deal. Both believed in work for work's sake. In a letter, Ruth Lee wrote, "I have always felt ... that the most important thing in life (aside from those old basics having to do with things like honesty and kindness, etc.) is to be able to pursue an occupation you love — and that the more passionately you love it the better."[29] The reward for this devotion was respect, prestige, the knowledge that they were making an important contribution, and the intrinsic pleasure of the work. Their colleagues thought very highly of them. Jeffrey D. Lanier said, "I truly think Dr. Thygeson is the greatest infectious disease clinician that has ever lived.... His basic principles of disease processes have held true all these years."[30]

In the course of their lives, Ruth Lee and Phil drew a great circle around the country: from West to East, from North to South, and then home to the San Francisco Bay area. Although they managed to acquire remarkably beautiful and valuable property in the form of land, they never had a lot of cash in the bank. Phil wrote late in life, "I was never a big earner. The most I ever made as a full professor was $30,000 a year. But Ruth Lee made this money go a long, long way. She provided for our old age." Phil also believed that Ruth Lee's willingness to work and her frugality enabled them to build their various homes. "She built a house in Tenafly, a cottage at Lake Tahoe, and a house on a hilltop in Los Altos.... Ruth Lee was a worker. She was never idle."[31]

In his nineties, Phil made the writing of essays on personal and medical topics a major life activity. "I wish that I had been born to be a great writer.... But that was not to be. I did not inherit the proper genes. There was been no great author in the Thygeson family." All the same, he wrote, "I suppose that I will die with a pen in my hand."[32] Phil cared deeply about leaving his story behind for others to read. "I have had a lot of interesting episodes in my life and I am trying to write them up. Someday some distant relative might read them."[33] At the age of ninety-three, Phil wrote, "There are some good things about old age. In my case, it is the fact that I knew ocular infectious disease and immunology before the development of the sulfonamides, the antibiotics, or the antiallergic drugs. And that has been a big thing in saving me from many mistakes. Later in life I know when the natural history of ocular disease [is] better than the treated history. And my first two teachers in ophthalmology, W. C. Finnoff and Edward Jackson, taught me when to treat and when not to treat."[34]

From the hindsight of old age, Phil could recount the ravages of overtreatment, especially eyes lost to the overzealous use of steroids in cases of herpes infection. He had also witnessed too much cauterization, too much surgery, and inappropriate use of X-rays as therapy. He believed that all too often treatment impeded the body's ability to heal itself. He believed the human immune system was the best possible tool whenever it could rise to the challenge. To that end, he wrote an essay entitled "Fever Therapy" to remind others that eliminating fevers meant knocking out one of the body's tried and true healing tools.[35] Phil came to believe that the most important aspect of the art of medicine was diagnosis. "Then comes prognosis," he wrote. "Treatment comes last."[36]

Late in life, Phil summed up his and Ruth Lee's teamwork and their different roles by saying, "We worked together, and our efforts were all directed to the prevention of blindness and impaired vision. I was a microbe hunter, and she participated in my work by way of advice, secretarial and editing skills."[37] On the personal front, Ruth Lee was like the approving mother he never had. "Ruth Lee was the inspiration for my work.... I wanted to make her proud of me. I wanted to do well just for her sake. I wanted to show that we made a team."[38] He gave her high praise: "She criticized constructively and saved me from some important errors. She was really a co-author in all my papers but she did not get proper credit for it."[39]

By the end of his life, Phil had been awarded some of the most prestigious honors and prizes available in ophthalmology. They included the Howe Medal from the American Ophthalmological Society, the Proctor Medal from the Association for Research in Ophthalmology, the Distinguished Service Award from the International College of Surgeons, the Chibret Gold Medal for Trachoma Research from the International Organization against Trachoma, an honorary LL.D. from UCSF, and the Castroviejo Medal from the Castroviejo Society. Ruth Lee was very proud of him and pleased to have been an essential part of his success, especially his work on reducing infection-caused blindness worldwide.

Trachoma has not been fully eradicated and it may be impossible to do so entirely. Still, there is great hope that nation by nation, trachoma will go the way of smallpox, becoming a bad memory of the past. The protocol that is the best current hope is known as SAFE. It consists of corrective surgery to help patients with advanced disease, antibiotics to treat active infection, face washing with clean water to reduce transmission among members of households, and environmental improvement to give access to clean water and improved sanitation.[40] Phil made a huge contribution to understanding the cause of trachoma and the disease process itself. This understanding, coupled with treatment, led to eradication of trachoma in many countries and the hope of eradication in many more.

In his final years, Phil wrote a series of essays about Ruth Lee. He also wrote about his hope of leaving the five acres of the Los Altos hilltop intact as a memorial and museum named for her and in her honor. He wanted to call it "The Ruth Lee Historical Hilltop" or the "Ruth Lee Thygeson Memorial Hilltop" and pointed out that it was one of only two remaining old orchards in Los Altos.[41] He never quite felt himself to be worthy of her. "How could a peasant like me have such a lovely wife?" he wrote.[42] Wistfully, he wrote, "Her spirit seems to pervade her little house on the hilltop. In future years I hope it can be kept much in the way she left it."[43] He remembered her as a person whose "beauty never faded."[44]

To Phil, the best way to honor Ruth Lee was to preserve the land and home she had loved. A Ruth Lee Thygeson Fund for Medical Education already existed. Phil hoped in addition to establish an annual Ruth Lee Thygeson Lecture.[45] "Gradually, the little old summer house on the hilltop began to accumulate artifacts from all over the world, so much so that there had to be a spillover into a barn," Phil wrote. "In a way, the house became a museum."[46] Why not preserve the Thygeson house, Phil reasoned, with its quality of being a memorial to medicine in the twentieth century?

When Ruth Lee died, his and Ruth Lee's marital trust became irrevocable. Phil could no longer make changes to it, which worried him. He also intermittently worried that one or both of his children would challenge his estate plans in court after his death, mainly because there was no provision for them in his will. There was plenty of talk in the family of his having bullied Ruth Lee into signing onto his estate plans, when in fact she wanted to leave some money to their children. As a matter of principle, Phil did not believe in children inheriting from parents. In his view, children were supposed to take care of themselves. He may have been forgetting those many early years when he and Ruth Lee depended on monthly support from his mother.

Neither Fritjof nor Kristin was written into the final testamentary plans, though in the end both children benefited from their parents' land wealth. In the 1980s, Phil and Ruth Lee legally deeded the Tahoe house and cottage to Kristin. She made Tahoe her primary home for years, but eventually sold both properties and moved to Colorado. Near the end of his life, Phil wanted to deed a half-acre of the hilltop to Fritjof, but the irrevocable trusts made that extremely difficult. Fritjof did, however, successfully petition the court for compensation after Phil's death.

Phil and Ruth Lee's beloved Los Altos property was worth millions of dollars. Phil was grateful that they had something of such value to give to the Proctor Foundation and other charitable causes after their deaths. Phil keenly believed in leaving a legacy for eye research and education. Indeed, some people say that his greatest legacy — in addition to his original research and teaching — was building the first foundation in the country "dedicated to ocular inflammatory infectious disease."[47] When he died, the Proctor Foundation was in good financial shape.

Phil believed in the value of "real dollars" from his youth, when it took at least an hour of his time to earn a dollar. "I believe that a child raised in genteel poverty has a much better chance of success in life than a child raised in luxury."[48] He thought his early childhood in St. Paul had been in some ways bad for him. The silver lining of his father's death was that he was forced to go out and find work at a young age. "Work did me a lot of good. I learned the value of money. I was never fired from a job for incompetence."[49] He had a favorite motto he wrote on postcards he mailed to friends and family: FILOLI. It stood for "Fight, love, live." He later amended it to: FILOLIWO. Fight, love, live, work.[50] He and Ruth Lee lived by the edict of Voltaire: "Work spares us from three great evils: boredom, vice, and need."[51]

The Los Altos hilltop has a very special feeling. Family friend and accountant Mary Leihy described it as an "incredible place." When you went there, it felt like "coming into a retreat.... Walking down the little brick steps into the house — it just wrapped you in its arms."[52] In addition to memorializing Ruth Lee, Phil not so secretly hoped his legacy would be treated much as Pasteur's had been — his home, his laboratory, his books all left intact. His obsession and passion in his final years was to try to ensure that after his death, the hilltop, with its five acres of apricot and peach orchards crowned

25. The End of the Journey

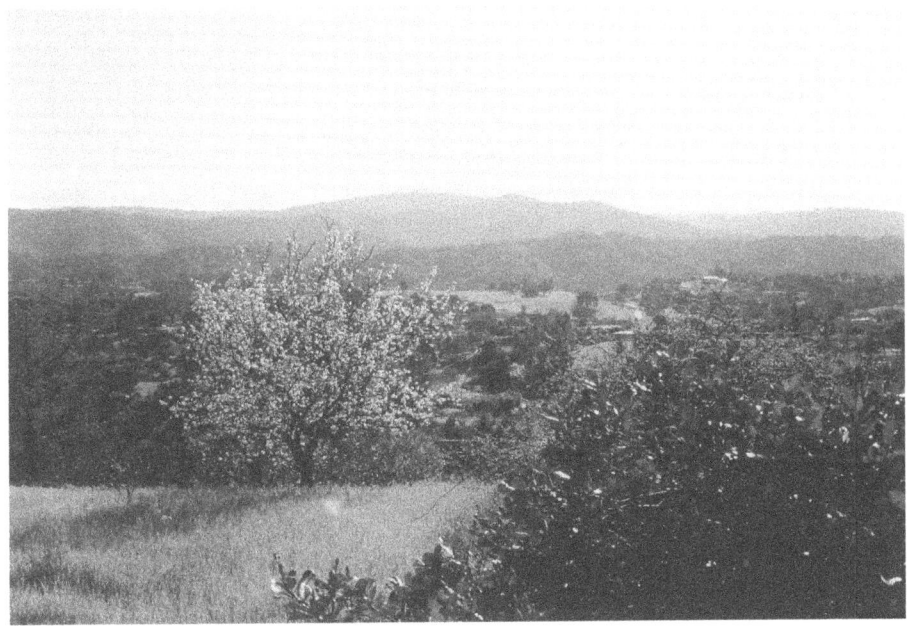

The view of the coastal hills and orchard country from the Los Altos hilltop.

by a sweeping view of their Northern California valley, would be preserved. The smallest bedroom in the house was known as the "Cubby." It housed what Phil and Ruth Lee had jokingly dubbed "The World's Smallest Indian Museum." It was full of Navajo rugs, baskets, pottery, kachina dolls, books, other artifacts. When questioned about the practicality of his wish to create a museum of sorts, Phil would say that what was done for Louis Pasteur could be done for the Thygesons, too. In an essay entitled, "My Ruth Lee: A Birthday Dream," he wrote, "I want to spend the rest of my life in making the Ruth Lee hilltop and library a shrine in her memory."[53] Phil Thygeson was more spiritual than he would admit.

Over the years, Ruth Lee and Phil had planted a series of memorial trees in the Los Altos orchard near the house. Many were planted before the deaths of the individuals they honored. They were thus a living legacy to the contributions of people involved with the Proctor Foundation, the Alta California Foundation, and Phil and Ruth Lee Thygeson. Ruth Lee was honored by a deodar that was once a living Christmas tree. Elizabeth C. Proctor was represented by a stately redwood and by camellias and rhododendrons that originated in her garden in Santa Fe. G. Richard O'Connor, and his work in uveitis, including toxoplasmosis, was embodied as an Italian cypress. Masao Okumoto was represented by a magnolia tree. Phil's long-term friends and former partners in the San Jose private practice were represented by a deodar for Daniel Vaughan and a cypress for Crowell Beard. Perhaps it all started with the Ludvig von Sallmann oak, which was given to Ruth Lee as a tiny sprig in the early 1970s.[54] It grew into a large oak with a wonderful canopy spreading over the fish pond. Mistletoe grew in the oak all year round. It was under this tree that Ruth Lee and Phil often entertained guests or sat alone together, holding hands and watching the sunset.

Phil had a major stroke in 1996 that affected the left side of his body. Unable to walk, he settled into his wheelchair and bed for his final years. He spent hours at his desk writing memorable essays about his medical career and life experiences. Due to his genetic stock and wonderful care by Earlene Chapman and others,[55] Phil was in remarkably good shape at the end, though he had been unable to walk for five years. He could hold a lucid conversation and still took an interest in life inside his house and beyond its walls. Fritjof was halfway through reading a biography of Abraham Lincoln aloud to his father, when Phil grew weak. Phil had always taken a rational, scientific approach to death. Yet, in his final days, he spoke of rejoining Ruth Lee and Lib. His last coherent words were about a farm. Perhaps he was thinking of his childhood farm on Lake Minnetonka. Finally, on July 27, 2002, Phil Thygeson performed his last great experiment, the results of which remain a mystery.

Chapter Notes

Introduction

1. Phillips Thygeson, M.D., *A Link with Our Past: External Eye Disease and the Proctor Foundation,* an oral history conducted in 1987 by Sally Smith Hughes, Ph.D., Regional History Office, University of California, in cooperation with The Foundation of the American Academy of Ophthalmology, 21.
2. The maxillary sinus, located below the eye, is accessed through the upper jaw above one of the patient's molar teeth. In the Caldwell Luc operation, a pocket is carved out to connect the maxillary sinus with the nose, thus improving sinus drainage. American Academy of Otolaryngology Head and Neck Surgery, www.entnet.org.

1. A Minnesota Childhood

1. Thygeson, *A Link with Our Past,* 1.
2. "Early Landowners in the Town of Martell, Pierce County, Wisconsin." http://piercebios.tripod.com/land.htm.
3. Thygeson, *A Link with Our Past,* 1.
4. Ibid.
5. Ibid.
6. Ibid.
7. Phillips Thygeson, "My Father," 1996.
8. Elling attended the Minnesota State Fair every year, giving a five-dollar gold piece to each of his grandchildren — Phil and his three older siblings. Phil never could have a conversation with his grandfather.
9. Thygeson, "My Father."
10. Sylvie Grace Thompson Thygeson, *The Suffragists,* an oral history conducted from 1972 to 1974 by Ralda Sullivan (Lee), Regional Oral History Office, University of California, Berkeley. http://ark.cdlib.org/ark:/13030/kt2h4n992z. Ralda Lee, Ph.D., Sylvie Thygeson's great-niece by marriage, was one of two scholars who interviewed Sylvie Thygeson in her final years and created a valuable oral history record.
11. Thygeson, *A Link with Our Past,* 46.
12. Sylvie Thygeson, *The Suffragists,* 4.
13. Kristin Thygeson, interview by Beret E. Strong, May 18, 2006.
14. Sylvie Thygeson, *The Suffragists,* 5.
15. Ibid, 6.
16. Ibid, 47.
17. Ibid, 6.
18. Ibid, 47.
19. Ibid, 7.
20. Nels Marcus Thygeson, M.D., interview by Beret E. Strong, May 12, 2005.
21. Sylvie Thygeson, *The Suffragists,* 6.
22. Ibid.
23. Ibid, 7.
24. Ibid, 10.
25. Ibid, 46.
26. Ibid, front matter.
27. Ibid., 9, 13–14.
28. Ibid., 8.
29. Ibid., 10.
30. Ibid., 12.
31. Ibid., 14.
32. Ibid., 12.
33. Ibid., 15.
34. Ibid., 24.
35. Ibid., 17.
36. Ibid., 25.
37. Ibid., 32.
38. Ibid., 18.

39. Ibid.
40. Thygeson, *The Suffragists*, 19 and front matter.
41. Ibid., 23.
42. Ibid., 25.
43. Nels Marcus Thygeson, interview by Beret E. Strong, May 12, 2005.
44. Michael T. Kaufman, "Stokely Carmichael, Rights Leader Who Coined 'Black Power,' Dies at 57," *New York Times* (November 16, 1998).
45. Ibid., 41.
46. Ibid, 42.
47. Ibid.
48. Ibid., 4.
49. Mary Thygeson Shepardson, interview by Beret E. Strong, 1991.
50. Ibid.
51. Phillips Thygeson, "Fili Guten — Good Boy," January 14, 1997.
52. Ibid.
53. Ibid., 1–2.
54. Thygeson, "Fili Guten — Good Boy," 1.
55. Ibid., 2.
56. Ibid., 2–3.
57. Phillips Thygeson, "Engines," n.d., 1.
58. Ibid.
59. Thygeson, "Fili Guten — Good Boy," 4.
60. Phillips Thygeson, "My Father Marcus," n.d., 5.
61. Ibid.
62. Thygeson, "Fili Guten — Good Boy," 3.
63. Ibid., 4.
64. Thygeson, "My Father Marcus," 6. Sylvie Thompson's Uncle Elmer ran for mayor of New York City as a socialist candidate and lost.
65. Ibid.
66. Phillips Thygeson, "Minnetonka Days," January 17, 1997, 3.
67. Ibid., 1.
68. Phillips Thygeson, "The Joy of a Farm on a Lake," September 28, 1996, 1.
69. Thygeson, "My Father Marcus," 4.
70. Ibid., 6.
71. Ibid., 5, and Thygeson, "The Joy of a Farm on a Lake," 2–3.
72. Thygeson, "The Joy of a Farm on a Lake," 1.
73. Thygeson, "Minnetonka Days," 5.
74. Thygeson, *A Link with Our Past*, 9.
75. Thygeson, "My Father Marcus," 7.
76. Ibid.
77. Fritjof Thygeson, interview by Beret E. Strong, November 6, 2004.
78. Phillips Thygeson, "The Winter of 1915," October 7, 1996, 1–2.
79. Ibid., 3.
80. Ibid., 4.
81. Nels Marcus Thygeson, interview by Beret E. Strong, May 12, 2005.
82. Thygeson, "My Father Marcus," 7.
83. Phillips Thygeson, "Father and Lala," February 5, 1998, 3.
84. Thygeson, "My Father Marcus," 7.
85. A generation later, the effects of Nel Marcus's premature death were still being felt. "The greatest tragedy of my father's life was that his father died when they were both too young for such a loss. My grandfather didn't have the opportunity to finish the task of teaching and guiding his son, and my father was too young to fully appreciate what his father had to give him. My father would have been a happier, more interesting, and more loving person if his father had simply lived longer." Fritjof Thygeson, communication with author, May 8, 2007.
86. Kristin Thygeson, interview by Beret E. Strong, November 1, 2004.

2. A San Francisco Childhood

1. Kristin Thygeson, interview by Beret E. Strong, November 1, 2004.
2. Ibid.
3. Esther was not the only stylish member of the family. Esther's rakish brother, known in the family as Uncle Billy, became a Hollywood actor who had a love affair with actress Billie Burke, who played Glinda the Good, the good witch of the North, in the famous 1939 film *The Wizard of Oz*, starring Judy Garland. Uncle Billy was a dashing lady's man in his early years. It is believed he died a homeless, alcoholic pauper on the streets of San Francisco decades later and that Phil would find him in the city morgue. As Phil and Ruth Lee's son Fritjof related, "My father dealt with his corpse.... He checked that name and he was 99 percent sure that this was ... his uncle-in-law. He died a hobo on the streets of San Francisco." Fritjof Thygeson, interview by Beret E. Strong, November 7, 2004.
4. Kristin Thygeson, interview by Beret E. Strong, November 1, 2004.
5. The voyage from England took over four months on three cramped, rickety ships.

The settlers' first winter was devastating because of freezing weather, shortage of food and water, infectious disease, and the fact that the local Algonquian Indians waged war upon them. Captain Smith returned to England briefly in 1608 and left the colonists to do their best to fend for themselves. This disastrous winter was known as the "starving time"; only 60 of the original 214 Jamestown settlers survived. The local Native Americans wished the settlers had never come and took advantage of opportunities to encourage them to return to England forever. "History of Jamestown," http://www.apva.org/history/.
    6. John Smith, *The Generall Historie of Virginia, New England & the Summer Isles*, vol. 1 (Glasgow, Scotland: James MacLehose and Sons, 1907), 203–04.
    7. William Box, n.d., "Jamestown Given New Life, 1610," http://lcweb2.10c.gov/learn/features/timeline/colonial/jamestwn/net.html. Also, a most likely fanciful novel describes Henry Spilman as being not over twenty-one years old when he, a "scapegrace, whose friends were willing to be rid of him," was most likely "shipped bound as an apprentice ... to be sold or bound out at the end of the voyage to pay his passage." This same novelist, who inaccurately represents some of the facts of John Smith's life, claims that Henry was the son of a distinguished antiquarian of Norfolk, England. Charles Dudley Warner, quoted from John Smith. John Smith, "Smith's Last Days in Virginia," http://www.readbookonline/net/read/194/6259/.
    8. "The Complete Book of Emigrants, 1607–1776. List of First Settlers at Jamestown Island, Virginia, in 1607 as Noted by Captain John Smith," n.d., http://www.runningdeerslonghouse.com/webdoc38.htm.
    9. "Path of the Parrish's," http://wwgeocities.com/awoodlief/parrishhist.htm?20053.
    10. Kristin Thygeson, interview by Beret E. Strong, November 1, 2004.
    11. James Spilman to Elizabeth Brewer, November 14, 1890.
    12. James Spilman to Elizabeth Brewer, November 18, 1890.
    14. James Spilman to Elizabeth Brewer, July 28, 1891.
    15. James Spilman to Elizabeth Brewer, July 5, 1891.
    16. Kristin Thygeson, interview by Beret E. Strong, November 1, 2004.
    17. Ibid.
    18. Emma Burke, *Overlook Magazine*, www.sfmuseum.net/1906/ew13.html.
    19. Ibid.
    20. Ibid.
    21. Donaldina Cameron, http://www.sfmuseum.net/1906/ew15.html.
    22. Ibid.
    23. "Mills Building," http://themillsbuilding.com/building/index.html.
    24. Emma Burke, *Overlook Magazine*, June 2, 1906. www.sfmuseum.net/1906/ew13.html.
    25. Peter Bacigalupi, *Edison Phonograph Monthly*, http://www.sfmuseum.net/1906/ew16.html.
    26. De Witt C. Baldwin, "Memories of the San Francisco Earthquake and Fire," http://www.sfmuseum.net/1906/ew8.html.
    27. James Spilman to Elizabeth Brewer, 27 April 1906.
    28. James Spilman to Elizabeth Brewer, April 29, 1906.
    29. James Spilman to Elizabeth Brewer, May 2, 1906.
    30. James Spilman to Elizabeth Brewer, April 29, 1906.
    31. James Spilman to Elizabeth Brewer, May 1, 1906.
    32. James Spilman to Elizabeth Brewer, May 3, 1906
    33. James Spilman to Elizabeth Brewer, June 20, 1909.
    34. Kristin Thygeson, interview by Beret E. Strong, November 1, 2004.
    35. Ibid.
    36. Kristin Thygeson, conversation with author, December 4, 2005.

3. A Death in the Family

    1. Thygeson, *A Link with Our Past*, 6.
    2. Kristin Thygeson, conversation with author, June 6, 2006.
    3. After World War I ended, Herbert Hoover, Sr., worked in Belgium with the Belgian Relief Commission.
    4. Thygeson, *A Link with Our Past*, 6.
    5. Ibid., 5.
    6. Nels Marcus Thygeson, interview by Beret E. Strong, May 12, 2005.
    7. Thygeson, *A Link with Our Past*, 5.
    8. Harry Helms, *All about Ham Radio* (San Diego, CA: High Text Publications, 1992), 7. Ham operators communicate with fellow hams. They are not allowed to seek financial benefit from the activity.
    9. Robert W. Peterson, *Boy Scouts: An American Adventure* (New York: American Heritage, 1984), 17.

10. Ibid., 23–25.
11. "Robert Baden-Powell as an Educational Innovator," http://www.infed.org/thinkers/et-bp.htm.
12. Ibid.
13. *Boy Scouts of America: Handbook for Boy* (1911), 240–41.
14. Ibid.
15. Ibid.
16. Nels Marcus Thygeson, interview by Beret E. Strong, May 12, 2005.
17. *Boy Scouts of America: Handbook for Boys*, 3.
18. Peterson, *Boy Scouts*, 56.
19. Ibid., 43.
20. Ibid., 89.
21. Ibid.
22. Ibid., 91.
23. Phillips Thygeson, "The High School Cadets," October 2, 1996.
24. *Boy Scouts of America: Handbook for Boys*, xii.
25. Ibid., 248.

4. Genteel Poverty and a Pandemic

1. Later in life, Lib and Ruth Lee sometimes donned surgical masks to avoid passing on colds and other minor illnesses to members of their families. This habit probably got its start in 1918 when contagion was a matter of life and death.
2. "The Influenza Epidemic of 1918," http://www.stanford/edu/group/virus/uda/.
3. Ibid.
4. Ibid.
5. Ibid.
6. David M. Morens and Jeffery K. Taubenberger, "1918 Influenza: The Mother of All Pandemics," *CDC*, http://www.cdc.gov/ncidod/EID/v0112n001/05-0979.htm
7. "The Influenza Epidemic of 1918."
8. "The Public Health Response," http://www.stanford.edu/group/virus/uda/fluresponse.html.
9. "Joseph Lister, 1st Baron Lister," http://en.wikipedia.org/wiki/Joseph_Lister.
10. A rhyme became popular among schoolchildren and even among adults who had to be reminded to wear their masks: "Obey the laws / And wear your gauze / Protect your jaws / From Septic Paws." The Public Health Response.
11. Ibid.
12. "The Medical and Scientific Conceptions of Influenza," http://www.stanford.edu/group/virus/uda/fluscimed.html.
13. Ibid.

5. Meeting at Stanford

1. Phillips Thygeson, "Vision," July 12, 1996.
2. Ruth Lee liked to say that Stanford began as a "poor boys school." That's actually something of a myth, though the university had great financial hardship in its early years and nearly everyone involved sacrificed to keep it going.
3. Edith R. Mirrielees, *Stanford: The Story of a University* (New York: Putnam's, 1959), 20.
4. "Stanford University History," n.d., http://www.stanford.edu/home/stanford/history/begin.html.
5. Ibid.
6. Ibid.
7. Mirrielees, *Stanford*, 23–24.
8. Ibid., 22–23.
9. Ibid., 63.
10. Ibid., 87.
11. Ibid., 88.
12. "Stanford University History: Stanford History by Presidency," n.d., http://www.stanford.edu/home/stanford/history/leader.html
13. Mirrielees, *Stanford*, 139–40.
14. Ibid., 140–41. Students in good academic standing were given credit for missing coursework.
15. Ibid., 141.
16. Ibid., 54–56.
17. Ibid., 61.
18. Ibid., 60–61.
19. Thygeson, *A Link with Our Past*, 5.
20. Mirrielees, *Stanford*, 191.
21. Ibid., 196.
22. Ibid., 191.
23. Ibid.
24. Ibid.
25. Ibid., 166–67.
26. Ibid., 178.
27. Ibid.
28. Ibid., 203. The advantage was in Stanford's court. In 1921, Stanford sent out a questionnaire to high school teachers and principals asking them to rate Stanford applicants on "scholarship, personality, industry, judgment, reliability, initiative, cooperation, native ability, leadership."

29. Thygeson, *A Link with Our Past*, 10.
30. Mirrielees, *Stanford*, 201.
31. Ibid., 184.
32. Ibid., 187.
33. Thygeson, *A Link with Our Past*, 10.
34. Ibid.
35. Ibid., 7. Ironically, Phil and Ruth Lee's son Fritjof would skip fifth grade and suffer a similar life-long inability to cope well with math.
36. Ibid., 10.
37. Mirrielees, *Stanford*, 166.
38. Thygeson, *A Link with Our Past*, 15.
39. Ibid., 13.
40. Ibid.
41. Ibid.
42. Ibid., 16.
43. Phillips Thygeson, "The Lady Ruth Lee," vol.1, n.d.
44. Nels Marcus Thygeson, interview by Beret E. Strong, May 18, 2005.

6. Courtship, a Wedding, and Victorian Values

1. Thygeson, *A Link with Our Past*, 17. The church was demolished long ago.
2. Nels Marcus Thygeson, interview by Beret E. Strong, May 18, 2005.
3. Thygeson, "The Lady Ruth Lee: Queen of the Ruth Lee Hilltop," v. 1.
4. Thygeson, "Vision."
5. Fritjof Thygeson, conversation with author, April 28, 2007.
6. Nels Marcus Thygeson, interview by Beret E. Strong, May 18, 2005. Marcus Thygeson tells a story of how he was made aware of the gap between his belief system and that of his grandmother. While in medical school at Harvard, Marcus told his grandmother about discovering that a friend's friend was a hit man for the mafia, as well as a good neighbor, businessman, and head of a family. As Marcus was about to say, "Isn't life fascinating? ... What do you do when you find out that this friend of yours has this dark side?" Ruth Lee looked at her grandson "with this look of horror on her face and said, 'And they still consider him their friend?' For her, there was no ambiguity. You don't associate with people like that. You call the police." Marcus concluded, "What a different world view."
7. Wayne Edward Oates, *Confessions of a Workaholic: The Facts about Work Addiction* (New York: World, 1971), 84.

8. Kristin Thygeson, conversation with author, December 4, 2005.
9. Their values tended to be largely secular. See, for example, Adrian Furnham, *The Protestant Work Ethic* (London: Routledge, 1990), 16. An eclectic set of values outlined by sociologist R. Williams includes achievement and success, work, morality and humanitarianism, efficiency and practicality, progress, science and rationalism, nationalism, individualism, democracy, racism, and group-supremacy.
10. Phillips Thygeson, "Great Books," January 17, 1997.
11. Peter Allan Dale, *In Pursuit of a Scientific Culture: Science, Arts, and Society in the Victorian Age* (Madison: University of Wisconsin Press, 1989), 11.
12. Walter E. Houghton, *The Victorian Frame of Mind, 1830–1870* (New Haven, CT: Yale University Press, 1957), 95.
13. Fritjof Thygeson, interview by Beret E. Strong, November 7, 2004.
14. Fritjof Thygeson, conversation with author, April 28, 2007.

7. Married and in Medical School

1. Thygeson, "The Lady Ruth Lee: Queen of the Ruth Lee Hilltop," v. 1.
2. Thygeson, *A Link with Our Past*, 15.
3. Ibid., 14–15.
4. Ibid., 16.
5. Ibid., 17.
6. Thygeson, "The Lady Ruth Lee: Queen of the Ruth Lee Hilltop," vol. 1.
7. Fritjof Thygeson, interview by Beret E. Strong, November 6, 2004.
8. Phillips Thygeson, "Stanford Medical School Days," 1997, 3.
9. Ibid.
10. Ibid, 5.
11. Ibid.
12. Thygeson, *A Link with Our Past*, 17.
13. Ibid.
14. Ibid., 18.
15. Ibid., 17.
16. Ibid., 11.
17. Ibid.
18. Thygeson, "Stanford Medical School Days," 4.
19. Thygeson, *A Link with Our Past*, 11.
20. Ibid., 12.
21. Kristin Thygeson, interview by Beret E. Strong, November 16, 2004.

8. Frontier Medicine in Colorado

1. Thygeson, *A Link with Our Past*, 25.
2. Thygeson, "The Lady Ruth Lee: Queen of the Ruth Lee Hilltop," v. 1.
3. Robert H. Shikes, *Rocky Mountain Medicine: Doctors, Drugs, and Disease in Early Colorado* (Boulder, CO: Johnson Books, 1986), 2.
4. Ibid.
5. Ibid.
6. W.H. Goode, in D.W. Blair, "The Early Diaries of Colorado," 79, master's thesis, University of Denver, 1944. Quoted in Ibid., 111.
7. Phillips Thygeson, "Dr. W.C. Finnoff," n.d.
8. Ibid., 25.
9. Ibid.
10. Thygeson, *A Link with Our Past*, 24.
11. Phillips Thygeson, "Edward Jackson," July 1, 1996.
12. Thygeson, *A Link with Our Past*, 25.
13. Thygeson, "Edward Jackson."
14. Nels Marcus Thygeson, interview by Beret E. Strong, May 18, 2005.
15. Thygeson, "Edward Jackson."
16. Ibid.
17. Ibid.
18. Thygeson, *A Link with Our Past*, 24.
19. Ibid.
20. Ibid., 26.
21. Shikes, 6.
22. Ibid.
23. Phillips Thygeson, "The Ideal Nurse: Lala and Earlene," June 28, 1996, 1.
24. Thygeson, "The Lady Ruth Lee: Queen of the Ruth Lee Hilltop," vol. 1.
25. Phillips Thygeson, "My Ruth Lee," vol. 1, September 24, 1996.
26. Phillips Thygeson, "The Natural History of Infectious Ocular Disease," July 8, 1996.
27. Shikes, *Rocky Mountain Medicine*, ix.
28. Ibid., 73.
29. Denver Quaker Cook Book (Denver, 1905), quoted in Ibid.
30. Shikes, *Rocky Mountain Medicine*, 22.
31. Ibid., 72.
32. Ibid., 23.
33. Ibid., 31.
34. Ibid., 36.
35. Ibid.
36. Lawrence N. Greenleaf, *King Sham, and Other Atrocities in Verse* (New York, 1868), quoted in Shikes, *Rocky Mountain Medicine*, 33.
37. Shikes, *Rocky Mountain Medicine*, 193.
38. City of Denver 3:16, 1914, quoted in Shikes, *Rocky Mountain Medicine* 194.
39. Shikes, *Rocky Mountain Medicine*, 194.
40. Ibid., 108.
41. Ibid.
42. Ibid., 109.
43. L.C. Boyd, "History of the Denver General Hospital, 1860–1924," quoted in Shikes, *Rocky Mountain Medicine* 59. In the 1860s, the indigent went to City Hospital and wealthy people received care at home. In the course of the decade, County Hospital opened its doors for the first time. It was only a hundred feet long and cost less than five thousand dollars to build.
44. Shikes, *Rocky Mountain Medicine*, 60.
45. Ibid.
46. Boyd, "History," in Shikes, *Rocky Mountain Medicine*, 61.
47. Ibid.
48. Ibid.
49. "Tuberculosis — Notification of Cases and Control of." Chap. 125, March 17, 1913," *Public Health Reports* 29:593, 1914. Quoted in Shikes, *Rocky Mountain Medicine*, 185.
50. Ibid., 187.
51. Ibid., 229.
52. Ibid.
53. Ibid., 230.
54. Ibid, 121.
55. Abraham Flexner, "Medical Education in the United States and Canada. A Report to the Carnegie Foundation for the Advancement of Teaching." *Bulletin No. 4*, Carnegie Foundation, New York, 1910. Quoted in Shikes, *Rocky Mountain Medicine*, 124.
56. Ibid., 125.
57. Biennial Report of the Regents of the University of Colorado, 1919–1920, quoted in Shikes, *Rocky Mountain Medicine*, 128.
58. Ibid., 228–29.
59. Ibid., 147.
60. Ibid., 156.
61. Ibid., 68.
62. *Denver Medical Times* 16:390, 1886, quoted in Shikes, *Rocky Mountain Medicine*, 68.
63. Ibid.
64. Ibid.
65. "Tuberculosis — Notification of Cases and Control of." Ch. 125, March 17, 1913," *Public Health Reports* 29:593, 1914. Quoted in Shikes, *Rocky Mountain Medicine,* 169.

66. *JAMA* 34:1430, 1900, quoted in Shikes, *Rocky Mountain Medicine,* 169.
67. Nels Marcus Thygeson, interview by Beret E. Strong, May 12, 2005.
68. Ibid.
69. Nels Marcus Thygeson, ibid.
70. Shikes, *Rocky Mountain Medicine,* 229.
71. Fritjof Thygeson, interview by Beret E. Strong, November 6, 2004.
72. Kristin Thygeson, interview by Beret E. Strong, November 1, 2004.
73. During the Depression, while living with Ruth Lee's sister Lib and husband Milton, Elizabeth Brewer Spilman had a reputation for never turning a hungry person away from her door. In keeping with the Protestant work ethic the family held dear, she would always accept the offers of itinerant men — essentially, hobos — to do a chore or two before she gave them a meal. One of the men showed up every year around the same time. He favored a certain kind of canned soup, so Elizabeth Spilman made sure she always had a can on hand. She'd say, "How about an egg to go with that?" And he'd respond, "An egg would go good, ma'am."
74. Kristin Thygeson, interview by Beret E. Strong, November 1, 2004.
75. Ibid.
76. Ibid.

9. Building a Real Log Cabin

1. James Lindberg, Patricia Raney, and Janet Robertson, *Rocky Mountain Rustic: Historic Buildings of the Rocky Mountain National Park Area* (Estes Park, CO: Rocky Mountain Nature Association, 1994), 12.
2. Lindberg et al., *Rocky Mountain Rustic,* 14.
3. Lindberg et al., *Rocky Mountain Rustic,* 65.
4. Lindberg et al., *Rocky Mountain Rustic,* 21.
5. Lindberg et al., *Rocky Mountain Rustic,* 129.
6. Lindberg et al., *Rocky Mountain Rustic,* 66.
7. http://www.cr.nps.gov/nr/twhp/wwwlps/lessons/410gcabins/4facts1.htm
8. Lindberg et al., *Rocky Mountain Rustic,* 128.
9. Lindberg et al., *Rocky Mountain Rustic,* 132.
10. Kristin Thygeson, interview by Beret E. Strong, November 16, 2004.
11. Thygeson, "The Lady Ruth Lee: Queen of the Ruth Lee Hilltop," vol. 1.
12. Nels Marcus Thygeson, interview by Beret E. Strong, May 12, 2005.
13. Hunt, 14.
14. Lindberg et al., *Rocky Mountain Rustic,* 19.
15. Hunt, 27.
16. Hunt, 41.
17. Hunt, 13.
18. Kristin Thygeson, interview by Beret E. Strong, November 16, 2004.
19. Kristin Thygeson, interview by Beret E. Strong, November 16, 2004.
20. Kristin Thygeson, conversation with author, December 4, 2005.

10. To Egypt in Search of Trachoma

1. "World Bank Trachoma at a Glance Pamphlet," www.trachoma.org. Since trachoma often renders its adult victims unable to work, it is estimated even now to cause lost human productivity in the amount of nearly three billion dollars per year. Children and the women who care for them are most at risk of infection. If a mother is blinded from trachoma, often her oldest daughter will leave school to take over her chores and wage work.
2. Phillips Thygeson, "Francis I. Proctor," January 12, 1997.
3. Ibid.
4. Hoslink, "Pioneers in Medical Laboratory Science," http://www.hoslink.com/history2.htm.
5. Thygeson, "Francis I. Proctor."
6. Phillips Thygeson, "Elizabeth C. Proctor: Our First Meeting," n.d.
7. Thygeson, *A Link with Our Past,* 30.
8. Ibid., 31.
9. Phillips Thygeson, "Roland P. Wilson," June 29, 1996.
10. Ibid.
11. Thygeson, *A Link with Our Past,* 31.
12. Ibid., 32.
13. Thygeson, "The Elizabeth C. Proctor Story," March 21, 1996.
14. Thygeson, *A Link with Our Past,* 32.
15. Ibid., 33.
16. Thygeson, "The Elizabeth C. Proctor Story."
17. Ibid.
18. Thygeson, "Roland P. Wilson."

19. Ibid.
20. Ibid.
21. Ibid.
22. This was Phillips Thygeson, "Bacterial Flora in Egyptian Trachoma," *American Journal of Ophthalmology* 14 (1931): 1104–07.
23. Thygeson, "Roland P. Wilson."
24. Wilson stayed on at the Giza Institute until called to serve in World War II. His role as director was eventually taken over by a friend and colleague of Phil's, Dr. Maxwell-Lyons.

11. Learning from a Nobel Laureate in Tunisia

1. "Charles Nicolle (1866–1936)," http://www.pasteur.fr/infosci/archives/nic0.html.
2. Thygeson, *A Link with Our Past*, 33.
3. Kristin Thygeson, interview by Beret E. Strong, November 1, 2004.
4. Fritjof Thygeson, interview by Beret E. Strong, November 6, 2004.
5. Thygeson, *A Link with Our Past*, 34.
6. Fritjof Thygeson, interview by Beret E. Strong, November 6, 2004.
7. Thygeson, *A Link with Our Past*, 36–37.
8. After their year in Tunis, Phil and Ruth Lee tried to keep up their French by speaking it at home and teaching it to Fritjof, but he had a hard time being an emerging speaker in two languages who could use only one of the languages with his little friends. Though Fritjof had learned French before he learned English, he became a monolingual English speaker, the dream of bilingualism abandoned. Fritjof Thygeson, interview by Beret E. Strong, November 6, 2004.
9. Ibid.
10. Thygeson, *A Link with Our Past*, 37.
11. Ibid., 35.
12. Ibid., 336.
13. Ibid., 52.
14. Ibid., 53.
15. Phillips Thygeson, "Charles Nicolle," June 19, 1996.
16. Ibid.
17. Thygeson, *A Link with Our Past*, 36.
18. Ibid., 34.
19. Phillips Thygeson, "Victor Morax," June 29, 1996. See also David V. Cohn, "The Life and Times of Louis Pasteur," http://www.louisville.edu/library/ekstrom/special/Pasteur/cohn.hmtl. Morax introduced him to the concierge of the Pasteur Institute, who was famous for having been bitten by a rabid wolf in 1886 as a child of nine. Due to his mother's impassioned pleading, the Alsatian boy had had the good fortune of being the first person to receive Pasteur's new vaccine for rabies. Pasteur wasn't a licensed physician and didn't want to offer a vaccine that hadn't been proven in humans, but the boy was badly mauled and was going to die. The boy, Joseph Meister, was the first person ever to be made immune to rabies. He returned as an adult for long years of work as concierge at the Pasteur Institute. He came to a tragic end, however, for when the Nazis occupied Paris in 1940, they demanded that he open Pasteur's crypt. Meister chose to kill himself to avoid carrying out the order.
20. Phillips Thygeson, "A Day with Victor Morax," February 2, 1998.
21. Thygeson, "Victor Morax."
22. Thygeson, "A Day with Victor Morax."
23. Thygeson, *A Link with Our Past*, 34.
24. Fritjof Thygeson, Interview by Beret E. Strong, November 6, 2004.
25. Thygeson, "Victor Morax."
26. Ibid.
27. Phillips Thygeson, "Microbiologist," September 27, 1996.
28. Paul De Kruif, *Microbe Hunters* (San Diego, CA: Harcourt, 1954), 1.
29. Ibid., 11.
30. Ibid., 6, 12–13.
31. Cohn., "The Life and Times of Louis Pasteur."
32. Ibid.
33. Ibid.
34. Ibid.
35. Ibid.
36. "Joseph Lister, 1st Baron Lister," http://www.absoluteastronomy.com/reference/joseph_lister_1st_baron_lister.
37. Ibid.
38. Frank Uwe, "Robert Koch — Beyond Postulates," *Virox-Solutions*, http://72.14.207.104/search?q=cache:rsJrRsUUIvkJ:www.virox.com/pdf/solutions_fall_05.pdf+robert+koch+ripe+apples+from+a+tree&hl=en&gl=us&ct=clnk&cd=2.
39. For one of the articles, Phil had a French-speaking first author, U. Lumbroso, who most likely took care of the language issues.
40. Thygeson, "The Lady Ruth Lee: Queen of the Ruth Lee Hilltop," v. 1.
41. Phillips Thygeson, "Vacations," n.d.

12. Research Idyll in Iowa City

1. "A Brief History of Ophthalmology at the University of Iowa," n.d., Department of Ophthalmology and Visual Sciences, University of Iowa Health Care, http://webeye.ophth.uiowa.edu/dept/LEGACY/History/history.htm.
2. Fritjof Thygeson, interview by Beret E. Strong, November 6, 2004.
3. Thygeson, *A Link with Our Past*, 38.
4. Ibid.
5. Carl A. Merry, "The Historic Period," 1996, University of Iowa, http://www.uiowa.edu/~osa/learn/historic/hisper.htm.
6. Ibid. The Meskwakis gave a lead mine to French-Canadian speculator Julien Dubuque in 1788, which he supplemented with a land grant from the Spanish governor of Louisiana. His operation was multiethnic and generally profitable, though it went through some lean times. When Dubuque died in 1810, possibly of lead poisoning, land speculators and creditors claiming debts swarmed in to try to take over his holdings. The Meskwakis burned all of the buildings of the mining and trade holding rather than let them be taken over by white speculators from the East.
7. Ibid.
8. "History of the University of Iowa," n.d., http://www.lib.uiowa.edu/spec-coll/Archives/chronohistory.htm.
9. Ibid.
10. Ibid.
11. Ibid.
12. Fritjof Thygeson, interview by Beret E. Strong, November 6, 2004.
13. Philip A. Jordan, "Adventures of a Student at Iowa," *Books at Iowa 28* (April 1978), University of Iowa, http://wwwlib.uiowa.edu/spec-coll/Bai/jordan3.htm.
14. Ibid.
15. Samuel Levey, *The Rise of a University Teaching Hospital, a Leadership Perspective: The University of Iowa Hospitals and Clinics* (Chicago: Health Administration Press, 1997), 48–49.
16. Ibid., 50.
17. Ibid., 444.
18. Ibid., 51.
19. Ibid., 449.
20. Ibid., 59.
21. Ibid., 146–59.
22. Ibid., 145.
23. Ibid., 148.
24. Ibid., 148–50.
25. Ibid., 165.
26. Chandler Dawson, "Phillips Thygeson, MD (1903–2002)," in *Chlamydial Infections: Proceedings of the Eleventh International Symposium on Human Chlamydial Infections*, June 2006, viii.
27. Ibid.
28. Fritjof Thygeson, interview by Beret E. Strong, November 6, 2004.
29. Ruth Lee Thygeson to Mara Thygeson, 16 April, 1975.
30. Levey, *University Teaching Hospital*, 68.
31. "A Brief History of Ophthalmology at the University of Iowa."
32. Levey, *University Teaching Hospital*, 101.
33. Ibid.
34. Ibid., 169.
35. Ibid., 170.
36. Thygeson, *A Link with Our Past*, 38.
37. Ibid.
38. Ibid., 38–39.
39. Ibid., 39.
40. Ibid.
41. Kristin Thygeson, interview by Beret E. Strong, November 1, 2004.
42. Thygeson, "The Lady Ruth Lee: Queen of the Ruth Lee Hilltop," v. 1.
43. Thygeson, *A Link with Our Past*, 40–41.
44. Ibid., 41.
45. Phillips Thygeson, "The Nature of the Elementary and Initial Bodies of Trachoma," *Archives of Ophthalmology* 12 (1934).
46. Thygeson, *A Link with Our Past*, 41.
47. Ibid.
48. Ibid., 42.
49. Ibid.
50. Thygeson, *A Link with Our Past*, 44.
51. Ibid, 45–46. Phil enjoyed telling stories of clinical and laboratory mishaps, partly because he found some humor in them and partly because some of them led to new insights. He told of a gynecologist who created a cotton obturator—what women might think of as akin to a tampon—attached a string to it, inserted it into a glass rod, and obtained samples of cervical secretions by this method. He managed to hit himself in the face with one of his obturators and came down with inclusion conjunctivitis. In New York, a resident delivering a baby infected himself in much the same manner by spanking a newborn too vigorously and getting secretions in his eye. This stimulated new re-

search during Phil's tenure at Columbia University.
52. Thygeson, *A Link with Our Past*, 49.

13. Fort Apache and the Great Experiment

1. Ibid., 50.
2. Ibid.
3. In Ruth Lee's kitchen, there were drawers of carefully folded plastic and paper bags for reuse, shards of Ivory soap put into a little metal device for the dishpan so that not even a remnant would go to waste.
4. Ibid., 26.
5. Ibid., 50.
6. "Images from the History of the Public Health Service, Introduction," National Library of Medicine, http://www.nlm.nih.gov/exhibition/phs_history/intro.html. A small bacteriology laboratory on Staten Island called the "Hygienic Laboratory" was opened in 1887 to help diagnose infectious diseases being brought to the United States by people—especially immigrants—arriving by ship. The laboratory changed locations in 1891, expanded, and later became the National Institutes of Health, considered the biggest biomedical research organization and facility in the world.
7. Thygeson, *A Link with Our Past*, 51.
8. The facilities at Fort Apache had been set up by the PHS at Dr. Proctor's request. Ibid., 54.
9. Ibid., 55.
10. Chandler Dawson, M.D., interview by Sally Smith Hughes, Ph.D., November 6, 1986, Regional Oral History Office, University of California, Berkeley, and American Academy of Ophthalmology. Dawson recalled Phil telling "this wonderful story about the local ranchers coming by looking for chimps, because they had never seen anything like it."
11. Phillips Thygeson, "Polk Richards," July 2, 1996.
12. Ibid.
13. Thygeson, *A Link with Our Past*, 51.
14. Thygeson, "Polk Richards."
15. "Arizona Apache Wars," http://www.geocities.com/zybt/awars.htm.
16. Ibid.
17. Thygeson, *A Link with Our Past*, 60.
18. Ibid.
19. Thygeson, "The Elizabeth C. Proctor Story."
20. Kristin Thygeson, conversation with author, December 4, 2005.
21. Thygeson, *A Link with Our Past*, 60.
22. Thygeson, "The Elizabeth C. Proctor Story."
23. Ibid., 62.
24. Ibid.
25. Ibid., 66.
26. Ibid., 63.
27. "The March toward War: The March of Time as Documentary and Propaganda," http://xroad.virginia.edu/~MA04/wood/mot/html/document.htm.
28. Ibid. Historian Raymond Fielding is quoted.
29. Ibid.
30. Thygeson, *A Link with Our Past*, 64.
31. Ibid., 64.
32. Paul De Kruif, "They Wait for Light," *Country Gentleman* 10–11 (September 1940): 10.
33. Ibid.
34. Ibid.
35. Ibid.
36. Ibid., 11.
37. Ibid., 33.
38. Thygeson, *A Link with Our Past*, 77.
39. Ibid., 78–79.
40. Ibid.
41. Ibid., 61.
42. Ibid.
43. Ibid.

14. The New York Chapter: Two Kinds of Politics

1. Ibid., 66–67.
2. Ibid., 67.
3. Ibid., 148.
4. Ibid., 69.
5. Ibid.
6. Ibid., 80.
7. Ibid.
8. Chandler Dawson, in Max Chernesky et al., eds., *Chlamydial Infections: Proceedings of the Eleventh International Symposium on Human Chlamydial Infections* (International Chlamydia Symposium, 2006), viii.
9. Thygeson, *A Link with Our Past*, 83.
10. Kristin Thygeson, interview by Beret E. Strong, November 1, 2004.
11. Thygeson, "The Lady Ruth Lee, Queen of the Ruth Lee Hilltop," v. 1.
12. Fritjof Thygeson, interview by Beret E. Strong, November 6, 2004.

13. Ibid.
14. Thygeson, *A Link with Our Past*, 103.
15. Nels Marcus Thygeson, interview by Beret E. Strong, May 18, 2005.
16. Fritjof Thygeson, interview by Beret E. Strong, November 6, 2004.
17. Kristin Thygeson, interview by Beret E. Strong, November 16, 2004.
18. Ibid.
19. Fritjof Thygeson, interview by Beret E. Strong, November 6, 2004.
20. Ibid.
21. Kristin Thygeson, interview by Beret E. Strong, November 1, 2004.
22. Ibid.
23. Mara Thygeson, interview by Beret E. Strong, June 29, 2005.
24. Kristin Thygeson, interview by Beret E. Strong, November 16, 2004.
25. Kristin Thygeson, interview by Beret E. Strong, November 1, 2004.
26. Ibid.
27. Thygeson, *A Link with Our Past*, 104.
28. Algernon B. Reese to Ruth Lee Thygeson, 1949.
29. Algernon B. Reese to Ruth Lee Thygeson, 1950.
30. Thygeson, *A Link with Our Past*, 104.
31. Colin Cherry, *On Human Communication* (Cambridge, MA.: Technology Press of M.I.T. Press, 1957), 19.
32. Thygeson, *A Link with Our Past*, 105.
33. Kristin Thygeson, interview by Beret E. Strong, November 1, 2004.
34. Ibid.
35. Ibid.
36. Fritjof Thygeson, interview by Beret E. Strong, November 6, 2004.
37. Ibid.
38. Ibid.
39. Clarence Lee Swartz, "What Is Mutualism?" 1927, http://www.panarchy.org/swartz/mutualism.9.html.
40. Fritjof Thygeson, interview by Beret E. Strong, November 6, 2004.
41. An interesting twist of fate is that both married Dwight Shepardson, M.D. Ruth, the older sister, married him and they had a daughter, Barbara. Ruth died of post-surgical hemorrhage when Barbara was fourteen. Mary came to care for her niece and eventually married her sister's widower.
42. Fritjof Thygeson, interview by Beret E. Strong, November 6, 2004.
43. Sylvie Thygeson, *The Suffragists*, 47–48.
44. Clarence R. Streit, *Union Now: A Proposal for a Federal Union of the Democracies of the North Atlantic* (New York: Harper & Brothers, 1939), http://www.constitution.org/aun/union_now.htm.
45. Ibid.
46. Ibid.
47. Ibid.
48. Ibid.
49. Ibid.
50. Fritjof Thygeson, interview by Beret E. Strong, November 6, 2004.
51. Eric Roark, "Herbert Spencer's Evolutionary Individualism," *Quarterly Journal of Ideology* 27, nos. 3 and 4 (2004): 6.
52. Quoted in "Herbert Spencer (1820–1903)," The Internet Encyclopedia of Philosophy, http://www.iep.utm.edu/s/spencer/htm.
53. Ibid.
54. Roark, "Evolutionary Individualism," 9.
55. Phillips Thygeson, "Families: The Story of Two Families," October 1, 1996, 1.
56. Phillips Thygeson, "The High School Cadets," October 2, 1996, 15.
57. Roark, "Evolutionary Individualism," 9.
58. Ibid., 13.
59. Quoted in Ibid., 25.
60. Quoted in Ibid., 26.
61. Phillips Thygeson, conversation with author, 1981.
62. David Weinstein, "Herbert Spencer," Stanford Encyclopedia of Philosophy, 2002, http://plato.stanford.edu/entries/spencer/.
63. Jonathan Marks, "Racism, Eugenics, and the Burdens of History" (paper presented at the IX International Congress of Human Genetics, Rio de Janeiro, August 20, 1996).
64. Ibid.
65. Ibid.
66. Ibid.
67. Ibid.
68. Phillips Thygeson, "My Children," September 27, 1996.
69. Ibid.
70. Phillips Thygeson, "Heredity," July 12, 1996.
71. Phillips Thygeson, "The Curse of Heredity," July 16, 1996.
72. Ibid.
73. Phillips Thygeson, "I Wasn't Programmed to Be a Father," September 29, 1996.
74. Kristin Thygeson, Conversation with author, December 4, 2005.
75. Thygeson, "I Wasn't Programmed to Be a Father."

76. Fritjof Thygeson, interview by Beret E. Strong, November 7, 2004.
77. Kristin Thygeson, interview by Beret E. Strong, March 1, 2005.
78. Thygeson, "Vision."
79. Kristin Thygeson, interview by Beret E. Strong, March 1, 2005.
80. Ibid.
81. Ibid.
82. Ibid.
83. Kristin Thygeson, interview by Beret E. Strong, November 16, 2004.
84. Thygeson, "I Wasn't Programmed to Be a Father."
85. G. Richard O'Connor, M.D., interview by Beret E. Strong, November 4, 2004.
86. Nels Marcus Thygeson, interview by Beret E. Strong, May 12, 2005.
87. Phillips Thygeson, "A Research Man," July 4, 1996.
88. Ibid.
89. Ibid.
90. Nels Marcus Thygeson, interview by Beret E. Strong, May 12, 2005.
91. Ralda Lee, Ph.D., interview by Beret E. Strong, May 28, 2005.
92. Mara Thygeson, interview by Beret E. Strong, June 29, 2005.
93. Nels Marcus Thygeson, interview by Beret E. Strong, May 12, 2005.
94. Phillips Thygeson, "I Am a Slave to Women," February 10, 1998, 1.
95. Thygeson, *A Link with Our Past*, 99.
96. Ibid., 100.
97. Ibid.
98. Ibid.
99. Thygeson, "A Research Man."
100. Thygeson, *A Link with Our Past*, 102.

15. World War II in the Army Air Corps

1. Fritjof Thygeson, interview by Beret E. Strong, November 7, 2004.
2. Phillips Thygeson, "Stability," July 20, 1996.
3. Ibid.
4. Ibid.
5. Thygeson, *A Link with Our Past*, 107.
6. Thygeson, "Stability."
7. Ibid.
8. Thygeson, *A Link with Our Past*, 109.
9. Ibid.
10. Fritjof Thygeson, interview by Beret E. Strong, November 6, 2004.
11. Phillips Thygeson, "Navajo Rugs," August 6, 1996.
12. Lou Cannon, "Profile, Carey Mcwilliams," California Journal http://www.californiajournal.org/news/features/_C.a.n.n.o.n/?3.
13. Mike Davis, "Optimism of the Will," *The Nation* (September 19, 2005), http://www.thenation.com/doc/20050919/davis.
14. Fritjof Thygeson, interview by Beret E. Strong, November 6, 2004.
15. Ibid.
16. Kristin Thygeson, interview by Beret E. Strong, November 16, 2004.
17. Ibid.
18. "Daughters of the American Revolution," http://www.americanrevolution.com/Daughters.htm.
19. Kristin Thygeson, interview by Beret E. Strong, November 16, 2004.
20. Ibid.
21. Fritjof Thygeson, interview by Beret E. Strong, November 6, 2004.
22. Kristin Thygeson, interview by Beret E. Strong, November 16, 2004.
23. Ibid.
24. Ibid.
25. Ruth Lee Thygeson to Mara Thygeson, December 13, 1982.
26. Ibid.
27. Kristin Thygeson, conversation with author, December 4, 2005.
28. Ralda Lee, interview by Beret E. Strong, May 28, 2005
29. Thygeson, *A Link with Our Past*, 110.
30. Ibid., 110–11.
31. Ibid., 112.
32. Ibid., 112–13.
33. Ibid., 114.
34. Ibid., 114–15.
35. Ibid., 115.
36. Ibid., 118.
37. Ibid., 116–17.
38. Ibid., 117.
39. Fritjof Thygeson, conversation with author, April 28, 2007.
40. Ibid.
41. Ibid., 118–19.
42. Ibid., 119.
43. Fritjof Thygeson, interview by Beret E. Strong, November 7, 2004.
44. Ibid.
45. Kristin Thygeson, interview by Beret E. Strong, November 16, 2004.
46. Thygeson, *A Link with Our Past*, 120.
47. Kristin Thygeson, interview by Beret E. Strong, November 16, 2004.

48. Jim Cadranell, "Classic Boats Call for Classic Books," *The Shorebird* (Fall 2004), http://www.bbyra.org/fleet/O_shorebird_fall_2004.pdf.
49. Ibid.
50. Kristin Thygeson, interview by Beret E. Strong, November 16, 2004.
51. Ibid.
52. Ibid. The pleasure of sailing had a lifelong impact on both of the children. When he came of age, Fritjof joined the navy and found himself living aboard a nuclear submarine. Kristin would later serve as crew with friends who rented bare boats to explore the Caribbean Islands and French Polynesia.
53. Nels Marcus Thygeson, interview by Beret E. Strong, May 18, 2005.
54. Fritjof Thygeson, interview by Beret E. Strong, November 6, 2004.
55. Ibid.
56. Ibid.
57. Ibid.
58. Kristin Thygeson, interview by Beret E. Strong, December 7, 2005.
59. Thygeson, *A Link with Our Past*, 119–20.
60. Ibid., 120–21.
61. Ibid., 124.
62. Kristin Thygeson, interview by Beret E. Strong, November 16, 2004.
63. Kristin Thygeson, interview by Beret E. Strong, March 1, 2005.
64. Kristin Thygeson, interview by Beret E. Strong, November 16, 2004.
65. Thygeson, *A Link with Our Past*, 122.

16. California and an Experiment in Private Practice

1. Phillips Thygeson, "The Ruth Lee Hilltop," n.d.
2. Phillips Thygeson, "My Hometown," February 5, 1998.
3. Phillips Thygeson, "Ruth Lee and Our Dream," January 17, 1997.
4. Elizabeth C. Proctor to Ruth Lee Thygeson, n.d.
5. Thygeson, "The Ruth Lee Hilltop."
6. Kristin Thygeson, interview by Beret E. Strong, March 1, 2005.
7. Thygeson, "The Ruth Lee Hilltop."
8. Kristin Thygeson, interview by Beret E. Strong, March 1, 2005.
9. Thygeson, *A Link with Our Past*, 123.
10. Daniel Vaughan, M.D., interview by Sally Smith Hughes, November 6, 1986, American Academy of Ophthalmology.
11. Thygeson, *A Link with Our Past*, 221.
12. Thygeson, "The Ruth Lee Hilltop."

17. The Francis I. Proctor Foundation for Research in Ophthalmology

1. Ibid., 131.
2. Ibid., 131–32.
3. Ibid., 133.
4. Ibid., 132–33.
5. Ibid., 134.
6. Ibid., 136–37.
7. Mathea R. Allansmith and G. Richard O'Connor, eds., *Phillips Thygeson and the Proctor Fellows* (n.p., 1972), 9.
8. Thygeson, *A Link with Our Past*, 134.
9. Ibid., 135.
10. "The Proctor Bulletin" 5, no. 1 (March 1982).
11. Phil guarded his relationship with Mrs. Proctor carefully and did not really share her with others. Chandler Dawson recalled going all the way to New Mexico with the Thygesons and visiting Mrs. Proctor. "I drove them to the door and waited outside for them, but they didn't invite me in to meet her." Chandler Dawson, M.D., interview by Sally Smith Hughes, November 6, 1986.
12. G. Richard O'Connor, M.D., interview by Sally Smith Hughes, December 15, 1986, American Academy of Ophthalmology.
13. Thygeson, *A Link with Our Past*, 222.
14. Nels Marcus Thygeson, interview by Beret E. Strong, May 12, 2005.
15. Kristin Thygeson, interview by Beret E. Strong, March 1, 2005.
16. Ibid.

18. Father and Son: From San Quentin to Steroids

1. Fritjof Thygeson, interview by Beret E. Strong, November 6, 2004.
2. Later in life, Fritjof reflected that his success as a public speaker and political leader was due to the "extraordinary education" he received from his mother. They read together, they discussed a vast range of issues, and he watched her embody her commitment to making the world a better and more just place

for everyone. Fritjof Thygeson, communication with author, May 8, 2007.
3. Ibid.
4. Ibid.
5. Ralda Lee, interview by Beret E. Strong, May 28, 2005.
6. Ibid.
7. Fritjof Thygeson, communication with author, May 8, 2007.
8. Ibid.
9. Fritjof Thygeson, communication with author, May 13, 2007.
10. Fritjof Thygeson, interview by Beret E. Strong, November 7, 2004.
11. Fritjof Thygeson, communication with author, May 13, 2007.
12. Khalid Tabbara, M.D., interview by Beret E. Strong, October 24, 2005.
13. Robert J. Brockhurst, B. Thomas Hutchinson, and S. Arthur Boruchoff, eds., *Controversy in Ophthalmology* (Philadelphia: W.B. Saunders, 1977), 458.
14. Ibid.
15. Ibid., 459.
16. The article in question is "Effect of Cortisone on Experimental Herpes Simplex Keratitis of the Rabbit," *American Journal of Ophthalmology* 34 (1951): 885–88.
17. Thygeson, *A Link with Our Past*, 246.
18. Ibid.
19. Jeffrey Lanier, M.D., interview by Beret E. Strong, January 7, 2006.
20. Ibid.
21. Fritjof Thygeson, interview by Beret E. Strong, November 6, 2004.
22. G. Richard O'Connor, interview by Sally Smith Hughes, December 15, 1986.
23. Lanier.
24. Brockhurst, *Controversy in Ophthalmology*, 460. By 1970, the problem had not gone away, but fortunately pharmaceutical companies were no longer allowed to give free samples of ocular steroid preparations to general practitioners and pediatricians.
25. Ibid., 463–65, 67–68.
26. *Twenty-fifth Anniversary of the Alta California Eye Research Foundation* (Los Altos: Alta California Eye Research Foundation, 1994), 173.
27. Thygeson, *A Link with Our Past*, 289.
28. *Twenty-fifth Anniversary of the Alta California Eye Research Foundation*, 174.
29. Frederick H. Verhoeff to Phillips Thygeson, October 9, 1951. Even the "heavenly" side of the drug brought Phil to some grief. In 1951, the text of Phil's Doheny lecture on phlyctenular keratitis appeared in the *American Journal of Ophthalmology*. The publication triggered an unhappy letter from a fellow ophthalmological luminary more than a generation older than Phil. Frederick H. Verhoeff called to Phil's attention his own paper on the same subject, published in the Ophthalmic Record in 1908. He complained to Phil: "In your lecture ... you make no mention of my paper. No doubt you have a good reason for not mentioning it, but I should like very much to know what this reason is. If you will look up my paper, you will see that my basis for the theory was substantially the same as you gave in your lecture." Alas, there is no record of Phil's response except a notation in Ruth Lee's hand on Verhoeff's letter. "Answered," it reads.
30. The article was published in *JAMA* 144 (1950): 1544–48.
31. Thygeson, *A Link with Our Past*, 244.

19. Mother and Daughter: World Federalist and Equestrienne

1. Kristin Thygeson, interview by Beret E. Strong, November 16, 2004.
2. Ibid.
3. Ibid.
4. Ibid.
5. Thygeson, "The Ruth Lee Hilltop."
6. Kristin Thygeson, interview by Beret E. Strong, March 1, 2005.
7. Ibid.
8. Ibid.

20. The Glory Days of Academic Medicine

1. Kristin Thygeson, interview by Beret E. Strong, December 7, 2005.
2. Nels Marcus Thygeson, interview by Beret E. Strong, May 18, 2005.
3. G. Richard O'Connor, interview by Beret E. Strong, November 4, 2004.
4. Thygeson, *A Link with Our Past*, 135.
5. *Phillips Thygeson and the Proctor Fellows*, 9.
6. Thygeson, *A Link with Our Past*, 141.
7. Ibid., 148.
8. Ibid.
9. Ibid.
10. *Phillips Thygeson and the Proctor Fellows*, 8.

11. Thygeson, *A Link with Our Past*, 137–38.
12. Ibid., 140–41.
13. Ibid.
14. Ibid., 147.
15. O'Connor, interview by Beret E. Strong, November 4, 2004.
16. Ibid.
17. Ibid.
18. O'Connor, interview by Sally Smith Hughes.
19. Ibid.
20. O'Connor, interview by Beret E. Strong, November 3, 2004.
21. Ibid.
22. Phillips Thygeson, "Eye Strain," July 23, 1996.
23. Thygeson, *A Link with Our Past*, 138.
24. Ibid.
25. Ibid., 141.
26. Ibid., 139.
27. Ibid., 149.
28. Dawson, in Chernesky et al., ix. In 1955, Phil and Ernest Jawetz began to collaborate with others on viral diseases of the eye, work that was supported by the NIH. "This collaboration resulted in the first isolation of adenovirus type 8, the cause of epidemic keratoconjunctivitis.... This group successfully isolated chlamydial agent from cases of neonatal conjunctivitis and trachoma.... This productive partnership continued for 25 years and included many studies on chlamydial, herpetic, adenoviral, and other eye infections."
29. Thygeson, *A Link with Our Past*, 150.
30. Ibid., 151.
31. Ibid., 143.
32. Ibid., 144.
33. Ibid., 143.
34. Ibid., 144.
35. Ibid., 145.
36. Nels Marcus Thygeson, interview by Beret E. Strong, May 18, 2005.
37. Thygeson, *A Link with Our Past*, 147.
38. Ibid., 146.
39. Ibid.
40. O'Connor, interview by Beret E. Strong, November 4, 2004.
41. Vaughan, interview by Sally Smith Hughes.
42. Ibid.
43. O'Connor, interview by Beret E. Strong, November 4, 2004.

21. World Health Organization and World Class Editing

1. The establishment in 1968 of the National Eye Institute, part of the National Institutes of Health, led to even more substantial federal funding for research at the Proctor Foundation.
2. Lanier. Other diseases of interest to the WHO were vitamin A deficiency and onchocerciasis.
3. Thygeson, *A Link with Our Past*, 230.
4. Ibid., 230–31.
5. Phillips Thygeson to Ruth Lee Thygeson, July 20, 1966.
6. Phillips Thygeson to Ruth Lee Thygeson, July 24, 1966.
7. Phillips Thygeson to Ruth Lee Thygeson, July 15, 1966.
8. Ibid.
9. Phillips Thygeson to Ruth Lee Thygeson, August 11, 1966.
10. Thygeson, *A Link with Our Past*, 233.
11. Ruth Lee Thygeson to Mara Thygeson, June 9, 1974.
12. Roger Nataf to Phillips Thygeson, April 3, 1957.
13. Phillips Thygeson to Roger Nataf, April 9, 1957.
14. Dawson, in Chernesky et al., ix.
15. Thygeson, *A Link with Our Past*, 232.
16. Ibid., 234.
17. Ibid., 235.
18. Ibid., 236.
19. Ibid., 136.
20. Mathea Allansmith, M.D., interview by Beret E. Strong, December 5, 2005.
21. O'Connor, interview by Beret E. Strong, November 4, 2004. Post-graduate fellows trained in those years had the opportunity to learn about the microscope from Lynette Feeny, a very skillful electron microscopist.
22. Dawson, interview by Beret E. Strong.
23. Ibid.
24. Thygeson, *A Link with Our Past*, 152–53.
25. Ibid., 153.
26. Dawson, interview by Beret E. Strong.
27. Ibid.
28. Thygeson, *A Link with Our Past*, 153.
29. Mike Ward and Bill Bishop, "Becoming Guinea Pigs to Avoid Poor Prison Care," in *Sick in Secret: The Hidden World of Prison*

Health Care, American-Statesman, December 17, 2001. http://www.statesman.com/specialreports/content/specialreports/prisons/17prisonmain.html.
30. Ibid.
31. "IOM Committee Considers Prison Research,"Alliance for Human Research Protection, July 24, 2005, http://www.ahrp.org/infomail/05/07/24.php.
32. Ward.
33. Thygeson, *A Link with Our Past,* 153.
34. O'Connor, interview by Beret E. Strong, November 4, 2005.
35. Ibid.
36. Thygeson, *A Link with Our Past,* 65.
37. Stephen J. Taylor, "Conscientious Objectors in World War II," Center on Human Policy, Syracuse University, 2003, www.google.com/search?q=cache:y5iW3brJJpgJ:www.disabilitystudiesforteachers.org/files/COS_WWII.pdf+world+war+II+conscientious+objectors+medical+experiments&hl=en&gl=us&ct=clnk&cd=2.
38. "History of Prison Research Regulation," *Advisory Committee on Human Radiation Experiments Report,* http://www.eh.doe.gov/ohre/roadmap/achre/chap9_4.html.
39. Ibid.
40. Thygeson, *A Link with Our Past,* 154.
41. The article is: L. Hanna, E. Jawetz, Y. Mitsui, P. Thygeson, S.J. Kimura, A. Nicholas, "Continuing Studies on the Association of Adenovirus type 8 with Epidemic Keratoconjunctivitis," *American Journal of Ophthalmology* 44 (1957): 66–74.
42. Thygeson, *A Link with Our Past,* 155–56.
43. J.B. de CM Saunders to Phillips Thygeson, 17 May, 1966.
44. Fritjof Thygeson, interview by Beret E. Strong, November 6, 2004.
45. O'Connor, interview by Beret E. Strong, November 4, 2004.
46. Ibid.
47. Ralda Lee, interview by Beret E. Strong, May 28, 2005.
48. O'Connor, interview by Beret E. Strong, November 4, 2004.
49. Vaughan, Interview by Sally Smith Hughes.
50. O'Connor, Interview by Beret E. Strong, November 4, 2004.
51. Thygeson, *A Link with Our Past,* 165.
52. Ibid., 193.
53. O'Connor, interview by Beret E. Strong, November 4, 2004.
54. Ibid.
55. Ibid.
56. Ibid.
57. Allansmith, interview by Beret E. Strong, December 5, 2005.
58. O'Connor, interview by Beret E. Strong, November 4, 2004.
59. Vaughan, interview by Sally Smith Hughes.
60. O'Connor, interview by Beret E. Strong, November 4, 2004.
61. Frederick C. Cordes to Ruth Lee Thygeson, 1951.
62. Algernon B. Reese to Ruth Lee Thygeson, 1951.
63. O'Connor, interview by Beret E. Strong, November 6, 2004.
64. *Twenty-fifth Anniversary of the Alta California Eye Research Foundation,* 11.
65. Giambattista Bietti to Ruth Lee Thygeson, December 31, 1954.

22. International Fellows and Fellowship

1. O'Connor, interview by Beret E. Strong, November 6, 2004.
2. Ibid.
3. Ibid.
4. Thygeson, *A Link with Our Past,* 207.
5. Paul Riordan-Eva, interview by Sally Smith Hughes, November 6, 1986, American Academy of Ophthalmology.
6. Thygeson, *A Link with Our Past,* 208.
7. *Phillips Thygeson and the Proctor Fellows,* 27.
8. Ibid., 28.
9. Allansmith, interview by Beret E. Strong, December 5, 2005.
10. *Phillips Thygeson and the Proctor Fellows,* 31.
11. Allansmith, interview by Beret E. Strong, December 5, 2005.
12. Ibid.
13. Ibid.
14. Jeffrey Lanier, interview by Beret E. Strong, January 7, 2006.
15. Allansmith, interview by Beret E. Strong, December 5, 2005.
16. Ibid.
17. Ibid.
18. Ibid.
19. Lanier.
20. Allansmith, interview by Beret E. Strong, December 5, 2005.
21. Ibid.

22. Elizabeth C. Proctor to chairman of Board of Trustees, Francis I. Proctor Foundation for Research in Ophthalmology, May 1957.
23. Allansmith, interview by Beret E. Strong, December 5, 2005.
24. Ibid.
25. Ibid.
26. Ibid.
27. Ibid.

23. Lake Tahoe and the Alta California Eye Research Foundation

1. "Vikingsholm," http://www.vikingsholm.com/history%200f%20eb.html.
2. The property was given to Kristin in the hope that it could continue to be used as the family vacation home, but was instead sold, as road, sewer, and water levies had become very expensive.
3. *Twenty-fifth Anniversary of the Alta California Eye Research Foundation*, 1.
4. Ibid.
5. Ibid., 2.
6. Ibid., 3.
7. Gary Holland, M.D., interview by Beret E. Strong, September 11, 2005.

24. Ripened Souls Tend Their Orchard

1. Ruth Lee Thygeson to Mara Thygeson, April 16, 1975.
2. Ruth Lee Thygeson to Mara Thygeson, March 1981.
3. Elizabeth C. Proctor to Ruth Lee Thygeson, n.d.
4. Phillips Thygeson to Ruth Lee Thygeson, July 28, 1966.
5. O'Connor, interview by Sally Smith Hughes.
6. O'Connor, interview by Beret E. Strong, November 4, 2004.
7. Ibid.
8. Phillips Thygeson, "My Children."
9. O'Connor, interview by Sally Smith Hughes.
10. O'Connor, interview by Beret E. Strong, November 5, 2004.
11. Emmett Cunningham, M.D., Ph.D., December 5, 2005.
12. Dawson, interview by Sally Smith Hughes.
13. Paul Riordan-Eva, interview by Sally Smith Hughes, November 6, 1986, Regional Oral History Office, University of California, Berkeley, and American Academy of Ophthalmology.
14. Jeffrey Lanier, interview by Beret E. Strong, January 7, 2006.
15. Phillips Thygeson, "Politics," July 4, 1996.
16. Khalid Tabbara, interview by Beret E. Strong, October 24, 2005.
17. Ibid.
18. Dawson, interview by Sally Smith Hughes.
19. Ruth Lee Thygeson to Mara Thygeson, November 11, 1986.
20. Thygeson, "Vision."
21. John Richardson, Jr., to Phillips Thygeson, July 25, 1973. When there was a student strike to protest the Vietnam War, Phil threatened to dismiss any Proctor fellows or staff who participated. According to Fritjof, none did, and Governor Ronald Reagan wrote a letter to commend Phil for his action. Fritjof Thygeson, conversation with author, April 28, 2007.
22. Mara Thygeson, interview by Beret E. Strong, July 1, 2005.

25. The End of the Journey

1. Quoted in Mara Thygeson, interview by Beret E. Strong, July 1, 2005.
2. Milo H. Fritz, to Phillips and Ruth Lee Thygeson, January 16, 1978.
3. Phillips Thygeson, "Our Dream. The Alta Foundation and the Hilltop," April 10, 1997.
4. Milo H. Fritz to Phillips and Ruth Lee Thygeson, January 16, 1978.
5. Mara Thygeson, interview by Beret E. Strong, June 29, 2005.
6. Ibid.
7. Vaughan, interview by Sally Smith Hughes.
8. This biography owes an enormous debt of gratitude to Sally Smith Hughes's oral history of Phillips Thygeson, for providing a solid chronology and a good deal of information not found elsewhere
9. Sally Smith Hughes, interview by Beret E. Strong, May 11, 2005.
10. Ibid.

11. Thygeson, "Our Dream. The Alta Foundation and the Hilltop."
12. Lindberg et al., 21.
13. Kristin Thygeson, interview by Beret E. Strong, March 1, 2005.
14. Ibid.
15. Mara Thygeson, interview by Beret E. Strong, June 29, 2005.
16. Margot and Gerry Lawrence, interview by Beret E. Strong, August 2, 2005.
17. Ibid.
18. Earlene Chapman, interview by Beret E. Strong, June 22, 2005.
19. Ibid.
20. Ruth Lee Thygeson to Mara Thygeson, November 11, 1986.
21. Thygeson, "Vision."
22. Sam and Jan Harwood, interview by Beret E. Strong, August 4, 2005.
23. Mary Leihy, interview by Beret E. Strong, September 20, 2005.
24. Harwood.
25. Quoted in Mara Thygeson, interview by Beret E. Strong, June 29, 2005.
26. At his memorial service, Chapman was quoted as saying, "Dr. T. was my friend." Fritjof Thygeson, conversation with author, April 28, 2007.
27. Chapman.
28. Ruth Lee Thygeson to Mara Thygeson, April 16, 1975.
29. Ruth Lee Thygeson to Mara Thygeson, November 11, 1986.
30. Jeffrey Lanier, interview by Beret E. Strong, January 7, 2006.
31. Phillips Thygeson, "The Joy of Beauty," January 13, 1997.
32. Phillips Thygeson, "The Art of Writing," January 13, 1997.
33. Phillips Thygeson, "Old Age," January 17, 1997.
34. Thygeson, "The Natural History of Infectious Ocular Disease."
35. Phillips Thygeson, "Fever Therapy," July 3, 1996.
36. Ibid.
37. Thygeson, "Our Dream. The Alta Foundation and the Hilltop."
38. Phillips Thygeson, "Life without Ruth Lee," October 4, 1996.
39. Phillips Thygeson, "My Ruth Lee: A Birthday Dream," March 28, 1994.
40. "About Trachoma: Safe Strategy," www.trachoma.org/safe.php.
41. Phillips Thygeson, "The Dream," February 23, 1994.
42. Phillips Thygeson, "Ruth Lee," 1996.
43. Phillips Thygeson, "A Proposal for a Ruth Lee Thygeson Lecture in the Alta Foundation," n.d
44. Thygeson, "The Joy of Beauty."
45. Thygeson, "The Dream."
46. Thygeson, "The Ruth Lee Hilltop."
47. Lanier.
48. Phillips Thygeson, "Genteel Poverty," January 14, 1997.
49. Ibid.
50. Phillips Thygeson, "Good and Bad," September 27, 1996.
51. Furnham, *Protestant Work Ethic*, 175.
52. Leihy.
53. Thygeson, "My Ruth Lee: A Birthday Dream."
54. *Twenty-fifth Anniversary of the Alta California Eye Research Foundation*, 13–14.
55. Phil's devoted team of care providers included Earlene Chapman, Fritjof Thygeson, Cheryl Stoll Thygeson, Ann Lottridge, Maria Anguiano and Renee Rosita. He deeply enjoyed the stimulation they provided and, as a doctor, appreciated their skillful nursing and care.

Bibliography

"About Trachoma: Safe Strategy." www.trachoma.org/safe.php.
Allansmith, Mathea. Interview by Beret E. Strong, December 5, 2005.
Allansmith, Mathea R., and G. Richard O'Connor, eds. *Phillips Thygeson and the Proctor Fellows.* n.p. 1972.
American Academy of Otolaryngology Head and Neck Surgery. www.entnet.org.
"Arizona Apache Wars." http://www.geocities.com/zybt/awars.htm.
Bacigalupi, Peter. *Edison Phonograph Monthly*, July 1906, http://www.sfmuseum.net/1906/ew16.html.
Baldwin, De Witt C. "Memories of the San Francisco Earthquake and Fire." n.d. http://www.sfmuseum.net/1906/ew8.html.
Bietti, G. B., to Phillips Thygeson, 31 December 1954, private collection.
Box, William. "Jamestown Given New Life, 1610." n.d. http://lcweb2.10c.gov/learn/features/timeline/colonial/jamestwn/net.html.
Boy Scouts of America: Handbook for Boys. 1911.
"A Brief History of Ophthalmology at the University of Iowa." n.d. Department of Ophthalmology and Visual Sciences, University of Iowa Health Care. http://webeye.ophth.uiowa.edu/dept/LEGACY/History/history.htm.
Brockhurst, Robert J., B. Thomas Hutchinson, and S. Arthur Boruchoff, eds. *Controversy in Ophthalmology.* Philadelphia, PA: W.B. Saunders, 1977.
Burke, Emma. *Overlook Magazine.* June 2, 1906. www.sfmuseum.net/1906/ew13.html.

Cadranell, Jim. "Classic Boats Call for Classic Books." Fall 2004. http://www.bbyra.org/fleet/O_shorebird_fall_2004.pdf.
Cameron, Donaldina. n.d. http://www.sfmuseum.net/1906/ew15.html.
Cannon, Lou. "Profile, Carey Mcwilliams." *California Journal.* http://www.californiajournal.org/news/features/_C.a.n.n.o.n/?3.
Chapman, Earlene. Interview by Beret E. Strong, June 22, 2005.
"Charles Nicolle (1866–1936)." http://www.pasteur.fr/infosci/archives/nic0.html.
Cherry, Colin. *On Human Communication.* Cambridge, MA: Technology Press of M.I.T. Press, 1957. Reprint, 2nd edition.
Cohn, David V. "The Life and Times of Louis Pasteur." February 11, 1996. http://www.louisville.edu/library/ekstrom/special/pasteur/cohn.html.
"The Complete Book of Emigrants, 1607–1776. List of First Settlers at Jamestown Island, Virginia, in 1607 as Noted by Captain John Smith." n.d. http://www.runningdeerslonghouse.com/webdoc38.htm.
Cordes, Frederick C., to Ruth Lee Thygeson, January 9, 1951, private collection.
Cunningham, Emmett, interview by Beret Strong, December 5, 2005.
Dale, Peter Allan. *In Pursuit of a Scientific Culture: Science, Arts, and Society in the Victorian Age.* Madison: University of Wisconsin Press, 1989.
"Daughters of the American Revolution." http://www.americanrevolution.com/Daughters.htm.
Davis, Mike. "Optimism of the Will." *The Nation.* September 19, 2005. http://www.thenation.com/doc/20050919/davis.

Dawson, Chandler. Interview by Beret E. Strong, March 10, 2005.

———. Interview by Sally Smith Hughes, November 6, 1986, Regional Oral History Office, University of California, Berkeley, and American Academy of Ophthalmology. Published with permission of the Museum of Vision and the American Academy of Ophthalmology, copyright © 1986.

De Kruif, Paul. *Microbe Hunters*. San Diego, CA: Harcourt, 1954.

———. "They Wait for Light." *Country Gentleman* 10–11 (September 1940): 33.

Fritz, Milo H., to Phillips and Ruth Lee Thygeson, January 16, 1978, private collection.

Furnham, Adrian. *The Protestant Work Ethic*. London: Routledge, 1990.

Harwood, Jan, and Sam Harwood. Interview by Beret E. Strong, August 4, 2005.

Helms, Harry. *All about Ham Radio*. San Diego, CA: High Text Publications, 1992.

"Herbert Spencer (1820–1903)." The Internet Encyclopedia of Philosophy. http://www.iep.utm.edu/s/spencer/htm.

"History of Jamestown." n.d. http://www.apva.org/history/.

"History of Prison Research Regulation." *Advisory Committee on Human Radiation Experiments Report*. February 1995. http://www.eh.doe.gov/ohre/roadmap/achre/chap9_4.html.

"History of the University of Iowa." n.d. http://www.lib.uiowa.edu/spec-coll/Archives/chronohistory.htm.

Holland, Gary. Interview by Beret E. Strong, September 11, 2005.

Hoslink. "Pioneers in Medical Laboratory Science." http://www.hoslink.com/history2.htm.

Houghton, Walter E. *The Victorian Frame of Mind, 1830–1870*. New Haven, CT: Yale University Press, 1957.

Hughes, Sally Smith. Interview by Beret E. Strong, May 11, 2005.

"Images from the History of the Public Health Service, Introduction." National Library of Medicine. http://www.nlm.nih.gov/exhibition/phs_history/intro.html.

"The Influenza Epidemic of 1918." n.d. http://www.stanford.edu/group/virus/uda/.

"IOM Committee Considers Prison Research." Alliance for Human Research Protection. July 24, 2005. http://www.ahrp.org/infomail/05/07/24.php.

Jordan, Philip A. "Adventures of a Student at Iowa." University of Iowa. April 1978. http://wwwlib.uiowa.edu/spec-coll/Bai/jordan3.htm.

"Joseph Lister, 1st Baron Lister." http://www.absoluteastronomy.com/reference/joseph_lister_1st_baron_lister.

"Joseph Lister, 1st Baron Lister." n.d. http://en.wikipedia.org/wiki/Joseph_Lister.

Kaufman, Michael T. "Stokely Carmichael, Rights Leader Who Coined 'Black Power,' Dies at 57." *New York Times*, November 16, 1998.

Lanier, Jeffrey. Interview by Beret E. Strong, January 7, 2006.

Lawrence, Gerry, and Margot Lawrence. Interview by Beret E. Strong, August 2, 2005.

Lee, Ralda. Interview by Beret E. Strong, May 28, 2005.

Leihy, Mary. Interview by Beret E. Strong, September 20, 2005.

Levey, Samuel. *The Rise of a University Teaching Hospital, a Leadership Perspective: The University of Iowa Hospitals and Clinics*. Chicago: Health Administration Press, 1997.

Lindberg, James, Patricia Raney, and Janet Robertson. *Rocky Mountain Rustic: Historic Buildings of the Rocky Mountain National Park Area*. Estes Park, CO: Rocky Mountain Nature Association, 1994.

"Louis Pasteur." Science and Technology Department, Embassy of France and Canada. http://www.ambafrance-ca.org/HYPERLAB/PEOPLE/_pasteur.html.

"The March toward War: The March of Time as Documentary and Propaganda." http://xroad.virginia.edu/~MA04/wood/mot/html/document.htm.

Marks, Jonathan. "Racism, Eugenics, and the Burdens of History." Paper presented at the IX International Congress of Human Genetics, Rio de Janeiro, Brazil, August 20, 1996.

Max Chernesky, et al., eds. *Chlamydial Infections: Proceedings of the Eleventh International Symposium on Human Chlamydial Infections*: International Chlamydia Symposium, 2006.

"The Medical and Scientific Conceptions of Influenza." n.d. http://www.stanford.edu/group/virus/uda/fluscimed.html.

Merry, Carl A. "The Historic Period." The University of Iowa. 1996. http://www.uiowa.edu/~osa/learn/historic/hisper.htm.

"Mills Building." http://themillsbuilding.com/building/index.html.

Mirrielees, Edith R. *Stanford: The Story of a University.* New York: Putnam's, 1959.

Morens, David M., and Jeffery K. Taubenberger. "1918 Influenza: The Mother of All Pandemics." *CDC*, January 2006, http://www.cdc.gov/ncidod/EID/v0112n001/05-0979.htm.

Nataf, Roger, to Phillips Thygeson, April 3, 1957, private collection.

Oates, Wayne Edward. *Confessions of a Workaholic: The Facts about Work Addiction.* New York: World, 1971.

O'Connor, G. Richard. Interview by Beret E. Strong, November 4 and 5, 2004.

———. Interview by Sally Smith Hughes, December 15, 1986, Regional Oral History Office, University of California, Berkeley, and American Academy of Ophthalmology. Published with permission of the Museum of Vision and the American Academy of Ophthalmology, copyright © 1986.

"Path of the Parrish's." n.d. http://wwgeocities.com/awoodlief/parrishhist.htm?20053.

Peterson, Robert W. *Boy Scouts: An American Adventure.* New York: American Heritage, 1984.

"The Proctor Bulletin" 5, no. 1 (March 1982).

Proctor, Elizabeth C., to chairman of Board of Trustees, Francis I. Proctor Foundation for Research in Ophthalmology, May 1957.

"The Public Health Response." n.d. http://www.stanford.edu/group/virus/uda/flure sponse.html.

Reese, Algernon B., to Ruth Lee Thygeson, May 27, 1949; May 29, 1950; February 19, 1951.

Richardson, John, Jr., to Phillips Thygeson, July 25, 1973, private collection.

Riordan-Eva, Paul. Interview by Sally Smith Hughes, November 6, 1986, Regional Oral History Office, University of California, Berkeley, and American Academy of Ophthalmology. Published with permission of the Museum of Vision and the American Academy of Ophthalmology, copyright © 1986.

Roark, Eric. "Herbert Spencer's Evolutionary Individualism." *Quarterly Journal of Ideology* 27, no. 3 and 4 (2004): 1–31.

"Robert Baden-Powell as an Educational Innovator." n.d. http://www.infed.org/thinkers/et-bp.htm.

Saunders, J.B. de CM, to Phillips Thygeson, May 17, 1966, private collection.

Shepardson, Mary Thygeson. Interview by Beret E. Strong, 1991.

Shikes, Robert H. *Rocky Mountain Medicine: Doctors, Drugs, and Disease in Early Colorado.* Boulder, CO: Johnson, 1986.

Smith, John. *The Generall Historie of Virginia, New England & the Summer Isles.* Vol. 1. Glasgow, Scotland: James MacLehose and Sons, 1907.

———. "Smith's Last Days in Virginia." http://www.readbookonline.net/read/194/6259/.

Spilman, James, to Elizabeth Brewer (Spilman), November 14, 1890; November 18, 1890; July 5, 1891; July 28, 1891; April 27, 1906; April 29, 1906; May 1, 1906; May 2, 1906; May 3, 1906; June 20, 1909; private collection.

"Stanford University History." n.d. http://www.stanford.edu/home/stanford/history/begin.html.

"Stanford University History: Stanford History by Presidency." n.d. http://www.stanford.edu/home/stanford/history/leader.html.

Streit, Clarence R. *Union Now: A Proposal for a Federal Union of the Democracies of the North Atlantic.* New York: Harper & Brothers, 1978. http://www.constitution.org/aun/union_now.htm.

Swartz, Clarence Lee. "What Is Mutualism?" 1927. http://www.panarchy.org/swartz/mutualism.9.html.

Tabbara, Khalid. Interview by Beret E. Strong, October 24, 2005.

Taylor, Stephen J. "Conscientious Objectors in World War II." Center on Human Policy. Syracuse University, 2003. http://www.google.com/search?q=cache:y5iW3brJJpgJ:www.disabilitystudiesforteachers.org/files/COS_WWII.pdf+world+war+II+conscientious+objectors+medical+experiments&hl=en&gl=us&ct=clnk&cd=2.

Thygeson, Fritjof. Interview by Beret E. Strong, November 6 and 7, 2004.

Thygeson, Kristin. Interview by Beret E. Strong, November 1 and 16, 2004; March 1, 2005; June 29, 2005; December 7, 2005; May 18, 2006.

Thygeson, Mara. Interview by Beret E. Strong, June 29, 2005.

Thygeson, Nels Marcus. Interview by Beret E. Strong, May 12 and 18, 2005.

Thygeson, Phillips. "The Art of Writing." January 13, 1997.

———. "Charles Nicolle." June 19, 1996.

———. "The Curse of Heredity." July 16, 1996.
———. "A Day with Victor Morax." February 2, 1998.
———. "Dr. W.C. Finnoff." n.d.
———. "The Dream." February 23, 1994.
———. "Edward Jackson." July 1, 1996.
———. "The Elizabeth C. Proctor Story." March 21, 1996.
———. "Elizabeth C. Proctor: Our First Meeting." n.d.
———. "Engines." November 15, 1996.
———. "Eye Strain." July 23, 1996.
———. "Families: The Story of Two Families." October 1, 1996.
———. "Father and Lala." February 5, 1998.
———. "Fever Therapy." July 3, 1996.
———. "Fili Guten—Good Boy." January 14, 1997.
———. "Francis I. Proctor." January 12, 1997.
———. "Genteel Poverty." January 14, 1997.
———. "Good and Bad." September 27, 1996.
———. "Great Books." January 17, 1997.
———. "Heredity." July 12, 1996.
———. "The High School Cadets." October 2, 1996.
———. "I Am a Slave to Women." February 10, 1998.
———. "I Wasn't Programmed to Be a Father." September 29, 1996.
———. "The Ideal Nurse: Lala and Earlene." June 28, 1996.
———. "The Joy of a Farm on a Lake." September 28, 1996.
———. "The Joy of Beauty." January 13, 1997.
———. "The Lady Ruth Lee: Queen of the Ruth Lee Hilltop 1." n.d.
———. "Life without Ruth Lee." October 4, 1996.
———. *A Link with Our Past: External Eye Disease and the Proctor Foundation*, an oral history conducted in 1987 by Sally Smith Hughes, Ph.D. Regional Oral History Office, University of California, Berkeley, and American Academy of Ophthalmology. Published with permission of the Museum of Vision and the American Academy of Ophthalmology, copyright © 1987.
———. "Microbiologist." September 27, 1996.
———. "Minnetonka Days." January 17, 1997.
———. "My Children." September 27, 1996.
———. "My Father." August 1, 1996.
———. "My Father Marcus." n.d.
———. "My Hometown." February 5, 1998.
———. Letter to Roger Nataf, April 9, 1957; private collection.
———. Letters to Ruth Lee Thygeson, July 20, 1966; July 24, 1966; July 25, 1966; July 28, 1966; August 11,1966; private collection.
———. "My Ruth Lee, 1." September 24, 1996.
———. "My Ruth Lee: A Birthday Dream." March 28, 1994.
———. "The Natural History of Infectious Ocular Disease." July 8, 1996.
———. "The Nature of the Elementary and Initial Bodies of Trachoma." *Archives of Ophthalmology* 12 (1934): 307–18.
———. "Navajo Rugs." August 6, 1996.
———. "Old Age." January 17, 1997.
———. "Our Dream. The Alta Foundation and the Hilltop." 10 April 1997.
———. "Politics." July 4, 1996.
———. "Polk Richards." July 2, 1996.
———. "A Proposal for a Ruth Lee Thygeson Lecture in the Alta Foundation." n.d.
———. "A Research Man." July 4, 1996.
———. "Roland P. Wilson." June 29, 1996.
———. "Ruth Lee." 1996.
———. "Ruth Lee and Our Dream." January 17, 1997.
———. "The Ruth Lee Hilltop." n.d.
———. "Stability." July 20, 1996.
———. "Stanford Medical School Days." January 16, 1997.
———. "Vacations." n.d.
———. "Victor Morax." June 29, 1996.
———. "Vision." July 12, 1996.
———. "The Winter of 1915." October 7, 1996.
Thygeson, Ruth Lee, to Mara Thygeson, June 9, 1974; April 16,1975; March 1981; December 13, 1982, November 11, 1986; private collection.
Thygeson, Sylvie Grace Thompson. "The Suffragists," an oral history conducted from 1972 to 1974 by Ralda Sullivan (Lee), Ph.D., Regional Oral History Office, University of California, Berkeley. http://ark.cdlib.org/ark:/13030/kt2h4n992z.
Twenty-fifth Anniversary of the Alta California Eye Research Foundation. Los Altos: Alta California Eye Research Foundation, 1994.
Uwe, Frank. "Robert Koch—Beyond Postulates." *Virox-Solutions*, Autumn 2005, http://72.14.207.104/search?q=cache:rsJrRsUUIvkJ:www.virox.com/pdf/solutions_fall_05.pdf+robcrt+kochıripe+apples+from+a+tree&hl=en&gl=us&ct=clnk&cd=2.

Vaughan, Daniel. Interview by Sally Smith Hughes, November 6, 1986, Regional Oral History Office, University of California, Berkeley, and American Academy of Ophthalmology. Published with permission of the Museum of Vision and the American Academy of Ophthalmology, copyright © 1986.

Verhoeff, Frederick H., to Phillips Thygeson, October 9, 1951, private collection.

"Vikingsholm." http://www.vikingsholm.com/history%200f%20eb.html.

Ward, Mike, and Bill Bishop. "Becoming Guinea Pigs to Avoid Poor Prison Care." *American-Statesman*. December 17, 2001. http://www.statesman.com/specialreports/content/specialreports/prisons/17prisonmain.html.

Weinstein, David. "Herbert Spencer." *Stanford Encyclopedia of Philosophy*. 2002, http://plato.stanford.edu/entries/spencer/

"Women and Victorian Values, 1837–1910." *Adam Matthew Publications*. http://www.adam-matthew-publications.co.uk/collections_az/Women+VV-2/contents-of-reels.aspx.

"World Bank Trachoma at a Glance Pamphlet." www.trachoma.org.

Index

Addis, Thomas 49
adenovirus 8, 188, 239
Africa 80–83
After 142–144
Alaska 164
All God's Children Got Wings 141
Allansmith, Mathea R. 195–198
Allen, James 96
Allenby, Edmund H.H. 74
Alliance for Human Research Protection 186
Alta California Eye Research Foundation 201–202, 216; memorial tree 223
American Board of Ophthalmology, board certification of 175–177
American Eugenics Society 123
American Medical Association (AMA), rules on human experimentation 187
American Ophthalmological Society (AOS), Ruth Lee's contribution to 96–97
American Samoa, trachoma treatment in 183
Andersen, Sigurd Ry 194
Anderson, Marian 136
Anguiano, Maria 242
anthrax 87
antisepsis, methods for 34
Appalachia, trachoma incidence in 101–102
Army Air Corps 132–134, 138–142
Australia, trachoma treatment in 183

Bacterium granulosis 57, 73, 82
Baden-Powell, Robert S.S. 30–31
Barkan, Hans 154
Basu, Prasanta Kumar 194
Beal, R. 98
Beard, Crowell 152, 156, 216; memorial tree 224
Benham, Rhoda Williams 111
Berkefeld filters 98
Bietti, Giambattista 181, 188

birth control, political activities of Sylvie Thygeson 11
Black Hawk Purchase 91
Blackburn, Sylvia 168
blepharitis 140
Boy Scouts of America 29–32
Brainard Lake (Colorado) 65
Braley, Alson E. 90–91, 96, 162, 206
Brazil, trachoma treatment in 183
Brothers Under the Skin 134–135
Browder, Earl 120
Brown, Clarence 105–107, 187
Brown, Scott 132

Calahan, H.A., *Learning to Sail* 143
Caldwell Luc operation 225
California, 1915 trip to 16
Cameron, Donaldina 24
Carmichael, Stokely 12
Carnegie archaeological excavation 72–74
Carrel, Alexis 111
Carter, Hodding, III 208
Carter, Jimmy 208
Carthage 80–81
Castroviejo, Roman 131
Cecilia Vaughan Memorial Fellowship 194
Cello, Robert 201
central serous retinopathy 139
Chandler, Loren 154
Chapman, Earlene 215, 218, 242
Chessman, Caryl 161
Chlamydia 93, 98, 100, 109, 175, 183; human experimentation with 185
Chlamydia trachomatis 4, 82, 84, 106; *see also* trachoma
cholera vaccine 87
Cibecue Massacre of 1881, 103–104
City Hospital (Denver) 230
Civil Rights movement 136, 207
Civilian Conservation Corps 64

249

Clearwater Beach, Florida 134–138
Clinton, William 208
Cogan, David G. 197
Colorado: medicine in the early years 54, 57–59
Colorado General Hospital 59
Columbia-Presbyterian Medical Center 111, 129–130
Columbia University 110
compromised host theory 163
conjunctivitis 161; allergic 77; follicular 77, 83; giant papillary (GPC) 195; inclusion 93, 98, 185; ophthalmia neonatorum 97; swimming pool 83, 99; vernal 195
Controversy in Ophthalmology 163
Cook, Robert 157
Cooperative Democracy Through Voluntary Association of the People as Consumers 119
Cordes, Frederick C. 154, 170, 174, 191
County Hospital (Denver) 59, 230
Cranston, Alan 166, 208
cross-cylinder refraction 56, 140

Darwin, Charles 122
Daughters of the American Revolution (DAR) 136
Davidson, Forrest 184
Dawson, Chandler 183, 185, 194
de Kruif, Paul: *Microbe Hunters* 83–84; "The Wait for Light" 107–108
de la Mora, Constancia, *In Place of Splendor* 119
dendritic keratitis 162
Denver and Gross College of Medicine 60
Dewey, John 116
Dibble General Hospital 152
disinfection, methods for 34
Dochez, Alphonse 109
Donaldson, David 173
Drew Field 134, 138–142
Dubuque, Julien 233
Duke-Elder, Sir Stewart 167
Dunnington, John 130, 154

Edward S. Harkness Eye Institute 110–111, 129–130
Egypt 74, 76–77
El Tobgy 77
electron microscopy 184
Elford, William J. 98
Elford collodion filters 98
Emerald Bay 200–201
estate 221–222
eugenics 122–123
S.S. *Exermont* 78–80

Fall River Road 63
Feeny, Lynette 239
filters 98
Finnoff, William C. 54–55, 73, 94, 220

Flexner, Abraham 60, 92
fluorescence microscopy 184
follicular conjunctivitis 77, 83
folliculosis 77
Forster, W.G. 109
Fort Apache 102–105, 157
Francis I. Proctor Foundation 170–175, 188, 204; establishment of 155; Fellows program 193–198; growth of 184; memorial tree 223; microscopy at 184; relationship of with UCSF ophthalmology department 174–175; Ruth Lee's role at 191–192; WHO Trachoma Reference Centre designation 183
Fritz, Milo H. 164, 167, 211
Fuchs, Ernst 112

genital trachoma *see* inclusion blennorrhea
George W. Hooper Foundation 154
germ theory 86
Geronimo 103–104
giant papillary conjunctivitis (GPC) 195
Giza Memorial Institute 74, 76
granulomatous uveitis, penicillin and 139
Guggenhime, Berthold 170

Halberstaedter-Prowazek (H.P.) inclusion body theory 82
Hallett, Joe 140–141
ham radio 29, 227
Hanna, Lavelle 175, 184
Harper, Frank 161
Harry Hind Research Library 184
Harwood, Jan 216
Heath, Harold 41
Heintz, Ralph 213
Heintz, Sophie 213
herpes simplex 161, 220
Hewlett, A.W. 49
Hind, Harry 184
Hogan, Michael J. 171–172, 206
Holland, Gary 201
Hollywood 16
Hooper Foundation *see* George W. Hooper Foundation
Hoover, Herbert 40
Hughes, Sally Smith 212–213
human experimentation 105–107, 184–188

immigrants, trachoma incidence in 101–102
In Place of Splendor 119
inclusion blennorrhea 97
inclusion bodies 82
inclusion conjunctivitis 93, 98, 161; human experimentation 185
Indian Health Service 147, 157; trachoma program 102
Indian Peaks 65
influenza pandemic 33–35
International Organization against Trachoma 78, 183

Iowa, early years 90–91
Ioway Indians 91
Irvine, Alexander Rodman 140
Ivy Committee, rules on human experimentation 187

Jackson, Edward 54–56, 140, 175, 220
Jamestown, Virginia settlement 19, 226–227
Jawetz, Ernest 185, 239
Jones, Barrie 165
Jordan, David Starr 11, 28, 37–40

keratoconjunctivitis 161, 239
Kerr, Clark 174
Knapp, Arnold 154
Knapp Foundation 130
Koch, (Heinrich Hermann) Robert 60, 87–88
Kochs Postulates 88

Lake Minnetonka, farm on 15
Lake Tahoe 199–202, 213
Lamarck, Chevalier de 121–122
Lancaster, Walter B. 140, 175
Lancaster device 140
Lang, Jack 177
Lanier, Jeffrey D. 196
Larsen, Anna (Lala) 12–13
Lawrence, Gerry 214
Lawrence, Margot 214
League of Nations 116
Learning to Sail 143
Le Bailly, Charles 78
Lee, Ralda 159
Leeuwenhoek, Antonie van 84
Leihy, Mary 214
Lilly, Walter 49
Lindner, Karl 74, 97
Lister, Joseph 34, 87–88
Loe, Fred 108–109
Los Altos hilltop 149–151, 167, 221–224
Lottridge, Ann 242
Lucien Howe Laboratory of Ophthalmology 155

MacCallan, H.F. 74, 76
MacLean, George E. 92
Mann, Dame Ida 167
"The March of Time" 107
marriage of Ruth Lee and Phillips Thygeson 43, 127–129, 180–181
maxillary sinus 225
Maxwell-Lyons, Peter 181
McWilliams, Carey, *Brothers Under the Skin* 134–135
Meister, Joseph 232
memorial trees 223–224
Mengert, W.F. 98
Meskwakis 90, 233
Meyer, Karl F. 49, 154–155, 175
microbe hunters 84

Microbe Hunters 83–84
military service 132–134, 138–142
miscegenation 141; Phils views on 219
Mitford, Jessica 186
Mitsui, Yuhihiko 188
Morax, Victor 83–84, 98
Mordhorst, Carl 194
Mosher, Clelia Duel 41–42, 113
Moulder, James W. 98
Mt. Edgecomb School 164

Nataf, Roger 82, 181–182
National Eye Institute 239
National Institutes of Health (NIH) 179; origin 234
Native Americans: human experimentation 186; trachoma incidence 72, 101–102
negative eugenics 122
Neisser, Max 82
Nicolle, Charles 78, 80, 82, 98, 108, 111, 183
1906 San Francisco earthquake 22–25, 38
1989 Loma Prieta earthquake 214
Nineteenth Amendment 37
95 Kirkham Street *see* Harry Hind Research Library
Nixon, Richard 208
Noguchi, Hideyo 72–73, 108
Nuremberg Code 186

O'Brien, Cecil Starling 90
O'Connor, G. Richard 98, 171, 190, 201, 204; memorial tree 223
ocular steroids, use of for herpetic keratitis 161–164, 238
The Officer's Wife 134
Okumoto, Masao 173, 189–190, 195–196; memorial tree 223
O'Neill, Eugene, *All God's Children Got Wings* 141
ophthalmia neonatorum 97
ophthalmology board certification 175–177
oral history 212–213, 225
Osler, William 49, 218
overtreatment 220

Paiute cabin 63, 66–71, 213
pannus 106
paratrachoma *see* inclusion blennorrhea
parenting 118–119, 124–127, 145
Paris, France, Pasteur Institute 83–84
Pasteur, Louis 83, 86–87, 232
Pasteur Institute: Paris 83–84; Tunis 78, 82
pasteurization 86–87
penicillin 139
phlyctenulosis 164
photography 173
physiological optics 56
Pischel, Dohrmann 154
placebo therapy 173–174
Plass, Everett 100

pneumonia 59
positive eugenics 122
positivism 45–46
Preventative Ophthalmology 172
preventative ophthalmology 171–172
Proctor, Elizabeth C. 74, 149, 150, 153–155, 183–184, 191, 201; final years 197; memorial tree 223
Proctor, Francis I. 72–74, 102, 108; estate 153–154
Proctor, Harrison 153–154
Proctor Bulletin 192
Proctor Foundation *see* Francis I. Proctor Foundation
psittacosis 188
pterygium 138
public health 54; preclinical thesis 50
Public Health Service (PHS) 102, 157

rabies vaccine 232
racial discrimination 134–136, 207
Rappleye, Willard C. 130, 147
red eye syndrome, treatment of with steroids 163
Reese, Algernon B. 116–117, 191
religious views 45–46
retirement years 210–213
Richards, Polk 74, 102–103, 108–109, 154
Roark, Eric 122
Rockefeller Foundation 56, 92, 111
Rockefeller Institute 72–73, 153
Rocky Mountain National Park 63
Roosevelt, Eleanor 136
Roosevelt, Franklin Delano 107, 116
Rosenfield, Milton Snyder 40, 113–114, 149
Rosita, Renee 242
rural public health 102

Sabin, Albert 111
SAFE protocol 221
sailing 142–144, 237
San Francisco earthquake 22–25, 38
Sanger, Margaret 11
sanitation 54; preclinical thesis 50
Saunders, John B. de C.M. 174
scanning ultra-microscopy 184
Schultz, Edwin 50
scientism 45–46
Seton, Ernest Thompson 30
Shepardson, Dwight 51, 235
SLATE 160
solar retinitis 139
Spanish flu pandemic 33–35
Spencer, Herbert 121–123
Spilman, Elizabeth (Lib) 22, 62, 149, 216, 218; editorial work 117; influenza 33–35; marriage 40
Spilman, Elizabeth Brewer 18, 231
Spilman, Esther 18, 226
Spilman, Henry 19

Spilman, James 18–19; courtship of Elizabeth Brewer 19–22; death 47–48
Spilman, Thomas 19
spontaneous generation 86
spotty keratitis 164
Stanford, Jane Lathrop 37
Stanford, Leland 37–38
Stanford, Leland, Jr. 37
Stanford University 154, 228; beginnings 37–39; School of Medicine 49
Stanford years 39, 41–42
Stanley, F.O. 63
sterilization 86–87, 172
steroid therapy 220; use for herpetic keratitis 161–164
Streit, Clarence 123; *Union Now* 120
Strong, Douglas 200
Strong, Peder 215
suffrage, political activities of Sylvie Thygeson 11
sulfanilamide 108–109
sulfonamides 220
Sun-Moon House 199–201
superficial punctate keratitis (SPK) 164
swimming pool conjunctivitis 83, 99
swimming pools, chlorination of 99–100
sympathetic ophthalmia, penicillin and 139

Tabbara, Khalid 206–207
Tenafly, New Jersey 112–113
Thompson, Mary 8–12
Thompson, Seymour Dwight 10
Thygeson, Cheryl Stoll 218, 242
Thygeson, Elling (brother) 31, 38
Thygeson, Elling (grandfather) 7, 225
Thygeson, Fritjof Peder 214, 222, 242; birth 62; political activism 158–161; relationship with parents 145; relationship with Phil 218; relationship with Ruth Lee 114, 118–119
Thygeson, Kristin 62, 136–137, 167–169, 214, 222; birth 93; relationship with Phil 218; relationship with Ruth Lee 118–119
Thygeson, Mara 128, 181, 203, 212, 219
Thygeson, Mary (sister) 12, 38–39, 128, 216, 218; communist views 120
Thygeson, Mary Nelson (grandmother) 7
Thygeson, Nels Marcus (father) 7–8, 10–12; death 17, 28–29, 226
Thygeson, Nels Marcus (grandson) 55, 61, 127, 145, 156, 170, 229
Thygeson, Phillips Baker (Phil): birth 7; board certification 176; childhood 12–17; clinical methods 172–174; directorship of the Proctor Foundation 188; estate 221–222; final years 217–224; ham radio activities 29, 48; high school education 28; honors 220–221; leadership style 204–206; medical internship 54–57, 61; medical school years 48–51; memorial tree 223; microscopy interests 5, 84; political views 121–124,

208–209; private practice 156–157; racial views 207, 218–219; scouting and 29–32; teaching methods 195–198; temperament 51–52, 115; Victorian values 44; views on contraception 123–124; views regarding family 124–125; war years (WWII) 132–134, 138–142, 146–148; WHO consultancy 179–183

Thygeson, Ruth (sister) 38; communist views 120

Thygeson, Ruth Lee Spilman: birth 18; care of Sylvie 204; childhood 22–27; editorial work 116–118, 190–192; education 127–128; estate 221–222; final years 214–217; memorial tree 223; parents' courtship 19–22; political activism 113–116, 166; political views 119–121; research collaboration 88–89, 96–97; Victorian values 44, 229; views regarding family 124–125; war years (WWII) 134–138, 146–148

Thygeson, Sylvie Grace Thompson (mother) 8–12, 48, 122; communist views 120, 166–167; final years 203–204; oral history 225

Thygeson's superficial punctate keratitis 164

USS *Tilefish* 160

Toxoplasma organism 111

toxoplasmosis 111

trachoma 72–74, 139, 188, 221; early research 73; early writings 57; effect of on family productivity 231; Egyptian research 76–77; etiology 82, 97–98, 106; filtering 98; incidence 4, 101–102; inoculation of human volunteer 105–107; MacCallan classification system 76; Proctor Foundation work 171; WHO committee 179–183

Tresidder, Donald B. 154

trichiasis 4

Trowbridge, Charles R. 63

tuberculosis 60–61; phlyctenulosis 164

Tunisia 80–83

typhoid 59

unilateral inclusion conjunctivitis *see* inclusion conjunctivitis

Union Now 114, 120

United Nations 166

University Hospital (Colorado) 59

University of California San Francisco (UCSF) 154

University of Colorado: medical school 60; ophthalmology at 55

University of Iowa 90–91; College of Medicine improvements 92; Department of Ophthalmology 91–92, 94; hospitals 93–94; medical research 94

uveitis 171

Vacaville prison 185

Valley Forge General Hospital 148

Vaughan, Daniel 152, 157, 177, 194, 216; memorial tree 224

Verhoeff, Frederick 177, 238

vernal catarrh 77

vernal conjunctivitis 195

Victorianism 44

Vikingsholm 200

Vivacious Lady 167–169

von Halberstaedter, Ludvig 82

von Prowazek, Stanslaus J.V. 82

von Sallman, Ludvig 112, 116, 131; memorial tree 224

"The Wait for Light" 107–108

Warbasse, James Peter, *Cooperative Democracy Through Voluntary Association of the People as Consumers* 119

Ward, Colorado 65

We Don't Like It Either 159

Wenhua 201

Wheeler, John 110–111, 129–130

Wilke, Wendell 116

Wilson, Roland P. 76

Wilson, Woodrow 102

Woman's Welfare League 11

world federalism 113–116, 120–121, 158–159, 166

World Health Organization (WHO) 179–183; Trachoma Reference Centres 183

World War I 40

zoonoses 201

www.ingramcontent.com/pod-product-compliance
Ingram Content Group UK Ltd.
Pitfield, Milton Keynes, MK11 3LW, UK
UKHW041935140426
5217IPUK00014B/487